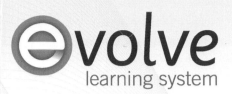

learning system

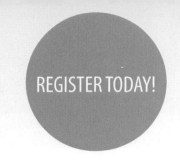

REGISTER TODAY!

To access your Learning Resources, visit:

http://evolve.elsevier.com/Papp

Register today to gain access to:

Evolve® Learning Resources for *Quality Management in the Imaging Sciences,* Fourth Edition, offers the following features:

Instructor Resources

- Instructor's Manual
- Testbank
- Powerpoint Slides
- Image Collection

Student Resources

- Critical Thinking Questions
- Documentation Forms
- Experiments
- Practice Exams

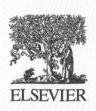

ELSEVIER

FOURTH EDITION

Quality Management

IN THE IMAGING SCIENCES

Jeffrey Papp, PhD, RT(R)(QM)
Professor of Physics and Diagnostic Imaging
College of DuPage
Glen Ellyn, Illinois

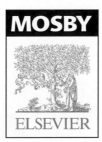

MOSBY

ELSEVIER

3251 Riverport Lane
St. Louis, Missouri 63043

QUALITY MANAGEMENT IN THE IMAGING SCIENCES,   ISBN: 978-0-323-05761-5
FOURTH EDITION

Notices

Knowledge and best practice in this field are constantly changing. As new research and experience broaden our understanding, changes in research methods, professional practices, or medical treatment may become necessary.

Practitioners and researchers must always rely on their own experience and knowledge in evaluating and using any information, methods, compounds, or experiments described herein. In using such information or methods they should be mindful of their own safety and the safety of others, including parties for whom they have a professional responsibility.

With respect to any drug or pharmaceutical products identified, readers are advised to check the most current information provided (i) on procedures featured or (ii) by the manufacturer of each product to be administered, to verify the recommended dose or formula, the method and duration of administration, and contraindications. It is the responsibility of practitioners, relying on their own experience and knowledge of their patients, to make diagnoses, to determine dosages and the best treatment for each individual patient, and to take all appropriate safety precautions.

To the fullest extent of the law, neither the Publisher nor the authors, contributors, or editors, assume any liability for any injury and/or damage to persons or property as a matter of products liability, negligence or otherwise, or from any use or operation of any methods, products, instructions, or ideas contained in the material herein.

Library of Congress Cataloging-in-Publication Data
Papp, Jeffrey.
  Quality management in the imaging sciences / Jeffrey Papp. – 4th ed.
    p. ; cm.
  Includes bibliographical references and index.
  ISBN 978-0-323-05761-5 (hardcover : alk. paper) 1. Diagnostic imaging–Quality control.
2. Radiography, Medical–Image quality. I. Title.
  [DNLM: 1. Diagnostic Imaging–standards. 2. Diagnostic Equipment–standards. 3. Quality Control.
WN 180 P218q 2011]
  RC78.7.D53P35 2011
  616.07′540685–dc22

                                                                    2009049812

Publisher: Jeanne Olson
Senior Developmental Editor: Rebecca Swisher
Publishing Services Manager: Hemamalini Rajendrababu
Project Manager: Sukanthi Sukumar
Senior Book Designer: Paula Catalano

Printed in the United States of America

Last digit is the print number: 9   8   7   6   5   4   3   2   1

To my daughter, Ashley Marie,
and all of my students, past, present, and future.

Lorrie Kelley, MS, RT(R)(MR)(CT)
Associate Professor
Director, CT/MRI Programs
Boise State University
Boise, Idaho

James M. Kofler, Jr, PhD
Assistant Professor of Radiologic Physics
Mayo College of Medicine
Department of Diagnostic Radiology
Mayo Clinic
Rochester, Minnesota

Joanne M. Metler, MS, CNMT
Assistant Professor
Coordinator, Nuclear Medicine Technology Program
College of DuPage
Glen Ellyn, Illinois

James A. Zagzebski, PhD
Professor
Departments of Medical Physics, Human Oncology,
    and Radiology
University of Wisconsin
Madison, Wisconsin

Laura Aaron, PhD, RT(R)(M)(QM)
Program Director and Associate Professor
Radiologic Sciences
Northwestern State University
Shreveport, Louisiana

Rex Allen Ameigh, MSLM, BSRT(R)
Director Radiologic Technology Program and Associate
  Professor
Austin Peay State University
Clarksville, Tennessee

Lori Balmer, MPA, RT(R)(MR)
Clinical Coordinator/Lecturer
Indiana University South Bend
South Bend, Indiana

Alberto Bello, Jr, MEd, RT(R)(CV)
Radiologic Technology Program Director
Danville Area Community College
Danville, Illinois

Mary Jo Bergman, Med, MS, RN, RT(R)
Program Director
MeritCare Health System
Fargo, North Dakota

Joseph R. Bittengle, MEd, RT(R)(ARRT)
Associate Professor and Division Director
Division of Radiologic Imaging Sciences
University of Arkansas for Medical Sciences
Little Rock, Arkansas

Deanna Butcher, MA, RT(R)
Program Director
St. Luke's College
Sioux City, Iowa

John H. Clouse, MSR, RT
Associate Professor
Owensboro Technical and Community College
Owensboro, Kentucky

Sandra Creaser, MM, RT(R)(N)(M)CNMT
Clinical Assistant Professor, Clinical Coordinator
MGH Institute of Health Professions
Charlestown, Massachusetts

M. Elia Flores, MEd, RT(R)
Program Director
Radiology Program
Blinn College
Bryan, Texas

Steve Forshier, MEd, RT(R)
APTR Online Clinical Director
Pima Medical Institute
Tucson, Arizona

Kerry Greene-Donnelly, MBA, RT(R)(M)(CT)(QM)
Assistant Professor
Upstate Medical University
Syracuse, New York

Ann M Hagenau, MS, RT(R)(M)
Instructor
Clarkson College
Omaha, Nebraska

Robert Hughes, RT (R)
Program Director
School of Radiography
Alegent Health Immanuel Medical Center
Omaha, Nebraska

Georgeann Jenkins, MEd, RT(R)(M)
Assistant Professor
Roxbury Community College
Boston, Massachusetts

Myke Kudlas, Med, RT(R)(WM)
Assistant Professor of Radiology
Mayo Clinic College of Medicine
Jacksonville, Florida

Angela M. Lambert, AS, BS, MS, ARRT, AFAA
Assistant Professor
Clinic Coordinator
Bluefield State College
Bluefield, West Virginia

Amy Freshley Lebkuecher, MS, RT(R)(T)
Associate Professor
Clinical Coordinator Radiologic Technology
Austin Peay State University
Clarksville, Tennessee

4. The latest changes in technology and current regulations have been updated throughout.

Quality Management in the Imaging Sciences continues to provide the wealth of information needed for instructors to guide students through quality management issues, for students and practitioners to prepare for the ARRT examination, and for technologists to succeed in the delivery of high-quality services.

INSTRUCTOR RESOURCES

Instructor ancillaries, including an ExamView Test Bank of over 400 questions; an electronic image collection of the images in the text; an Instructor's Manual of chapter outlines, teaching tips, and teaching strategies; and a new PowerPoint lecture presentation are all available at http://evolve.elsevier.com.

Jeffrey Papp, PhD, RT(R)(QM)

Quality management and its associated topics, quality assurance and quality control, are vitally important in modern diagnostic imaging departments. Government and accreditation agencies mandate procedures to ensure that equipment is functioning within accepted standards and that it is operated properly. Such procedures also must be appropriately documented. Because these responsibilities have been delegated to technologists, they need additional knowledge. The American Registry of Radiologic Technologists (ARRT) recognized this need by offering an advanced level examination in quality management in March 1997.

I have been teaching a course in quality assurance/quality management since 1983 and had never required a textbook because I could not find one single book that contained all of the necessary material. Instead, I had to reserve different books and government publications in our library for students to consult as reference sources or suggest that they consult individual chapters, research papers, and literature from various equipment manufacturers and suppliers. During discussions with other radiologic science educators, I discovered that most of them had the same problem in teaching this topic. I also had been besieged with requests from practicing technologists for study material for the Quality Management Advanced Level Examination. Previously, I could respond only by supplying a listing of several reference books.

From these many years of frustration came the impetus to write the first edition of *Quality Management in the Imaging Sciences*. The first three editions were very well received, so I am particularly pleased to offer this fourth edition, which will again fill several needs. Radiography educators find it to be a tailor-made text for instruction in quality management. It also serves as a practical reference for day-to-day consultation by practitioners responsible for implementing quality management programs in diagnostic imaging departments. Additionally, this comprehensive resource allows those practicing technologists studying for the Quality Management Advanced Level Examination to use a single reference book. The material contained in Chapters 12, 13, 14, and 15 pertains to specialized areas of imaging (CT, MRI, sonography, and nuclear medicine) and is not covered on the Advanced Level Examination offered by the ARRT. Those readers preparing for the examination will find the material available in Evolve Resources particularly useful because it contains two sample tests based on the content outline developed by the ARRT for the Quality Management Examination.

Quality Management in the Imaging Sciences includes the most up-to-date information available on the quality management aspects of darkrooms, processing, equipment and accessories, fluoroscopic and advanced imaging equipment, artifacts, repeat analysis, and silver recovery. Quality assurance organizations and their websites are listed in Appendix B, and full-page documentation forms are available in Evolve Resources.

The following special features are included, as in the first three editions:

- Federal regulations are set in boldface type in the text, and the symbol Ⓖ appears beside them.
- Procedures are highlighted as separate elements with step-by-step guidelines.
- Key terms are identified at the beginnings of chapters, set in boldface type, and explained within chapters.
- Learning objectives, chapter outlines, and chapter review questions (with answers) are provided as study tools.
- Key term definitions are collected in a glossary.

NEW TO THE FOURTH EDITION

Additional updates continue to benefit the reader:

1. Revisions to the mammography chapter correspond with new standards outlined in the Mammography Quality Standards Act, as well as new digital mammographic systems.
2. The material on Evolve Resources that accompanies the text offers these features:
   - Two 165-question mock examinations to encourage self-testing that are particularly convenient for those readers preparing for the ARRT Advanced Level Examination in Quality Management
   - Full-size sample documentation forms that can be used "as is" or modified to meet the needs of a particular department
   - Student experiments and analyses of them to correspond with appropriate chapters that have been modified for digital-only departments
   - Questions for analysis and critical thinking that challenge the reader to prepare for real-life situations
3. Expanded material for digital imaging and quality control procedures for electronic image monitors is provided.

Just as with the first three editions of this text, the production of this fourth edition has required the help and input of many people. I must start with my associates in the Diagnostic Medical Imaging program at the College of DuPage, namely, Gina Carrier, Pam Jankovsky, Rosanne Paschal, and Shelli Thacker, for all of their support and understanding while I was preoccupied with writing this text. It is also important to include my Dean, Thomas Cameron, and my Associate Dean, Karen Solt. I also wish to thank Patty Holvey of Good Samaritan Hospital in Downers Grove, Illinois; Janet Petersen of Elmhurst Memorial Hospital, Elmhurst, Illinois; and Pam Verkuilen of Saint Alexius Medical Center in Hoffman Estates, Illinois, for all of their help in gathering information on digital imaging.

I am deeply indebted to my contributing authors, Lorrie Kelley, Program Director for CT/MRI at Boise State University; James M. Kofler, Assistant Professor, Department of Diagnostic Radiology, Mayo Clinic; Joanne M. Metler, Coordinator for Nuclear Medicine at the College of DuPage; and James A. Zagzebski, Professor of Medical Physics at the University of Wisconsin, Madison.

I would also like to thank Jeanne Olson, Rebecca Swisher, Mary Pohlman, Karen Baer, and everyone at Elsevier for their help, support, and patience in the production of this text and the accompanying material found in the Evolve Resources.

Finally, I must thank Professor Gerard Lietz of DePaul University for giving me the knowledge, inspiration, and love of medical physics that allowed me to be successful in this profession.

Jeffrey Papp, PhD, RT(R)(QM)

CONTENTS

CHAPTERS

APPENDICES

Introduction to Quality Management

KEY TERMS

action
aggregate data
    indicator
appropriateness of care
benchmarking
brainstorming
concurrent data
continuity of care
cost of quality
critical path
customer
Deficit Reduction Act

effectiveness of care
efficacy of care
efficiency of care
expectation
FMEA
focus group
FOCUS-PDCA
HIPAA
indicators
input
Mammography Quality
    Standards Reauthorization Act

output
process
quality assessment
quality assurance
quality control
quality improvement team
Safe Medical Devices Act
Six Sigma
sentinel event indicator
supplier
SWOT analysis
system

OBJECTIVES

At the completion of this chapter the reader should be able to do the following:
- Identify the need for quality management in diagnostic imaging
- Discuss the impact of government regulation and The Joint Commission accreditation on quality management
- Explain the differences between quality assurance, quality control, and quality management
- Identify the five steps of a process
- List the various tools of group dynamics
- Explain TJC 10-step monitoring and evaluation process and cycle for improving performance

OUTLINE

Diagnostic imaging is a multistep process by which information concerning patient anatomy and physiology is gathered and displayed with the use of modern technology. Unfortunately, numerous sources of variability, in both human factors and equipment factors, can produce subquality images if not properly controlled. This can result in repeat exposures that increase both patient dose and department cost and possibly decrease the accuracy of image interpretation. This in turn can result in decreased customer satisfaction (customers being physicians, vendors, insurance companies, employees, and patients) that ultimately costs the healthcare provider lost business and revenue. The purpose of a quality management program is to control or minimize these variables as much as possible. In a diagnostic imaging department, these variables include equipment; image receptor; processing; viewing conditions; and competency of the technologist, support staff, and the observer or interpreter.

When discussing the *quality* of particular goods or services (or in our case, the quality of patient care and the diagnostic images that we produce), one must keep in mind the three levels on which quality is determined:

1. *Expected quality.* This is the level of quality of the product or service that is expected by the customer and may be influenced by outside factors such as prior word of mouth from friends and relatives. A diagnostic imaging professional would likely have the least amount of impact on this level of quality because it is present before the patient comes into the imaging department.
2. *Perceived quality.* This is the customer's perception of the product or service. It is based on the customer's perception of the product or service and is highly subjective and more difficult to measure quantitatively. For patients undergoing diagnostic imaging, their experience (such as how long they had to wait or how they were treated) during the procedures greatly influences their perception of quality. Therefore how well an imaging professional performs his or her respective responsibilities will have the greatest impact on this level of quality. Because perceived quality is often what brings patients back to a hospital or imaging center, it can be more important than the actual quality.
3. *Actual quality.* This level of quality uses statistical data to measure outcomes and considers all factors that can influence the final outcome (e.g., the quality of the image, accuracy of diagnosis, timeliness of report to primary physician). It also can compare the quality of the product or service with that of a competitor.

Since the early 1980s, healthcare delivery in the United States has undergone dramatic changes that have affected diagnostic imaging departments and their ability to provide quality care. These changes include the following:

- *Advances in technology, equipment, and procedures.* The digitization of radiography, along with expensive technologies such as magnetic resonance imaging (MRI), spiral computed tomography (CT), electron beam tomography, positron emission tomography (PET), digital radiography and fluoroscopy, and single photon emission computed tomography (SPECT), has increased the cost of equipment acquisition, installation, and maintenance.
- *Legislation and government regulations.* Legislation such as the **Safe Medical Devices Act (SMDA)** of 1990, the Mammography Quality Standards Act (MQSA) of 1992, and the **Mammography Quality Standards Reauthorization Act (MQSRA)** of 1998 has increased the responsibility of diagnostic imaging department managers and staff to document proper equipment operation and procedures. This is in addition to requirements from the Occupational Safety and Health Administration (OSHA), the Environmental Protection Agency (EPA), and the Food and Drug Administration (FDA) that affect matters ranging from blood-borne pathogens to disposal of processing chemicals.
- *The Joint Commission Accreditation Procedures.* The accreditation procedures of The Joint Commission (TJC) have gone from the philosophy of quality assurance (QA) to one of total quality management (TQM) (explained in more detail later in this chapter).
- *Corporate buyouts and mergers.* Since 1980, more than 1000 hospitals have closed in the United States. Many others have been purchased by "for profit" healthcare organizations or have merged to condense costs or reduce competition, or both.
- *Methods of reimbursement for services rendered.* The previous method of "fee for service" reimbursement of healthcare expenses is rapidly being replaced by managed care plans such as health maintenance organizations (HMOs) and point of service plans such as preferred provider organizations (PPOs). The lower rate of reimbursement from these plans has reduced the operating budgets of many diagnostic imaging departments. In addition, many insurers are now employing radiology benefits management companies (RBMs) to determine the necessity of various diagnostic imaging orders.

These changes have made a quality management program essential to the operation and survival of a diagnostic imaging department. The cost of such a program in the form of personnel time and test equipment is more than offset by the savings from lower repeat rates, less equipment downtime, film and chemical savings in nondigital departments, greater department efficiency, and increased customer satisfaction because waiting time can be reduced. When assessing the effectiveness of a quality management program, one must consider the **cost of quality**. This is defined as the expense of not doing things right the first time. In diagnostic imaging departments, this could be considerable because the result could lead to lost business at the very least or the injury or death of a patient at the very worst.

HISTORY OF QUALITY MANAGEMENT IN RADIOLOGY

One of the earliest known methods of evaluating the quality of clinical healthcare by assessing patient outcomes was carried out by Florence Nightingale in the 1860s. She was one of the first to use a systematic approach to collecting and analyzing mortality rates in hospitals. The origins of modern quality management can be traced back to the early 1900s, to the work of an industrial engineer named Frederick Winslow Taylor. Taylor is considered the "Father of Scientific Management" because of his philosophy that the planning function and the execution stage be separate and that numerous individuals be assigned specific tasks within the production process to minimize the complexity of the task. With complexity minimized, the hope was to maximize efficiency because, theoretically, fewer mistakes would occur. Job tasks were broken down into simple, separate steps that could be performed over and over again (i.e., assembly lines). Only specific persons were assigned the task of quality control inspection. This philosophy was common practice, both in American industry and in healthcare settings (including diagnostic radiology), until the 1980s.

During the 1980s, the concept of quality improvement began to gradually replace the concept of scientific management. This concept is credited to W. Edwards Deming and Joseph Juran, who used the quality improvement philosophy to revitalize the economy of Japan after World War II. This concept combines quality control with an overall management philosophy that gives input to all persons involved in the process of creating the specific good(s) or service(s). This concept is discussed in further detail later in this chapter. Many diagnostic imaging departments have been systematically monitoring their equipment and procedures (quality control) since the 1930s, independent of any government regulation or accreditation agency. The main motivations were to save money and increase efficiency and quality of care. Since then, governmental action and policies mandated by the TJC have all but required that an extensive quality management program be implemented by diagnostic imaging departments.

Governmental Action

The federal government's first step toward requiring that diagnostic imaging departments implement quality management programs came in 1968 with the Radiation Control for Health and Safety Act. This law required the U.S. Department of Health, Education, and Welfare (now called Health and Human Services) to develop and administer standards that would reduce human exposure to radiation from electronic products. The Bureau of Radiological Health (BRH) (now called the National Center for Devices and Radiological Health) was given the responsibility for implementing this act. The BRH set forth regulatory action, beginning in 1974, with several amendments to control the manufacture and installation of medical and dental diagnostic equipment to reduce the production of useless radiation. These regulations are contained in the document Title 21 of the Code of Federal Regulations Part 1020 (21 CFR 1020). Title 21 refers to the FDA. In 1978 the BRH published the "Recommendations for Quality Assurance Programs in Diagnostic Radiology Facilities." The Joint Commission, along with most state public health agencies, has adopted these recommendations into its various policies governing diagnostic imaging departments.

In 1981 the Consumer-Patient Radiation Health and Safety Act addressed issues such as unnecessary repeat examinations, quality assurance techniques, referral criteria, radiation exposure, and unnecessary mass screening programs. It also established minimum standards for accreditation of educational programs in the radiologic sciences and for the certification of radiographic equipment operators. This law motivated many states to enact licensure laws for radiologic technologists. However, there is no legal penalty for noncompliance contained within the law and eight states, plus the District of Columbia, currently have no minimum educational or certification criteria for healthcare workers who perform radiologic procedures. As of the writing of this edition, the eight states are Alabama, Alaska, Georgia, Idaho, Missouri, North Carolina, Oklahoma, and South Dakota. The states of Michigan and Nevada license mammographers but not radiographers, while Wisconsin does not license radiographers but does require American Registry of Radiologic Technologists certification. In September 2000, the Consumer Assurance of Radiologic Excellence (CARE) Act was first introduced in Congress by Rep. Rick Lazio (R-NY) as H.R. 5624. In 2006, the CARE bill was retitled the Consistency, Accuracy, Responsibility and Excellence in Medical Imaging and Radiation Therapy Bill because many of the imaging disciplines included in the CARE legislation are not directly related to radiology. The CARE Act mandates educational and training requirements for all technologists performing imaging procedures (thereby mandating the standards contained in the Consumer-Patient Radiation Health and Safety Act of 1981). In addition to improving the quality of care nationwide, enacting the CARE Act also would save considerable money each year. According to the Radiologic Society of North America (RSNA) journal,

Radiology, approximately 130 million diagnostic radiology procedures are performed on 36 million Medicare enrollees per year. Over $10 billion is spent by Medicare on medical imaging procedures each year (according to the Medicare Payment Advisory Commission MedPAC). If the national repeat examination rate is between 4% and 7% (averaging 5.5%) and the CARE bill can lower repeat rates from 5.5% to 4.5%, enacting education and credentialing standards could save Medicare over $100 million a year. As of the printing of this text, the CARE Act has yet to be enacted. In July of 2008, Congress passed the Medicare Improvements for Patients and Providers Act of 2008 (MIPPA), which mandates that any non-hospital institution performing advanced diagnostic services (such as nuclear medicine and PET) must be accredited (by January 1, 2010) in order to receive federal funding (Medicare reimbursement). Should the CARE bill be adopted, the same provisions would be in place for hospital based services.

In the mid-1980s, the Occupational Safety and Health Administration (OSHA), in response to the outbreak of human immunodeficiency virus (HIV) and hepatitis B virus (HBV), amended the existing federal regulations concerning infection control in the workplace and mandated a policy on blood-borne pathogens. All workplaces had to implement these new regulations by the spring of 1992. This policy states that an exposure control plan must be in place for all industries in which workers may come in contact with blood and other infectious materials. Included in this policy are standard precaution procedures (also known as *Tier 1 procedures*), education programs for employees, free hepatitis B immunization for staff who might be exposed to blood or body substances, follow-up care to any staff member accidentally exposed to blood or bodily fluids through needle sticks and so on, personal protective equipment supplied by the employer (including gloves, gowns, laboratory coats, face shields, eye protection, pocket masks, and ventilation devices), and disposal procedures. These infection control procedures also must include transmission-based precautions (also known as *Tier 2* or *category-specific precautions*) that are used in addition to Tier 1 or standard precautions. They are used when a specific communicable disease is suspected or confirmed and are designed to place a barrier between the patient with the disease and everyone else. They are specifically geared toward preventing infection by minimizing the three specific modes of disease transmission—air, droplet, and contact. The complete OSHA policy on infection control blood-borne pathogens can be found in the Federal Register under Title 29 of the Code of Federal Regulations Part 1910 (29 CFR 1910). OSHA also is responsible for monitoring the workplace environment including the requirements for occupational exposure to radiation and to chemicals found in processing solutions. OSHA also has proposed an Ergonomics Standard with the objective of reducing the rising incidence of work-related injury and workers' compensation claims.

The Safe Medical Devices Act (SMDA) of 1990 was enacted in order to increase the amount of information the FDA and device manufacturers receive about problems with medical devices. Under the act, medical facilities must to report to the FDA and the manufacturer, if known, any medical devices (e.g., malfunctioning bed, nonworking defibrillator, nonworking pacemaker, malfunctioning radiation therapy unit) that have caused the death or serious injury of a patient or employee. Facilities also must report device-related serious injuries to the device manufacturer or to the FDA if the manufacturer is not known. In addition, the SMDA requires that device user facilities must submit to the FDA, on a semiannual basis, a summary of all reports submitted during that time period. It also authorizes civil penalties to healthcare workers or facilities that do not report defects and failures in medical devices. When any incidents of unsafe medical devices are reported to the FDA, Form 3500 should be used for voluntary reporting and Form 3500A should be used for mandatory reporting. Mandatory reporting requirements for user facilities are shown in Table 1-1.

In 1992 the MQSA mandated quality assurance programs for all facilities that want to perform mammographic procedures to obtain FDA approval. Specific requirements were designed for dedicated equipment, physicians interpreting the images, medical physicists, and technologists. Most of these standards were formulated by or in conjunction with the American College of Radiology and were in use by many facilities before enactment of the MQSA. This law became effective October 1, 1994. The MQSA was replaced by the MQSRA of 1998. As part of the new law, final FDA regulations concerning mammographic procedures became effective April 28, 1999, replacing interim regulations

TABLE 1-1	Mandatory Reporting Requirements for User Facilities		
Category	**Report Form**	**To Whom**	**When**
Death	FDA 3500 A	FDA and manufacturer	Within 10 working days
Serious injury	FDA 3500 A	Manufacturer; FDA only if manufacturer is unknown	Within 10 working days
Annual report of death and serious injury	FDA 3419	FDA	January 1

FDA, Food and Drug Administration.

that were used during the original law. The final regulations emphasize performance objectives rather than specify the behavior and manner of compliance. More specific information on the MQSA can be found in Chapter 11.

The Health Insurance Portability and Accountability Act (**HIPAA**) of 1996 (also known as the Kennedy-Kassebaum Act or Public Law 104–191) was enacted to simplify healthcare standards and save money for healthcare businesses by encouraging electronic transactions, but it also requires new safeguards to protect patient security and confidentiality. HIPAA established national standards for healthcare e-commerce that include the following:

1. Electronic patient record system security requirements (security standard): This created a new national standard for the administrative, technical, and physical safety of protected health information (PHI).
2. Standard electronic formats for insurance transactions such as enrollment, encounters, and claims (transaction standard): This standard requires the implementation of a uniform set of codes and forms, such as the American National Standards Institute (ANSI) ASC X12N format for electronic healthcare transactions or professional and institutional claims.
3. Standard identifiers and codes for institutions, personnel, diagnoses, and treatments (national identifier standard): This created national numbers to identify employers (EIN), health plans (Payer ID) and healthcare providers (National Provider Identifiers or NPI). It also contains a set of codes that are used to encode all healthcare data. The four categories of these codes are (a) diseases (ICD-9); (b) injuries (ICD-10); (c) actions taken to prevent, diagnose, treat, or manage diseases (CPT-4); and (d) substances, equipment, and supplies (HCPCS).
4. Patient information, confidentiality, and privacy rules (privacy standard): This created a new national standard for privacy of protected health information.

The Department of Health and Human Services first issued proposed regulations for these standards in November 1999, with final rules approved in December 2000. They took effect April 14, 2001, and all healthcare organizations had to comply and implement them by April 14, 2005. All medical records and patient information, whether electronic, on paper, or oral, are covered by these final rules.

Failure to comply with these standards can result in significant penalties. For example, any person who violates the privacy standard of HIPAA is subject to a penalty of not more than $100 for each violation, not to exceed $25,000 in any one calendar year. For wrongful disclosure of individually identifiable health information, such as a person who knowingly uses or causes to be used a unique health identifier, obtains individually identifiable health information relating to an individual; or discloses individually identifiable health information to another, that

person shall be fined not more than $50,000, imprisoned not more than 1 year, or both. If the offense is committed under false pretenses, the person shall be fined not more than $100,000, imprisoned not more than 5 years, or both. If the offense is committed with the intent to sell, transfer, or use individually identifiable health information for commercial advantage, personal gain, or malicious harm, the person shall be fined not more than $250,000, imprisoned not more than 10 years, or both.

This means that healthcare administrators must formulate new policies and procedures including establishing a system of security and confidentiality, training all personnel in these policies, and appointing a staff member to act as a security officer who will monitor compliance with these policies. This is discussed further in Chapter 2. Complete HIPAA guidelines can be found in the Federal Register under Title 45 of the Code of Federal Regulations Parts 160-164 (45 CFR 160-164).

The **Deficit Reduction Act** of 2005 (DRA) was enacted to help make $11 billion in cuts from 2007 (when the DRA went into effect) to 2015 in Medicare and Medicaid programs. One aspect of the program is to reduce payments for freestanding diagnostic imaging centers by capping some current procedural terminology (CPT) codes that were higher than hospital outpatient rates and freezing CPT codes already lower than hospital outpatient rates. Current procedural terminology codes were developed by the American Medical Association (AMA) and adopted by the federal government and private insurance providers to classify medical, surgical, and diagnostic services. The DRA also requires imaging centers to have quality control standards in place in order to receive reimbursement.

Having an effective quality management program also has become necessary as a condition of receiving reimbursement for services by the federal government. The United States Department of Health and Human Services, through its sub-branch, the Centers of Medicare and Medicaid Services (CMS), emphasizes effective quality management procedures be documented in order for healthcare facilities to receive reimbursement for any healthcare service, and many private insurance companies have followed this practice.

The Joint Commission

In the 1970s, The Joint Commission (TJC, formerly known as the Joint Commission for the Accreditation of Healthcare Organizations or JCAHO) began requiring hospitals and other healthcare providers to perform and document specific quality management procedures in order for these facilities to obtain accreditation. This accreditation is voluntary, but hospitals and medical centers that do not have it may not possess Medicaid certification, hold certain licenses, have a residency program for training physicians, obtain reimbursements from insurance companies, or receive malpractice insurance. However, some hospitals may choose not to be accredited by TJC and instead have inspections by their state public health departments. These hospitals include many rural hospitals that may be critical access hospitals and would still receive Medicaid and Medicare reimbursements. TJC accredits not only hospitals but also facilities for long-term care, ambulatory care, mental health, and chemical dependency. These quality management procedures are extensive and specific in nature. For example, any equipment that is inspected daily (Monday through Friday) also must be inspected on Saturday and Sunday if the opportunity exists that a patient would need that piece of equipment on the weekend. Second, refrigerators that contain medical supplies must have a thermometer, and a log of the daily recorded temperature (including weekends) must be kept. TJC also requires accredited institutions to have a process in place for correcting customer complaints (a process known as *service recovery*). This means that proper performance and documentation of quality management procedures are essential to pass TJC inspections. Standards set by TJC to receive accreditation require that healthcare organizations have a planned, systematic, and organization-wide approach for monitoring, evaluating, and improving the quality of care, as well as those of management, governance, and support activities. TJC standards also require that healthcare organizations must perform routine inspections of all equipment, devices, and supplies.

Before 1991, TJC used the concepts of quality assurance and quality control requiring systematic monitoring and evaluation, with the responsibility left to the medical director or department head. Because these concepts now have been incorporated into the newer quality management philosophy, an understanding of quality assurance and quality control is still important and is discussed in the following paragraphs.

Quality Assurance. Quality assurance (QA) is an all-encompassing management program used to ensure excellence in healthcare through the systematic collection and evaluation of data. The primary objective of a QA program is the enhancement of patient care; this includes patient selection parameters and scheduling, management techniques, departmental policies and procedures, technical effectiveness and efficiency, in-service education, and image interpretation with timeliness of reports. The main emphasis of the program is on the human factors that can lead to variations in quality care. Quality assurance should not be confused with **quality assessment,** which is the measurement of the level of quality at some point in time with no effort to change or improve the level of care.

Quality Control. Quality control is the part of the QA program that deals with techniques used in monitoring and maintaining the technical elements of the systems that affect the quality of the image. Therefore quality control is the part of the QA program that deals with instrumentation and equipment. A quality control program includes the following three levels of testing:

Level I: Noninvasive and Simple. Noninvasive and simple evaluations can be performed by any technologist and include tests such as the wire mesh test for screen contact and the spinning top test for timer accuracy.

Level II: Noninvasive and Complex. Noninvasive and complex evaluations should be performed by a technologist who has been specifically trained in quality control procedures. This is because more sophisticated equipment, such as special test tools, meters, or the Noninvasive Evaluation of Radiation Output (NERO) computerized multiple function unit, is used. Many educational programs now include this level of competency for graduation, so the number of technologists with these skills is increasing. The American Society of Radiologic Technologists (ASRT) includes quality control and QA duties in its practice standards for radiographers, sonographers, nuclear medicine technologists, computed tomography (CT) technologists, magnetic resonance imaging (MRI) technologists, mammographers, interventional radiographers, and bone densitometry technologists. The American Registry of Radiologic Technologists (ARRT) offers an advanced level certification exam for technologists wishing to document their knowledge of QA and quality control procedures and protocols. This can be used to verify qualification for a quality management technologist position.

Level III: Invasive and Complex. Invasive and complex evaluations involve some disassembly of the equipment and are normally performed by engineers or physicists. This textbook focuses on levels I and II of quality control testing. The following are the three types of quality control tests on various levels:

- Acceptance testing is performed on new equipment or equipment that has undergone major repair to demonstrate that it is performing within the manufacturer's specifications and criteria. It also can detect any defects that may exist in the equipment. The results obtained during acceptance testing also are used to establish the baseline performance of the equipment that is used as a reference point in future quality control testing.

- Routine performance evaluations are specific tests performed on the equipment in use after a certain amount of time has elapsed. These evaluations can verify that the equipment is performing within previously accepted standards and can be used to diagnose any changes in performance before becoming radiographically apparent.

- Error correction tests evaluate equipment that is malfunctioning or not performing at the manufacturer's specifications and also are used to verify the correct cause of the malfunction so that the proper repair can be made.

Continuous Quality Improvement. The older QA/quality control program ensured that a certain level of quality was met; it required monitoring only periodically for maintenance. It was segmented in approach because each department in a facility monitored and evaluated its own structural outcomes, creating a tendency to view individual performances rather than the process or system in which that individual was functioning. In turn, the program was externally motivated because its emphasis was on demonstrating compliance with externally developed standards. As long as the standards were met, no further work was required to improve the system.

In 1991, TJC began incorporating the concepts of continuous quality improvement (CQI), also referred to as *total quality management (TQM)*, *total quality control (TQC)*, *total quality leadership (TQL)*, *total quality improvement (TQI)*, and *statistical quality control (SQC)*, to replace the older QA/quality control philosophy into their program for accreditation of healthcare organizations. This concept is based on the "14 Points for Management" developed by W. Edwards Deming (Box 1-1) and the Japanese management style.

The CQI concept does not replace the concept of quality assurance/quality control but incorporates it at a higher conceptual level. Instead of just ensuring and maintaining quality, it continually improves quality by focusing on improving the system or process in which individual workers function rather than on the individuals themselves. For these processes to improve, it is essential to focus on the organization as a whole, rather than on individual departments. It also promotes the need for objective data to analyze and improve processes. Every employee should be actively involved in CQI (rather than just management or the quality control technologist) for the program to be successful. In this way, CQI can be internally motivating because employees will see that their involvement is tied to the success of the hospital, creating an atmosphere in which employees are motivated to do better because they are participating actively. Management must take the responsibility to promote this atmosphere, effectively allocate resources needed for improvement, treat employees as assets and not expenses, and work together toward shared goals. For healthcare institutions, this should allow the ultimate focus to be on improving patient care, which should build a satisfied customer base and benefit the institution in the long term.

PROCESS IMPROVEMENT THROUGH CONTINUOUS QUALITY IMPROVEMENT

As mentioned earlier, CQI focuses on the process in which employees operate rather than on the employees themselves. The rationale is that problems and variability with the process are the main cause of poor quality. The concept of process improvement through CQI is based on the following premises:

- 85/15 Rule—the process or system in place is the cause of problems 85% of the time, and the people or personnel within the process are the cause of problems 15% of the time.
- 80/20 Rule—80% of the problems are the result of 20% of the causes.
- Workers who are closest to the problem probably know what is wrong with the process and are better able to fix it.
- Structured problem-solving processes that use statistical means to verify performance produce better long-term solutions than processes that are not structured.
- Improving quality is the responsibility of everyone within an organization because all are a part of the process.

For healthcare organizations, most of the processes should be oriented toward the deliverance of high quality care and the achievement of customer satisfaction. A **process** is an ordered series of steps that help achieve a desired outcome or all the tasks directed at accomplishing one particular outcome grouped in a sequence. A **system** is a group of related processes. The parts of any process include a supplier, input, action, output, and the customer.

BOX 1-1 | Fourteen Points of Management

1. Create constancy of purpose toward improvement of product and service, with the aim to become competitive and stay in business and provide jobs.
2. Adopt a new philosophy.
3. Cease dependence on mass inspection to achieve quality. Build quality into the product in the first place.
4. End the practice of awarding business on the basis of price alone. Instead, minimize total cost. Move toward a single supplier for any one item because of a long-term relationship built on loyalty and trust.
5. Improve constantly and forever the system of production and service to improve quality and productivity and thus constantly reduce costs.
6. Institute training on the job.
7. Institute leadership to help people do the job better.
8. Drive out fear so that everyone can work effectively for the good of the organization.
9. Break down barriers among departments.
10. Eliminate slogans, exhortations, and targets for the work force.
11. Eliminate work quotas. Substitute leadership.
12. Eliminate merit rating systems.
13. Institute a vigorous program of education and self-improvement.
14. Involve everyone in the organization in the transformation of total quality improvement (TQI).

From Deming WE: *Out of the crisis,* Cambridge, Mass, 1986, Center for Advanced Educational Services, MIT Press.

- A **supplier** is an individual or entity that furnishes input to a process (e.g., person, department, organization) or one who provides the institution with goods or services. For diagnostic imaging departments, examples may include imaging equipment vendors and referring physicians.
- **Input** is information or knowledge necessary to achieve the desired outcome. For diagnostic imaging departments, examples may include patient information, examination requested, knowledge of procedures, and workload.
- **Action** is the means or activity used to achieve the desired outcome. Examples for diagnostic imaging departments may include computer entry and form completion and assignment of patients to appropriate rooms.

These first three steps are variable factors that influence the next portion of the process called the *output*.

- **Output** refers to the desired outcome, product, or characteristics that satisfy the customer. In diagnostic imaging departments, examples may include completed paperwork and completed diagnostic examination.
- **Customer** refers to a person, department, or organization that needs or wants the desired outcome.

According to Deming, the customer determines what constitutes quality. This can be broken down into the following groups:

- *Internal customers:* Generally, these are individuals or groups from within the organization such as referring physicians, hospital employees, departments, and department employees.
- *External customers:* These are individuals or groups from outside the organization such as patients and their families, third-party payers, and the community.

The satisfaction of the customer, both internal and external, is the driving force behind CQI because it focuses on the needs and expectations of customers and the continuous improvement of the product or service. By continually meeting or exceeding customer satisfaction, the process is considered to be successful.

Key Quality Characteristics

Key quality characteristics (KQCs) are those qualities or aspects that have been identified as being most important to the customer. These characteristics must be constantly measured and improved in order for customer satisfaction to increase. Examples in diagnostic imaging departments would be availability of a procedure (e.g., MRI, positron emission tomography [PET]), accurate report of image findings delivered promptly to the ordering physician, and minimal waiting time for patients.

Key Process Variables. Key process variables (KPVs) are the components of any process that may affect the final output of the process. There are five major categories of key process variables: manpower, machines, materials, environment, and policies.

- *Manpower* refers to the personnel involved in the process.
- *Machines* refers to the equipment used in the process.
- *Materials* refers to the type and quality of materials used in the process.
- *Environment* refers to the physical and psychological aspects on people involved in the process.
- *Policies* refers to the steps in the procedure or policy manual that have been used in the process.

Problem Identification and Analysis

Group Dynamics. For the continual improvement of the processes involved in customer satisfaction, several tools must be used to identify and analyze the data obtained. Groups or teams of individuals who are familiar with or are using the processes are generally the most successful in helping with problem identification in CQI. This is because a single individual may not have enough knowledge or experience, or both, with all of the aspects of a process. A team consists of at least two persons. For healthcare organizations, the ideal number for most teams or groups is between 6 and 12 persons. To be effective, these teams should be goal oriented, share equal responsibility, and be empowered by management. By working together, team members not only can improve older processes and develop new and better ones but also develop a sense of ownership within the organization (and therefore be more productive workers). Group dynamic tools that can be used in quality management include brainstorming, focus groups, quality improvement teams, quality circles, multi-voting, consensus, work teams, and problem-solving teams.

Brainstorming. Brainstorming is a group process used to develop a large collection of ideas without regard to their merit or validity. For example, a department meeting of all staff could be used to solicit ideas or suggestions for a particular topic. The leader of this session should encourage participation by everyone, not criticize any contribution made, and record all ideas for future assessment. It is also important to announce the topic to be discussed to all team members before the session. It also may be more effective for the leader to review the particular subject at the beginning of the session and then phrase the topic that will be discussed in the form of a question. However, the discussion should be relevant to the topic being discussed, and the leader must direct members to adhere to this topic.

Focus Groups. A focus group is a small group that focuses on a particular problem and then hopefully derives a solution. Generally, the applicable ideas on a particular problem obtained from brainstorming are considered in this smaller group, which can come to a consensus. Focus groups also may be responsible for obtaining additional data such as the interviewing of customers and patient surveys. This may add to a higher implementation cost for focus groups as compared with other group dynamic tools. A focus group must have a skilled facilitator to be successful.

Quality Improvement Team. A quality improvement team is a group of individuals who implement the solutions that were derived by the focus group. This may or may not include members of the focus group. Ideally, quality improvement teams should have six or seven members who are key customers or suppliers, or both, of the steps in the process (i.e., the people who actually do the steps in the process). It is best to avoid teams of managers only because they usually do not have detailed knowledge of the process. Input from other customers and suppliers should be sought by the team.

Quality Circles. This type of group dynamic tool is normally composed of supervisors and workers who are from the same department or who may have the same function in a similar department. Quality circles should be scheduled to meet regularly and have the specific function to identify potential problems with departmental processes and then formulate solutions. Levels of productivity and quality of images produced within a department are possible issues that may be discussed by quality circles.

Multi-voting. This method is normally used after a brainstorming session to dismiss nonessential or non-realistic ideas and then concentrate on those that can realistically solve the problem. All members of the brainstorming session are given a list of all of the ideas that were formulated and are then asked to vote on which one they consider the most important. The ideas with the fewest votes are discarded and the process repeated (thus the name, *multi-voting*) until just one key idea remains. This method reduces a large number of ideas or options to a manageable few judged important by the participants.

Consensus. This is another method that can follow a successful brainstorming session. After the initial ideas are formulated during the brainstorming session, the group members, through discussion and teamwork, come to an agreement on the most important idea to be addressed. Total agreement within the group is unnecessary, but any decision should at least be acceptable to all group members.

Work Teams. These teams focus on solving a complete problem or completing an entire task, rather than focusing on any one particular step in a process. Some work teams, known as *self-managed teams (SMTs)* are composed of 6 to 18 persons and are empowered by management to take any corrective action necessary to solve the assigned problem or task. The SMT members should be highly trained in the particular area in which they are working. The teamwork created by these teams is highly successful in facilitating CQI and solving potential problems.

Problem-Solving Teams. These teams work on specific tasks and meet to solve particular problems. They normally function to identify, analyze, and then solve both quality and productivity issues. Problem-solving teams must have a knowledgeable facilitator who is responsible for teaching team members the appropriate problem-solving tools for guiding them through the process.

5 Whys. This is a question-asking method developed by the Toyota Corporation that is used to explore the cause/effect relationships that may underlie a particular problem. Its ultimate goal is to determine the root cause of a problem. For example:

The department waiting time is excessive. (the problem)

1) Why? - One of the five x-ray rooms in the department is always malfunctioning.
2) Why? - The unit in the room is used 24 hours a day/seven days a week.
3) Why? - The unit is 10 years old.
4) Why? - It is beyond its useful service life and has never been replaced.
5) Why? - Administration will not approve the purchase of a new unit.

Once the root cause is identified, a solution can then be devised to solve it.

Thought Process Map (TPM). This tool is one of the first tools that should be employed for a process improvement project. It presents thoughts, ideas, and questions at the beginning of a project to help a team or person identify all information and progress. There are five basic steps to create a TMP:

- Define the project's goal(s). The project improvement team needs to clearly define what needs to be accomplished or what problem needs to be solved. Brainstorming among the group is a good way to define the goal.
- List the knowns and unknowns. The team leader should use a large poster board or easel pad and make two columns—one for what the team knows and one for what the team does not know. This can help identify the amount and type of data necessary to complete the project.
- Ask grouped questions or questions that define, measure, analyze, improve, or control (DMAIC). Focusing on the unknowns from step 2, create questions from the categorical perspectives of DMAIC. These perspectives are discussed in more detail later in this chapter.
- Sequence and link the questions. The questions in step 4 are now linked together using a flowchart (discussed in Chapter 2).

- Identify possible tools to be used. This step involves identifying potential tools that can be used to answer the questions posed in step 3. The most effective way to accomplish this step is to create a four-column matrix that assigns a column for the question, the tool or method, who is responsible, and the due date.

Specific Quality Management Quality Improvement Processes

TJC 10-Step Process. In 1985, TJC introduced the 10-step monitoring and evaluation process as the mechanism for satisfaction of accreditation. Although it is still in use today, the emphasis of some of its steps has changed from QA to CQI.

Step 1: Assign responsibility for the department's monitoring and evaluation activities. In QA, the medical director is ultimately responsible, but the task is usually delegated to a supervisor or QA technologist. With CQI, both intradepartmental and interdepartmental committees work together with hospital management participation. A separate quality management department is found in many healthcare facilities, while others use a unit or section within the diagnostic imaging area for QM responsibilities. Regardless, each department or committee is responsible for documenting the effectiveness of its quality management activities and for reporting such activities to the organization-wide program. Staff members who perform quality management responsibilities also should make sure that the overall organizational program is functional and effective.

Step 2: Delineate the scope of care and service provided by the department. With the QA model, the major services of a particular department are listed (e.g., imaging modalities offered, types of patients served, credentials of staff), whereas under CQI, the scope of care or service for the hospital as a whole is defined.

Step 3: Identify important aspects of care and service. Under QA, specific departmental tasks or functions are identified, with emphasis on high volume (chest radiography), high risk (mammography interpretations and angiography), and high risk/problem prone (intravenous pyelography [IVP] and examinations requiring intravenous [IV] contrast media). With CQI, the entire hospital determines the key functions to be monitored. This should include important functions relating to patients, care of patients, leadership, use of medications, use of blood and blood components, and determination of the appropriateness of admissions and continued hospitalization.

Step 4: Identify indicators or performance measures. The Joint Commission defines an **indicator** as a valid and reliable quantitative process or outcome measure related to one or more dimensions of performance. There are two important types of indicators.

Sentinel Event Indicator. A sentinel event is an unexpected occurrence involving death or serious physical or psychological injury, or the risk thereof. Serious injury specifically includes loss of limb or function. The phrase "or the risk thereof" includes any process variation for which a recurrence would carry a significant chance of a serious adverse outcome. The events are called "sentinel" because they signal the need for immediate investigation and response. A **sentinel event indicator** identifies an individual event or phenomenon that is significant enough to trigger further review each time it occurs. These events are undesirable and occur infrequently, such as the death of a patient during a diagnostic examination as a result of contrast media reaction, suicide of a patient in a setting where the patient receives around-the-clock care, unanticipated death of a full-term infant, infant abduction or discharge to the wrong family, sexual assault of a patient, hemolytic transfusion reaction involving administration of blood or blood products having major blood group incompatibilities, and surgery on the wrong patient or wrong body part.

Aggregate Data Indicator. An **aggregate data indicator** quantifies a process or outcome related to many cases. It may occur frequently and may be desirable or undesirable. Examples include the number of cesarean sections and the number of reported medication errors.

Using QA, each department identifies indicators, whereas under CQI, an interdisciplinary team identifies indicators that focus more on the process of care. The performance indicators that are most relevant to healthcare organizations would include the following:

- **Appropriateness of care** is whether the type of care (i.e., specific test, procedure, or service) that has been requested is necessary. In other words, is it relevant to the patient's clinical needs, given the current state of knowledge (Are you doing the right thing?).
- **Continuity of care** is the degree to which the care/intervention for the patient is coordinated among practitioners or organizations, or both, over time.
- **Effectiveness of care** is the level of benefit when services are rendered under ordinary circumstances by average practitioners for typical patients, as defined by K.N. Lohr.* It also may be defined as the degree to which the care/intervention is provided in the correct manner, given the current state of knowledge, in order to achieve the desired/projected outcome for the patient.
- **Efficacy of care** is the level of benefit expected when healthcare services are applied under ideal conditions and the best possible circumstances or the degree to which the care/intervention has been shown to accomplish the desired outcome (i.e., Are

---

*From Lohr KN: Outcomes measurement: concepts and questions, *Inquiry* 25:37–50, 1988.

you doing the right thing well?). Most healthcare systems deliver care that is somewhere between effectiveness and efficacy. QA attempts to bring effectiveness to efficacy, whereas CQI goes a step further in allowing for continued improvement once effectiveness has been reached.

- **Efficiency of care** refers to the outcome obtained when the highest quality of care is delivered in the shortest amount of time, with the least amount of expense, and with a positive outcome for the patient condition.

An aggregate data indicator involves the relationship between the outcomes (results of care) and the resources used to deliver patient care.

- **Respect and caring** is defined as the degree to which the patient or a designee is involved in his or her own care decisions and to which those providing services do so with sensitivity and respect for the patient's needs, expectations, and individual differences. Respect and caring refers to how well patients are treated during the delivery of healthcare service, what the patient's level of satisfaction is, and how well a patient's complaints are handled by staff and management.
- **Safety in the care environment.** This is the degree to which the risk of an intervention and the risk in the care environment are reduced for the patient and others, including the healthcare provider. Safety in the care environment includes equipment functioning and operation, application of universal precautions, and competency of staff.
- **Timeliness of care.** This is defined as the degree to which the care/intervention is provided to the patient at the most beneficial or necessary time. Timeliness of care refers to the delivery of healthcare within a reasonable amount of time, with minimal waiting time.
- **Cost of care.** Cost of care refers to the delivery of healthcare that is reasonable for the current marketplace.
- **Availability of care.** This is defined as the degree to which appropriate care/intervention is available to meet the patient's needs. Availability of care refers to the availability at the clinical facility of the type of care or procedure required by the patient. A good example would be how early a patient who has a breast lump would be able to have a mammogram.

Step 5: Establish a Means to Trigger Evaluation. Under QA, a level of **expectation** is to be identified for each indicator. TJC identifies a level of expectation (formerly known as a *threshold*) as a pre-established level of performance applied to a specific indicator. The levels can be determined internally (on the basis of past performance of the facility) or externally (on the basis of federal and state regulations or professional guidelines such as those of TJC). As long as the indicator is below the expectation level in a negative event or condition, no further action or evaluation is required. For a highly desirable condition or event, the level of expectation is set at 100%. Under CQI, interdisciplinary teams use statistical methods to determine levels or patterns that trigger evaluation.

Step 6: Collect and Organize Data. Under QA, the department determines the protocol for data collection. First, the method of collection is determined. These data must be collected systematically and on important processes and outcomes that are related to the care of the patient or the functions of the healthcare organization. Options for collection include the following:

- *Patient surveys and questionnaires.* These should be sent to patients 3 to 7 days after discharge or on service dates for outpatients. These are the simplest mechanisms for obtaining customer/patient information. These should be brief (completed in 15 minutes or less, to generate a high response rate), have responses that can be measured quantitatively (such as multiple choice or Likert scale), and be clearly worded so that patients understand what is being asked of them.
- *Patient records.* Information such as sentinel events or other data is easily obtained.
- *Staff reports.* These include patient care logs, diaries, drug reaction reports, medication variance reports, and so on.
- *Focus groups.* As previously discussed, these small groups collect data that focus on finding a solution to a specific problem.
- *Computer database.* Considerable patient information and relevant data from across the country may be available in some computer databases. However, privacy concerns such as those addressed in the HIPAA (previously discussed) may limit access to database information.

Next, the size of the sample is determined (e.g., how many patients, cases). Then the frequency of collection is determined (e.g., concurrently, daily, weekly, monthly). **Concurrent data** are any data collected during the time of care. Data that should be collected and processed on a continuous basis include patient deaths (dependent on the patient mix and regional factors) and serious complications to treatment. The frequency at which data are collected for a specific indicator is reviewed annually to indicate whether the data are adequately capturing the desired information. The final task is to analyze the data and determine how they are manipulated for comparison with the level of expectation or with pre-established criteria. Under CQI, an interdisciplinary team determines the protocol for data collection from various areas of the hospital.

Step 7: Initiate Evaluation. With QA, the staff evaluates the level of performance for an indicator by comparing it with the expectation level. With CQI, the leaders identify areas for evaluation according to the data collected.

Step 8: Take Actions to Improve Care and Service. With QA, individuals are evaluated as to whether expectation levels were achieved and corrective action taken accordingly. The CQI method looks at the process used in providing the care or service rather than at the individual.

Step 9: Assess Effectiveness of Actions and Maintain Improvements. The QA method examines whether the actions taken in Step 8 are effective in ensuring quality, whereas the CQI method shows that improvement is continually being sustained. Documentation of these methods is important.

Step 10: Communicate Results to Affected Individuals and Groups. With the QA method, all results are given to a QA committee and then shared with the department staff and hospital QA committee, whereas with CQI, all results are reported to the leaders and other affected individuals. All data collected must be consolidated for distribution in a final report. A common method of presenting such results is with a storyboard (Fig. 1-1). A storyboard can summarize a whole report or process with photographs and graphs and a minimum of text. The final report should include a description of a process identified for improvement, the method used to identify that process; the department involved; the source of all data collected; any cause of variation that is identified; any corrective action that was taken; the person or persons who implemented this action; the timetable for implementation; whether or not the process was actually improved; future plans to monitor the process; and any plans to restudy, if applicable.

TJC Cycle for Improving Performance. The Joint Commission 10-step monitoring and evaluation process is still valid and is the basis of their "Cycle for Improving Performance," which identifies the steps *design, measure, assess,* and *improve.*

Design. Systematic planning and implementation are key to the design of any function or process. When new functions and processes are being designed and planned, the following factors should be considered:

- The organization's overriding purpose (mission), view of its future (vision), and strategies for carrying out its mission and fulfilling its vision (strategic plan)
- Needs and expectations of patients, staff, accrediting agencies, and payers (customers and suppliers)
- Current knowledge about organizational and clinical activities from both inside and outside the organization
- Current and relevant data, such as the number of patients receiving diagnostic imaging examinations per month, the department repeat rate, and the number of practicing physicians
- Availability of resources such as funds, staff time, and equipment

Measure. A *measure* is defined by TJC as a collection of valid and reliable data to demonstrate the effectiveness and efficiency of care and performance improvement. These data can be collected by various means including focus groups and quality improvement teams.

Assess. *Assessment* is defined by TJC as translating data collected during measurement into information that can be used to change processes and improve

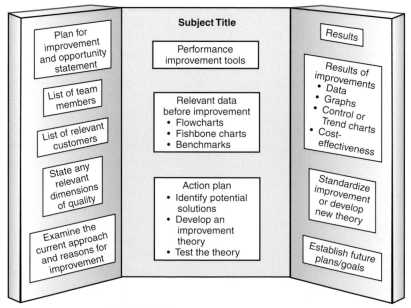

FIGURE 1-1 Model for a storyboard.

performance. Proper assessment usually requires comparing data with a reference point or standard. This includes the following:

Internal:

- *Historical patterns of performance in the organization* (also called *baseline performance*). This is a comparison of current performance levels with those occurring previously such as comparing current department repeat rates with those of the previous year.
- *Desired performance limits.* The patient population and referring physicians expect a certain level of performance. This should be compared with the level achieved, as indicated by the current data. The healthcare organization also may establish its own control limits, targets, and specifications that can be compared with the data obtained.

External:

- *Practice guidelines and parameters.* These procedures, developed by professional societies, expert panels, or in-house practitioners, represent a consensus of the best practices for a given diagnosis, treatment, or procedure. These are usually described in the form of a **critical path** that documents the basic treatment or action sequence in an effort to eliminate unnecessary variation. A critical path defines the optimal sequence and timing of intervention by healthcare practitioners for a particular diagnosis or process.
- *Performance measurement system.* A performance measurement system is an entity consisting of one or more automated databases that facilitates performance improvement in healthcare organizations through collection and dissemination of process or outcome measures of performance, or both. These systems allow an organization to compare its performance with that of other organizations using information such as patient outcomes, costs, lengths of stay for certain treatments, and mortality and morbidity rates. Examples are the TJC Indicator Measurement System (IMS) and databases maintained by federal and state governments and third-party payers.
- *Benchmarking.* **Benchmarking** involves comparing one organization's performance standards with that of another; however, it focuses on the other organization's key processes that achieve performance rather than the numbers and statistical data obtained in an aggregate external reference database. Two main types of benchmarking exist: internal and external. Internal benchmarking compares performance with the best practices within one's own organization. External benchmarking compares an organization's performance with other organizations. External benchmarking can be further broken down into two types, competitive and world-class. Competitive external benchmarking involves comparing an organization to competitors marketing the same product or service. The American College of Radiology (ACR) publishes a National Radiology Data Registry (NRDR) that contains regional and national benchmarks for various diagnostic imaging modalities. This can be accessed online at **http://nrdr.acr.org/**. World-class external benchmarking involves benchmarking against organizations outside of one's specific industry. A good example might be comparing the billing and collection practices of a healthcare organization with those of a bank or department store.

Improve. Once knowledge is gained through measurement and analysis, action can be taken to improve processes by refining or redesigning a process to improve its level of performance. This cycle of design, measure, assess, and improve should be continuously repeating in a CQI program (Fig. 1-2).

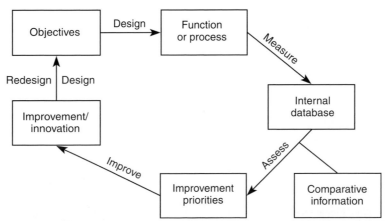

FIGURE 1-2 Cycle for improving performance, showing the important steps, including inputs and outputs, of a systematic approach to improvement. *(From Joint Commission Resources: Forms, charts, & other tools for performance improvement, Oakbrook Terrace, Ill, 1994, JCAHO. Reprinted with permission.)*

Other Quality Management/Quality Improvement Models

The following are some of the other specific quality management/quality improvement models that are currently in use:

- Evangelical Health Systems CQI Monitoring System
- FADE was created by Organizational Dynamics, a private consulting firm (Fig. 1-3).
- The Five-Stage Plan was developed by Joiner and Associates, a quality consulting group.
- The **SWOT analysis**, developed at Stanford Research Institute in California from 1960–1970, analyzes the internal and external environment of a healthcare organization. The environmental factors internal to the organization can be classified as strengths (**S**) or weaknesses (**W**), and those external to the organization can be classified as opportunities (**O**) or threats (**T**). The SWOT analysis provides information that can be helpful in matching a healthcare organization's resources and capabilities to the competitive environment in which it operates. The organization's strengths are its resources and capabilities such as a good reputation among customers, expertise of physicians and staff, or advanced equipment that may not be available at competing imaging departments. Weaknesses are usually the absence of certain strengths such as a poor reputation among customers or lack of availability of latest equipment and procedures. Opportunities for growth might include obtaining the latest equipment or hiring physicians with advanced skills. Threats to the healthcare organization may include competition from a nearby facility or new regulations or reimbursement procedures.

- The **FOCUS-PDCA** (Fig. 1-4) approach was developed by the Hospital Corporation of America (HCA) in the 1980s that adapted the "plan, do, check, and act" (PDCA) cycle used by Deming in Japanese industry. The PDCA cycle was initially developed by Walter A. Shewhart and may be referred to as either the Shewhart cycle, Deming cycle, or PDCA cycle. The Hospital Corporation of America included the preliminary steps of FOCUS. This model consists of the following tenets:

F   Find a process to improve or a problem to solve.
O   Organize a team that knows the process and work on improvement.
C   Clarify the problem and current knowledge of the process.
U   Understand the problem and the causes of process variation.
S   Select the method to improve the process.
P   Plan to implement a new method to improve the process.
D   Do the implementation and measure the change.
C   Check the results of the change.
A   Act to hold the improvements and continue further improvements.

- A **Failure Mode and Effects Analysis (FMEA)** is a procedure for analysis of potential failure within a system, classifying the severity or determining the failure's effect upon the system and helping determine remedial actions to overcome these failures. It was first used by the U.S. Armed Forces in the late 1940s and expanded by NASA in the 1960s to help put a man on the moon. In the late 1970s, the Ford Motor Company implemented FMEA into the automotive industry. Before conducting FMEA, it is

FADE

Phases of FADE problem solving

Focus–

choose a problem and describe it

Analyze–

learn about a problem by collecting and analyzing pertinent data

Develop–

develop a solution and a plan

Execute–

implement the plan, monitor the results, adjust as needed

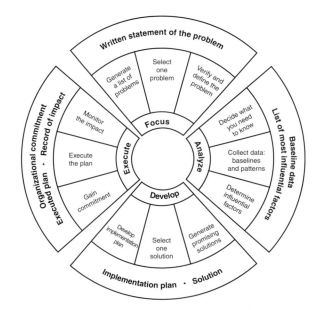

FIGURE 1-3 Phases of FADE problem solving. *(Printed with permission from* Quality Action Teams: Team Members Workbook, *Organizational Dynamics, Inc. 1987, www.odionline.com.)*

FOCUS-PDCA

Hospital Corporation of America

Expands on the PDCA Cycle by including
"preliminary steps," i.e., FOCUS.

- **F**ind process improvement opportunity
- **O**rganize a team that knows the process
- **C**larify current knowledge of the process
- **U**ncover root causes for process variation
- **S**tart improvement cycle

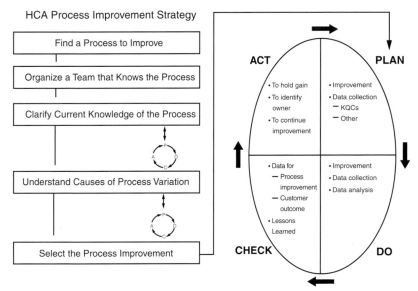

FIGURE 1-4 The FOCUS-PDCA Model. *(Reprinted with permission from Hospital Corporation of America, Nashville, Tennessee, 1989).*

necessary to describe the process or system being evaluated. This is best done by using a flowchart (described in the next chapter). The analysis itself occurs in 3 steps:

Step 1: Severity. Determine all failure modes and their effects. Each effect is given a **severity number (S)** ranging from 1 (no danger) to 10 (important). If the severity of an effect has a number of 9 or 10, actions are considered to eliminate the failure mode (such as using only nonionic contrast media). A severity rating of 9 or 10 is usually reserved for effects that would cause injury or result in litigation.

Step 2: Occurrence. In this step, it is necessary to look at the cause of a failure and how often it occurs. All potential causes for failure should be identified and documented. A failure mode is given a **probability number (O)**, which also ranges from 1 to 10. Actions need to be determined if an occurrence is high (meaning greater than 4 for non-safety failure and greater than 1 when the severity number from Step 1 is 9 or 10).

Step 3: Detection. Whenever actions are taken to minimize failure, it is important to see how efficiently failures can be detected in the system to prevent further failure. Each combination from

the first 2 steps receives a **detection number (D)**, which represents the ability of tests and inspections to detect failure modes.

- Once these three steps are completed, **Risk Priority Numbers (RPN)** are calculated by multiplying the numbers from each step: RPN = S × O × D. This number is generally used as a threshold value in the evaluation of any action to reduce failure.

- **Six Sigma** is a management strategy that seeks to identify and remove the causes of errors in business processes. It was originally developed by Motorola in 1986 and is now used in a variety of applications including healthcare management. The term is derived from statistics (discussed in the next chapter) where the word Sigma (the lower case Greek letter σ) is used to represent the standard deviation (a measure of variation) of a statistical population. Six sigma comes from the concept that if there are three standard deviations on either side of the mean of a process and the nearest limit (covering 99% of all variables), then there will be virtually no items that fail to meet the specifications. It allows you to measure how many errors you may have in a process so you can systematically figure out how to eliminate them. This procedure was inspired by Deming's PDCA cycle and consists of these five steps:

Define process improvement goals that are consistent with customer demands and the institution's strategy.

Measure key aspects of the current process and collect relevant data.

Analyze the data to verify cause-and-effect relationships. Determine what the relationships are and attempt to ensure that all factors have been considered.

Improve or optimize the process based on data analysis.

Control the process to ensure that any deviations from the target are corrected before they result in errors or failure.

SUMMARY

In modern diagnostic imaging departments, the radiologists, department administrators and supervisors, technologists, and support staff should work together to ensure that adequate processes are in place to properly care for the patient, achieve the highest quality image possible, and obtain the correct diagnosis from that image. These processes also are necessary to meet accreditation standards or government requirements, or both. The processes also should be reviewed continuously by all parties and modified as the need arises. Any quality management plan should have specific objectives (what the program is intending to achieve), an outline of the chain of command and responsibilities within the organization, the scope of the program, a mechanism for monitoring various aspects of patient management, evaluation of the program's effectiveness in meeting the objectives, and the efficacy of the program. Having an effective quality management program also has become necessary as a condition of receiving reimbursement for services by the federal government and many private insurance companies.

REVIEW QUESTIONS

1. Which levels of quality control testing can usually be performed by a quality assurance/quality management technologist: level I, level II, or level III?
   a. I and II
   b. I and III
   c. II and III
   d. I, II, and III

2. Which government agency mandates a policy on exposure to blood-borne pathogens?
   a. FDA
   b. EPA
   c. OSHA
   d. CDRH

3. Which of the following terms best describes information or knowledge necessary to achieve a desired outcome?
   a. Supplier
   b. Input
   c. Action
   d. Output

4. How many basic steps are involved in the creation of a TPM?
   a. 3
   b. 5
   c. 7
   d. 10

5. A procedure to identify potential failure within a system is
   a. SWOT
   b. FMEA
   c. Six Sigma
   d. FOCUS-PDCA

6. Which of the following terms best describes a person, department, or organization that needs or wants a desired outcome?
   a. Supplier
   b. Input
   c. Action
   d. Customer

7. Who is considered to be the "Father of Scientific Management"?
   a. W. Edwards Deming
   b. Joseph Juran
   c. Raymond Smith
   d. Frederick Winslow Taylor

8. Which of the following groups is usually responsible for implementing the solutions that the focus groups have determined will improve a particular process?
   a. Quality circle
   b. Work team
   c. Quality improvement team
   d. Problem-solving team

9. Which of the following terms best describes a valid and reliable quantitative process or outcome measure related to one or more dimensions of performance?
   a. External customer
   b. Indicator
   c. Level of expectation
   d. Sentinel event

10. The highest quality of care delivered in the shortest amount of time with the least amount of expense and a positive outcome is termed _____ of care.
    a. appropriateness
    b. continuity
    c. effectiveness
    d. efficiency

Quality Management Tools and Procedures

OBJECTIVES

At the completion of this chapter the reader should be able to do the following:

- Describe the four main components of a quality management program
- List and define the basic terms used in statistical analysis
- Discuss the seven types of graphs and charts used to organize and present data in total quality management

- List the basic administrative responsibilities of a quality management program
- Describe the various components of a risk management program
- Describe the radiation safety protocols for patients and radiation personnel

OUTLINE

A comprehensive quality management program consists of many different components, depending on the size and complexity of the healthcare organization. Programs for diagnostic imaging departments, regardless of the size, should contain at least the following components:

- *Equipment quality control.* This aspect of a quality management program involves evaluation of equipment performance to ensure proper image quality, as well as patient and operator safety. These procedures are covered extensively in Chapters 3 through 15.
- *Administrative responsibilities.* This aspect of the quality management program involves the establishment of various processes to accomplish the specific departmental tasks that are required such as departmental procedure manuals for performing diagnostic examinations or procedures for scheduling and routing of patients. It also involves data collection and analysis to continuously improve these processes. Other responsibilities include cost control, management of personnel, education of personnel (education for newly hired personnel and continuing education for existing workers), equipment acquisition, communication with various vendors, communication with other departments within the healthcare organization, and various other activities.
- *Risk management.* The ability to identify potential risks to patients, employees, and visitors at the healthcare institution and establish processes that would minimize these risks is extremely important to healthcare organizations. Civil litigation and workers' compensation judgments can severely deplete the financial resources of even the largest healthcare organization.
- *Radiation safety program.* This is to ensure that patient exposure is kept as low **as reasonably achievable (ALARA)** and that department personnel, medical staff, and members of the general public are protected from overexposure to ionizing radiation.

INFORMATION ANALYSIS

To implement the various components of a quality management program, a considerable amount of data must be collected and analyzed, which requires the use of statistics. Statistics is the mathematical science pertaining to the collection, analysis, interpretation, and presentation of data. This data then can be used to verify the success of organizational processes or provide justification for changing and improving these processes.

To assist in the implementation of a quality management program, diagnostic imaging personnel need a basic knowledge of the terminology and data presentation tools used in statistical analysis.

Terminology Used in Statistical Analysis

Population. A **population** comprises the entire set or group of items being measured. Identifying the population to be measured is one of the first steps in performing a statistical analysis. For example, if you perform a statistical analysis of the number of repeat chest radiographs during a particular month, you focus on just the patients receiving chest examinations (that particular population) rather than each patient receiving each type of radiographic procedure.

Sample. A **sample** is the number of items actually measured from a population. Some populations may be extremely large and therefore difficult to study. Sampling involves choosing a portion or evaluating a subset of the population that makes data collection more practical, timely, and efficient. An example of sampling is the nationwide measurement of persons watching particular television programs. Only certain persons have their television viewing patterns actually monitored by the ratings services, and the results are extrapolated to be indicative of the entire population. This is known as *statistical inference.* Sampling must be performed carefully to ensure that the sample chosen is representative of the entire population.

Data Set. A **data set** is the information or measurements acquired by evaluating the particular sample.

Frequency. The **frequency** is the number of times a particular value of a variable occurs or the number of observations of an event. For example, during a repeat study of chest examinations, 37 chest views had to be repeated during a particular month. Therefore the frequency of repeated chest views for that month was 37.

Dependent Variables. **Dependent variables** are those variables that are observed in statistical studies to change in response to independent variables and are not controlled during the study. The dependent variable also can be referred to as response variables, measured variables, or output variables. For example, if one were to study how different brands of contrast media cause allergic reactions in diagnostic imaging patients, a researcher could compare the frequency and intensity of a reaction to the different brands of contrast media. In this study, the frequency and cause of allergic reactions would be the dependent variables.

Independent Variables. Independent variables are those that are deliberately manipulated to invoke a change on the dependent variables. Independent variables also may be referred to as predictor variables or input variables. In the example presented under dependent variables comparing how different brands of contrast media cause allergic reactions in diagnostic imaging patients, the different brands of contrast media given to diagnostic imaging patients would be the independent variable.

Continuous Variables. Continuous variables are those variables being studied that have an infinite range of possible mathematical values. Examples might include the age of patients, weight of patients, height of patients, and time of a particular event.

Dichotomous Variables. Dichotomous variables are those variables being studied that have only two opposing choices, such as male or female and on or off.

Central Tendency. The central tendency is the central position of a sample frequency. In statistical analysis, there are several possible measures of central tendency, three of which are the mean, the median, and the mode.

- *Mean.* The **mean** is the average set of observations and can be denoted by either μ, $\overline{X}$, or M. The mean provides the greatest reliability of the three measures of central tendency.

$$\text{Mean} = \frac{\text{Sum of observed values } (\Sigma)}{\text{Total number of values } (N)}$$

For example, if the values 7, 3, 6, and 4 are observed, the mean is determined by taking 20 (the sum of the observed values) divided by 4 (the total number of values observed), which yields a mean of 5.
- The **median** is a point on a scale of measurement above which are exactly one half of the values and below which are the other half. In other words, it is the numeric middle. For example, if the values 4, 6, 8, 10, and 12 are observed, the median is 8.
- The **mode** is the one value that occurs with the greatest frequency in the data set. For example, if the values 2, 3, 4, 4, 4, 5, and 5 are observed, the mode is 4. The mode provides information about the most typical occurrence, but this is usually just a rough estimate of central value.

Reliability. Reliability refers to the consistency of repeated measurements of the same thing or the reproducibility of a result and is sometimes known as *precision*. Many factors, such as the sample size (larger samples are usually more reliable), the design of the data collection process (e.g., Are the questions on a survey worded in a "biased" way?), and the collection and interpretation of the data (e.g., Is the person collecting the data including all of the information given?), can affect the reliability of statistical information. A new quality management program may have unreliable data at first because of the "start-up effect." This effect can cause an unusually high or low data result because the human tendency is to be hyperaware when new studies are begun. To counteract the start-up effect, a sufficient period of time needs to elapse to allow the data to change and stabilize before reliable data analysis is obtained. Reliability or precision does not imply accuracy.

Accuracy. Accuracy refers to the ability to measure what is purported to be measured and is sometimes referred to as **validity.** In other words, do the data collected reflect the reality of the situation being studied? One also can think of accuracy as how well a value that has been studied and measured agrees with the true value.

Bias. Bias is a systematic or nonrandom difference between the true value of a property and individual measurements of that property or the presence of a systematic error. Sometimes bias in a statistical context is thought of as being synonymous with the term **prejudice.** This is an incorrect assumption because prejudice refers to an individual's state of mind that would create a desire for a particular outcome.

Error. *Measurement error* refers to the difference between the measured value and the true value of the variable being measured. Errors of measurement can be divided into two categories, systematic errors and random errors. Systematic errors, also known as determinate errors, result from factors such as malfunctioning equipment, not correcting all outside influences, and poor design of the data collection process. Examples in imaging would include equipment not calibrated properly or incorrect exposure factors selected by a technologist. Random errors, also known as indeterminate errors, are caused by statistical fluctuations or uncertainties such as quantum mottle.

Range. Range refers to the difference between the highest and lowest values and is a measure of the dispersion of the data distribution.

Standard Deviation. The **standard deviation** is the range of variation or dispersion of a set of values surrounding the mean, or the spread or distribution of a data set. It can apply to a random variable, a population, a probability distribution, or a multiset. This can be symbolized by the capital letters *SD* or the small Greek letter *sigma* (σ). It is defined as the root-mean-square (RMS) deviation of the values from their mean. Since standard deviation is a measure of statistical dispersion, it measures how widely spread the values in a data set are from the mean. If many data points are close to the mean, then the standard deviation is small; if many data points are far from the mean, then the standard deviation is large. If all data values are equal, then the standard deviation is zero.

$$\sqrt{SD = \frac{\Sigma x^2}{M}}$$

The small letter x is the amount of deviation of a value X from the mean (M). $x = X - M$. For example, with the values 7, 3, 6, and 4, the mean is 5. The standard deviation is determined with the following equation:

$$SD = \sqrt{\frac{(7-5)^2 + (3-5)^2 + (6-5)^2 + (4-5)^2}{5}}$$

The standard deviation is 1.41.

When a large standard deviation is obtained (i.e., a large variation has occurred from the mean), it is important to analyze why this has occurred. Possibilities to consider include that this may be a normal occurrence and that the data are valid. It is also possible that the ways in which the measurements were obtained, calculated, or determined were not correctly performed. The validity of the standard deviation value must be determined before the results of the study being performed can be considered valid.

Variance. Variance is the square of the standard deviation and is used to determine if the separate means of several different groups differ significantly from each other (e.g., between male and female patients, different age groups). Like standard deviation, it is used as a measure of the dispersion of a set of values.

Poisson Distribution. A **Poisson distribution** is a random distribution in which the variance is equal to the mean. This distribution is generally asymmetrical for low mean values (<10). In Poisson statistics, the standard deviation can be estimated by taking the square root of the mean. For example, if a sample has a mean of 144, the standard deviation is 12. This method is used in nuclear medicine.

Gaussian Distribution. A **Gaussian distribution** is also known as a *normal distribution* and creates a bell-shaped curve that is continuous with both tails extending to infinity (Fig. 2-1). The distribution is symmetric about the mean value of the measurement set with the spread of the measurements characterized by the

standard deviation of the measurements. With this distribution, 68% of all values will fall within 1 standard deviation on either side of the mean, 95% will fall within 2 standard deviations, and 99% will fall within 3 standard deviations. (This is the basis of **Six Sigma,** discussed in the last chapter, whereby 99% of all variables are covered.)

Variation. **Variation** refers to anything that would cause a process to deviate from acceptable standards. Sources of variation in diagnostic imaging might include materials and supplies, equipment, procedures and methods, personnel, and management. Two basic types of variation are encountered in diagnostic imaging, special cause variation and common cause variation. Common cause variation is generally due to the process or system in place, as well as the people within the system (i.e., personnel or patient population). Special cause variation is assignable to a specific cause or causes and arises because of special circumstances.

Validity. As mentioned previously, validity is sometimes referred to as *accuracy.* In survey measurement, there are three main types of validity of concern: construct validity, content validity, and criterion validity. Construct validity is the extent to which a measure would agree with other survey instruments that have been used to measure the same parameters and have a proven accuracy. Content validity is the extent to which a survey will cover all of the content area. Criterion validity compares the results obtained in a survey to an established criterion measure.

Information Analysis Tools

As mentioned previously, total quality management (TQM) is devoted to process improvement so that goods and services can be delivered more efficiently to increase customer satisfaction. This means that data must be collected about how well the various processes are being implemented; customer satisfaction surveys and repeat

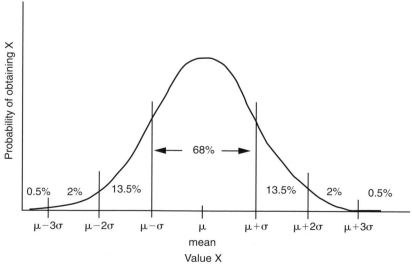

FIGURE 2-1 Gaussian probability (normal) distribution.

analysis of radiographic images are examples of data collection. Once these data are collected, they then must be organized and presented in a format that is easy to analyze. Seven basic statistical tools can be used to display data for interpretation and analysis: flowcharts, cause-and-effect diagrams, histograms, Pareto charts, scatter plots, trend charts, and control charts.

Flowchart. A **flowchart** is a pictorial representation of the individual steps that can be contained in a process. It is designed to present the sequence of events in the process from its beginning point to its end point. When correctly constructed, it can demonstrate potential problem areas, inconsistencies, or redundancies that can produce variations in the output of the process, which may result in system failure. It also can help document current processes, redesign current processes, and design new processes. Flowcharts are relatively easy to construct but are best developed by persons who are directly involved or have knowledge of the particular process to be presented.

Before constructing a flowchart, one must identify all of the inputs, outputs, and actions within the process, as well as the sequence in which they occur. Then the appropriate symbol must be chosen to characterize each step within the process. For an explanation of the symbols used in a flowchart, see Box 2-1. Computer software programs are available for help in constructing a satisfactory flowchart. An example of a flowchart is shown in Figure 2-2.

Cause-and-Effect Diagram. A **cause-and-effect diagram** is a causal analysis tool (also called a *fishbone chart* or *Ishikawa diagram,* in honor of the person credited with its development). It is used to demonstrate graphically the causes and effects of different variables or conditions on a key quality characteristic and thereby, potential areas for improvement.

To construct a cause-and-effect diagram, you must first determine the key quality characteristic to be improved. Then potential causes of the effect must be identified so that they are included in the chart. Brainstorming by a quality improvement team or similar group may be helpful in this identification. The main ideas are listed on branches flowing toward the main branch of the diagram and grouped according to categories. All possible problems or causes for each of these main ideas must then be listed as subcauses within each branch. An example of a cause-and-effect diagram is shown in Figure 2-3.

Histogram. A **histogram** is a data display tool in the form of a bar graph that often plots the most frequent occurrence of a quantity in the center. A histogram differs from a bar graph in that it is the area of the bar/s that denotes the value and not the height of the bars. The distribution of continuous data is often best accomplished with a histogram. It also can help demonstrate the amount of variation within an individual process. Histograms often are used in diagnostic imaging to depict such continuous variables as the monthly repeat rate of a department or the number of examinations performed monthly. They also are programmed into computerized radiography systems to create satisfactory images (see Chapter 9). Software programs such as *Microsoft Excel* can generate histograms from information contained in a spreadsheet. Figure 2-4 shows an example of a histogram.

Pareto Chart. A **Pareto chart** is a causal analysis tool that is named after Wilfredo Pareto, an Italian political economist. The Pareto chart is a variation of the histogram or bar graph, which prioritizes the most frequent problems at the y-axis (far left) of the graph and the other problems in decreasing order to the right. The Pareto chart was developed to illustrate the 80/20 Rule (that 80% of the problems stem from 20% of the causes). The horizontal axis, or x-axis, indicates the factors or problems to be evaluated, whereas the vertical axis, or y-axis, demonstrates the frequency of occurrence. Pareto charts also may include a horizontal reference, or norm (normal occurrence). The Pareto chart is useful in identifying the main causes of problems and in demonstrating the results of improvement strategies that have been implemented. An example of a Pareto chart is shown in Figure 2-5.

Scatter Plot. A **scatter plot** (also called a *scatter diagram*) is a traditional two-axis graph (x-axis and y-axis), with several data points that have been plotted throughout. It is designed to determine whether a relationship

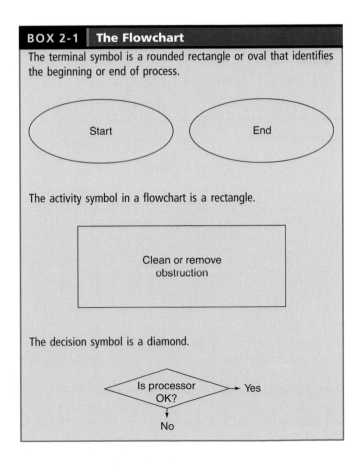

BOX 2-1 | The Flowchart

The terminal symbol is a rounded rectangle or oval that identifies the beginning or end of process.

Start

End

The activity symbol in a flowchart is a rectangle.

Clean or remove obstruction

The decision symbol is a diamond.

Is processor OK? → Yes

No

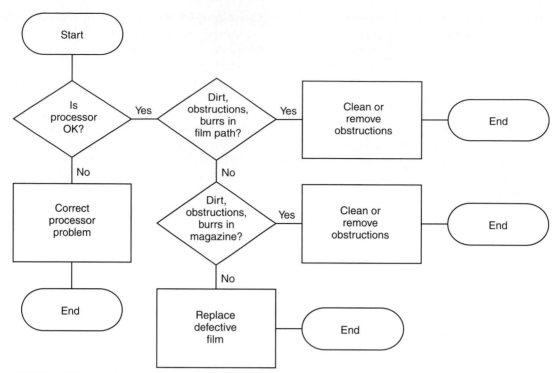

FIGURE 2-2 Flowchart diagrams the process of eliminating scratches on images caused by film processors.

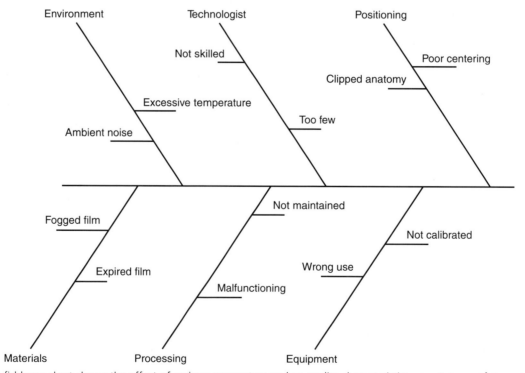

FIGURE 2-3 A fishbone chart shows the effect of various parameters on key quality characteristics or outcomes of proper image quality.

exists between two different variables in a process. Once the data points are plotted, the scatter plot then is examined to see if these points are scattered in any particular pattern. If so, a correlation may exist between the two variables. A positive correlation is indicated when both the x and y values increase in relation to each other. A negative correlation is demonstrated when there is an increase in the x variable in relation to a decrease in the y variable. An example of a scatter plot is shown in Figure 2-6.

Trend Chart. A **trend chart** (also called a *run chart* or *run-sequence plot*) pictorially demonstrates whether key indicators are moving up or down over a given period of time. Trending refers to the evaluation of data

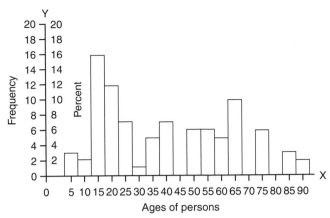

FIGURE 2-4 Histogram. Frequency of occurrence is demonstrated on the y-axis, and category or class interval is demonstrated on the x-axis. This example plots percentage of patients undergoing diagnostic procedures versus ages of patients.

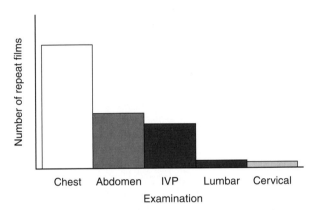

FIGURE 2-5 A Pareto chart indicates specific areas that cause unsatisfactory outcomes, so that improvement actions can be appropriately directed. IVP, Intravenous pyelography.

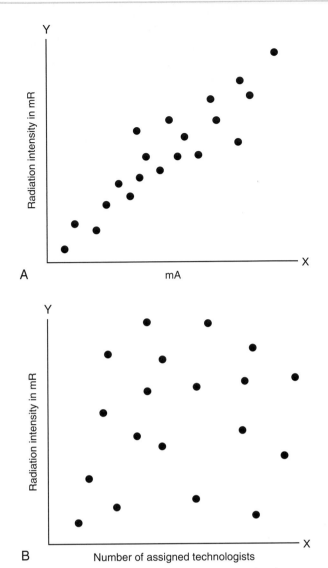

FIGURE 2-6 A scatter plot graph shows relationship between a key outcome or characteristic (y-axis) and a key process variable (x-axis). Graph **A** indicates a positive correlation between two values, and graph **B** indicates that no correlation exists. *mA*, Milliampere; *mR*, milliroentgen.

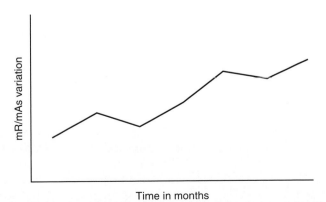

FIGURE 2-7 A trend graph displays amount of variation of indicator (radiation emitted from an x-ray generator) as a function of time. *mAs*, Milliampere-second; *mR*, milliroentgen.

collected over a period of time for the purpose of identifying patterns or changes. The variable being measured is placed on the vertical axis, or y-axis, and the time factor is placed on the horizontal axis, or x-axis. Often, some measure of central tendency (mean or median) of the data is indicated by a horizontal reference line. The trend chart can display the performance of, and any variation in, a process over a given period of time. For a trend chart to be constructed, the measurement or indicator to be measured must first be identified. Then all relevant data must be collected and analyzed. Next, all data points are plotted and connected with a linear line.

Once the chart has been constructed, the plotted points and lines must be analyzed to determine the degree of variation within the indicator. If there are no large spikes (upward or downward) and the line is relatively flat, then the process is considered to be under control. If unusual trends are observed, then the potential causes must be investigated and corrected. Trend charts cannot determine the source of any problem within a process, only if and when they have occurred. An example of a trend chart is shown in Figure 2-7.

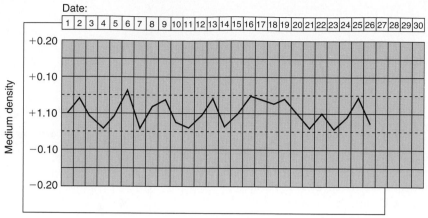

FIGURE 2-8 A control graph displays amount of variation of indicator (speed or medium density value from a sensitometry film) as a function of time, with upper and lower control limits indicated.

Control Chart. A **control chart** is a modification of the trend chart, in which statistically determined upper and lower control limits are placed with a central line that indicates an accepted norm. If the plotted data points fall above or below these control limits, then the process is considered unstable. The control chart was invented by Walter A. Shewhart while working at Bell Labs in the 1920s, so it is sometimes referred to as the Shewhart chart or process/behavior chart. Like the trend chart, the control chart cannot identify a specific cause of a problem, but rather if and when they have occurred. The control chart is often used for demonstrating the performance of automatic film processors over time (see Chapter 5). An example of a control chart is shown in Figure 2-8.

MISCELLANEOUS ADMINISTRATIVE RESPONSIBILITIES

In Chapter 1, a distinction between quality assurance (which deals with human factors) and quality control (which deals with equipment factors) is made. Merging these entities in a TQM program requires certain administrative procedures (Box 2-2) to be implemented by radiologists, department administrators, quality control technologists (Box 2-3), quality improvement committees, and radiographers (since they have direct patient contact and are therefore on the front line in demonstrating quality of care). Some of the more important administrative procedures follow.

BOX 2-2	**Administrative Procedures**

Establish thresholds of acceptability
Establish an effective communication network
Provide for patient comfort
Ensure accepted performance of diagnostic imaging personnel
Develop a record-keeping system
Establish corrective action procedures

BOX 2-3	**Quality Management Technologist Duties**

1. Ensures that services are performed in a safe environment in accordance with established guidelines
2. Ensures that equipment maintenance and operation comply with established guidelines
3. Assesses equipment to determine acceptable performance on the basis of established guidelines
4. Ensures that protocol and procedure manuals include recommended criteria and are reviewed and revised on a regular basis
5. Performs quality assurance activities on the basis of established quality protocols
6. Provides evidence of ongoing quality assurance activities
7. Monitors image production to determine variance from established quality standards
8. Obtains assistance from appropriate personnel to implement a quality assurance action plan
9. Maintains knowledge of, observes, and enforces the practice of standard precautions
10. Develops and implements a modified action plan when testing results are not in compliance with guidelines
11. Provides timely, concise, accurate, and complete documentation that adheres to current protocol, policy, and procedures

Data from American Society of Radiologic Technologists: *Practice standards for medical imaging and radiation therapy*, Albuquerque, 2000, ASRT.

Threshold of Acceptability

The threshold of acceptability includes levels of accuracy, sensitivity, and specificity of diagnosis (see Chapter 11). It also should include such items as the number of radiographs per examination, the amount of radiation per examination, and the performance thresholds of the equipment. These should be established according to both external factors (such as federal and state guidelines or professional and accrediting agencies) and internal factors, which are based on the needs and resources of the individual department.

Communication Network

Proper communication among all members of a diagnostic imaging department is essential for a successful quality management program. Items such as the proper radiographic examination ordered for a particular patient must be supplied to the technologist from the ordering physician and office support staff. The technologist also must communicate the appropriate patient history to the radiologist and ensure proper film identification and marking. Administrative personnel and radiologists must then communicate with technologists about proper procedures and guidelines for patient care and image parameters. Diagnostic imaging departments also should have proper communication with other departments within the healthcare setting such as the emergency department staff or floor nurses so that the patient can be cared for properly. Proper communication also includes report dictation, transcription, and distribution to the ordering physician and other interested parties. Modern imaging departments rely on electronic reporting and electronic record keeping, so a major administrative responsibility is making sure that all personnel have competency in computer usage and knowledge of HIPAA requirements.

Patient Comfort

Patient comfort, convenience, and privacy should be provided within reasonable limits in diagnostic imaging departments. Factors such as patient scheduling, preparation, waiting time, ambient room temperature, and politeness and consideration of personnel should be monitored regularly. This is best accomplished by a patient survey or questionnaire, which should be sent to patients 3 to 7 days after the procedure for maximum reliability. As mentioned in Chapter 1, respect and caring and timeliness of care are key clinical performance indicators that require measurement by The Joint Commission (TJC).

Personnel Performance

Policies should be developed to ensure that diagnostic personnel are performing their duties within accepted professional standards for areas such as proper equipment operation, critical thinking, and interaction with patients and other personnel. Information obtained from repeat analysis studies and patient surveys can be useful in assessing performance. Documentation of data, periodic review of these data, and any corrective actions that have been taken also should be included. Personnel education programs also should be offered and documented to improve performance and maintain staff competency.

Record-Keeping System

A record-keeping system is necessary to document that quality control procedures are being implemented and that they are in compliance with accepted norms. Items that should be included are processor control charts, equipment checklists, examination requisitions, room logs, incident reports, personnel dosimetry reports of radiation exposure, and image interpretation reports.

Corrective Action

If equipment or personnel are not performing to accepted standards, corrective action must be taken and documented. Equipment downtime and failure should be documented in a logbook. In-service education or other corrective action procedures may be necessary for department personnel. A flowchart is a useful tool in demonstrating corrective actions for possible problems.

RISK MANAGEMENT

An important aspect of a quality management program for diagnostic imaging departments is **risk management.** This is the system or process for the identification, analysis, and evaluation of risks and the selection of the most advantageous method for minimizing them. Other names for risk management include *safety and loss prevention, total loss control,* or *loss control management.* The purpose of a risk management program is to maintain quality patient care and a safe environment for employees and visitors, while conserving the healthcare institution's financial resources. The overall responsibility for risk management may lie with a risk management coordinator, a risk management team, the individual department manager, or the department quality management person, depending on the size and structure of the institution. However, all employees must be made aware of their role in the risk management process. This includes proper education in both departmental and institutional policies and procedures, awareness of safety issues, and the immediate reporting of incidents and hazardous conditions to the appropriate person.

Risk Analysis

The first step in developing risk management policies and procedures for diagnostic imaging departments is to perform a risk analysis. This means identifying the potential risks to patients, employees, students, and visitors to the diagnostic imaging department.

- *Risks to patients.* The potential risks to patients in diagnostic imaging departments are considerable. For example, patients may slip and fall, be hit by equipment, have a reaction to contrast media, have entered the department with a traumatic injury and be improperly manipulated, and receive the wrong diagnostic procedure. Other more subtle risks can include excess radiation exposure (due to failure to adequately shield the patient from repeat images), exposure to infectious disease (due to failure of the technologist to maintain room cleanliness), and breach of confidentiality (due to technologists discussing patient information near waiting areas or other unauthorized persons). These potential risks can be reduced by having the appropriate policies and procedures in place and making sure that employees have knowledge of and follow these procedures. The Joint Commission publishes extensive safety guidelines for patients for various types of healthcare institutions on their website, www.jointcommission.org. Documentation of adherence to these guidelines is essential in obtaining and maintaining TJC accreditation.

- *Risks to employees and medical staff.* Risks to employees and professional staff include injuries from falls, back injury from lifting patients or heavy equipment, repetitive stress injuries, needle sticks, exposure to infectious diseases, exposure to ionizing radiation, and exposure to toxic chemicals such as processing solutions. Most of the risks to employees and medical staff (like those to the patient) also can be reduced by implementing appropriate policies and procedures. Information concerning work-related employee injuries and illness is available in the Occupational and Safety Health Administration (OSHA) 2000 Log. This report must be posted at the work site each year during the month of February. These reports may be maintained by the human resources department, risk manager, or employee health department, depending on the institution.

- *Risk to others.* This category includes such persons as students, visitors, and volunteers and is probably the most difficult category to assess. This is due to the potential size of this group and the variety of persons that can be included. Another potential difficulty is that the individuals within this group probably have little or no knowledge of the policies and procedures of the healthcare institution. The greatest potential risks to members of this group are injuries from falling and exposure to infectious disease. It is imperative to have appropriate policies and procedures in place to address these risks and to encourage employees (because they should have been educated in risk management) to report any hazardous conditions (e.g., liquid spills) immediately.

- Once a risk analysis is performed and policies and procedures have been created to reduce any potential risks, the next step in a risk management program is to create an investigation procedure for any incidents that may occur. An **incident** is any occurrence that is not consistent with the routine care of a patient or the normal course of events at a particular facility. Facilities should have some type of "incident report" form that is to be completed as soon as possible after an incident. The completed reports should be reviewed immediately by the department manager and then forwarded to the risk manager for additional review. The risk manager should then determine if any follow-up

action is necessary. This can include additional investigation, notification of government agencies (e.g., the Food and Drug Administration [FDA], OSHA, the Nuclear Regulatory Commission [NRC], the Environmental Protection Agency [EPA]), or the obtainment of legal counsel. A risk management program also should include policies and procedures addressing claims prevention and loss potential. **Loss potential** refers to any activity that costs a facility either money or its reputation. Educating employees on safety policies and procedures, emphasizing quality patient care, and communicating effectively within the healthcare facility can greatly reduce the occurrence of incidents and therefore the cost of defending any claims that may result from these incidents. With these policies in place and documentation that they are being implemented, loss potential can be reduced, first by minimizing the chance of an incident and second by showing that the healthcare facility did all that it could to minimize risk, which should cast a more favorable opinion if litigation becomes necessary.

Policies and Procedures

Finally, if an incident does occur, a risk management program should have policies and procedures in place that address responsibility of the healthcare institution for the outcome of the incident, for example, paying the medical bills for a patient or employee who is injured in a diagnostic imaging department. Having effective policies and procedures addressing this type of responsibility and loss can often prevent the filing of a claim or reduce the amount of a claim after litigation. As with all quality management components, keeping proper records of all incidents, documents, reports, and policies is imperative for the process to be successful. The following list summarizes the key concepts of an effective risk management program:

1. *Risk analysis*—to identify all potential hazards and risks that can occur
2. *Written policies and procedures*—to reduce all risks and deal with incidents as they occur
3. *Employee education*—to inform employees of all policies and procedures, as well as seek input from employees (such as a brainstorming session) to identify and reduce further risks
4. *Periodic inspection*—to make sure that all policies and procedures are being implemented
5. *Record keeping*—to document that all policies and procedures have been implemented

RADIATION SAFETY PROGRAM

Diagnostic imaging procedures (with the exception of magnetic resonance imaging and sonography) contribute the largest single exposure to artificial radiation (more than 90%) in the United States. The average effective dose equivalent for diagnostic radiographs is 39 millirem (mrem) (0.39 millisievert [mSv]) and 14 mrem (0.14 mSv) for nuclear medicine procedures. This is in addition to the 360 mrem (3.6 mSv) per year that is received from natural sources such as cosmic radiation (from outer space), terrestrial radiation (from the earth, air, and drinking water), and internal radiation (from our own body tissues). The 360 mrem (3.6 mSv) per year is an average for the United States and can vary considerably from one location to the next. Persons who live in areas where the altitude is high or where exposure to radon-222 is common may experience considerably more than 360 mrem per year. It is therefore imperative that patients, visitors, hospital staff, and radiographers themselves receive as little radiation exposure as possible. It is the primary responsibility of each radiographer to ensure that this indeed occurs. A quality management program should have radiation safety policies and procedures in place to make sure that all employees who administer ionizing radiation to patients are aware of this responsibility. The NRC (or state radiation governing body) and TJC require a Radiation Safety Committee, administered by a Radiation Safety Officer, to implement these policies. Additional responsibilities of this committee would include creating policies and procedures for the safe handling and disposal of radioactive materials, radiation accidents, and care of patients exposed to radiation.

Implementation of proper radiation safety protocols is mandated by the federal government and most state governments. The more important federal laws are described in Chapter 1. The enactment of the laws mentioned in Chapter 1 means that radiographers may have to interact with one or more regulatory agencies that oversee compliance. These federal agencies include the following:

- *The FDA.* As mentioned previously, the FDA, through the Center for Devices and Radiological Health (CDRH), regulates the design and manufacture of x-ray equipment. These regulations are contained in the document Title 21 of the Code of Federal Regulations Part 1020 (21 CFR 1020). Title 21 refers to the FDA. The FDA also must certify the administrative, professional, and technical aspects of mammographic services in order to obtain Medicare and most private insurance reimbursement. The FDA uses three classifications of all medical devices:

  Class I—General Controls: Class I devices are subject to the least regulatory control and present minimal potential for harm to the user. Examples would include image receptors, grids, and lead aprons.

  Class II—Special Controls: Class II devices are those for which general controls alone are insufficient to assure safety and effectiveness. In addition to complying with general controls, class II devices also are subject to special controls. Examples would include collimators, pressure injectors for contrast media, and barium enema tips.

  Class III—Premarket Approval: Class III is the most stringent regulatory category for devices. Class III devices are those for which insufficient information exists to ensure safety and effectiveness solely through general or special controls. Class III devices are usually those that support or sustain human life; are of substantial importance in preventing impairment of human health; or present a potential, unreasonable risk of illness or injury. Examples include angioplasty catheters and cardiovascular stents.

- *The NRC.* This agency is responsible for enforcing both equipment standards and radiation safety practices. This information is published in Title 10 of the Code of Federal Regulations Part 20 (10 CFR 20). Title 10 refers to the Department of Energy, which contains the NRC. In some states called *agreement states,* the NRC allows the state to have the responsibility to enforce equipment standards and radiation safety practices. The reader can check with his or her state department of public health to see if a particular state is an agreement state.

- *OSHA.* This agency is responsible for establishing standards for safety and monitoring the workplace environment including the requirements for occupational exposure to radiation, handling and disposal of hazardous materials, universal precautions (Tier 1) for protection of employees from infectious diseases, and personal protective equipment. This information is contained in Title 29 of the Code of Federal Regulations Part 1910 (29 CFR 1910). Title 29 refers to OSHA.

Patient Radiation Protection

Radiographic Examinations. The federal government recommends that the "As Low As Reasonably Achievable" (ALARA) concept be used during all diagnostic x-ray procedures. ALARA is covered in detail in the National Council on Radiation Protection (NCRP) Report #107. Some of the main recommendations of the ALARA program for radiographic examinations include the following:

1. *Use of high kilovolt (peak) (kVp) and low milliampere-second (mAs) exposure factors.* This is the most effective method of reducing patient exposure because milliampere-second selection is the primary control of the quantity of radiation emitted by the x-ray source. This is even more critical with computerized radiographic (CR) systems and direct-to-digital radiographic (DR) systems. With these systems, the computer can compensate for overexposure to radiation when it

creates the final image on the monitor. This can lead technologists to become careless in their milliampere-second selection; they can overexpose the patient. It is extremely important to adhere to your system's recommended exposure indicator values (e.g., the S-numbers in the Fuji CR system, logM in Agfa CR system, etc.) to avoid overexposure to your patient. The radiographer must keep in mind that the kilovolt (peak) that is used must be kept in an optimum range for the particular part of the body that is being radiographed because excessive kilovolt (peak) can produce images that may be of poor diagnostic quality (especially with film/screen image receptors).

2. *Use of high-speed image receptor systems.* This is the second most effective method of reducing patient exposure because a faster speed system requires a lower mAs value to obtain a diagnostic image. With conventional film/screen imaging systems, most departments use rare-earth phosphors that are high speed and demonstrate acceptable recorded detail. When deciding which image receptor to use, one must consider that faster speed film/screen systems can demonstrate poorer resolution than slower speed systems. Most current CR and DR systems possess a system speed that is comparable to a 200- to 300-speed film/screen system.

3. *Use of proper filtration.* Filtration removes lower energy x-rays from the primary beam before contact with the patient. This can reduce the patient's entrance skin dose by as much as 90%. There is usually a certain amount of inherent filtration (filtering performed by the window of the x-ray tube, as well as any cooling oil) present and added aluminum between the x-ray tube window and the top of the collimating device.

4. *Use of the smallest field size possible, along with proper collimation.* This reduces the amount of the patient's body that is exposed to radiation, thereby reducing the total dose. The effect of field size can be seen by calculating a value known as the **dose area product (DAP)**; this calculation incorporates the total dose of radiation along with the area of field that is being used. The units used to measure this value are either roentgen (R) × square centimeter or coulomb per kilogram (C/kg) × square centimeter. For example, a field size of 5 × 5 cm (25 cm^2) can receive a dosage of 4 R, yielding a DAP of 100 R × square centimeter. A field size of 20 × 20 cm (400 cm^2) can receive a much lower dose of only 0.25 R but still yield the same DAP of 100 R × square centimeter because of the increase in the size of the x-ray field.

5. *Use of optimum processing conditions.* Regardless of whether one is using film/screen radiography or a digital radiographic imaging system, proper image processing must exist in order to obtain consistent image quality. Automatic film processor quality control is extremely important in lowering the patient dose in conventional film/screen radiography. For example, if the developer temperature were too low, the resulting radiographs would appear to lack optical density. This can lead to a repeat image (increasing the dose for that particular patient) or to an increase in technical factors for subsequent images (increasing patient dose for all subsequent patients). For CR and DDR systems, proper manipulation of both preprocessing and post-processing software factors by the radiographer is necessary to obtain a proper image.

6. *Avoidance of repeat examinations.* The ideal overall repeat rate for diagnostic imaging departments is no greater than 4% to 6% (2% for mammographic procedures). This figure can vary depending on the patient population and acceptance standards of a particular imaging department but should never exceed 10% to 12%. Proper patient instructions, along with correct positioning and technique selection by the radiographer, should help reduce the need for repeat examinations. Digital radiographic systems can reduce the repeat rate due to technique error because post-processing software can yield some correction of image brightness (optical density in film/screen imaging) and image gray scale (contrast in film/screen imaging). Proper positioning is extremely important when automatic exposure control (AEC) devices are used with conventional film/screen imaging (to be sure the correct portion of the anatomy is over the cell that has been selected) and with CR and DDR systems (because the computer must compare the image obtained with its preprogrammed ideal image to obtain the correct image).

7. *Use of a posteroanterior (PA) projection instead of an anteroposterior (AP) projection for scoliosis series on young female patients.* Normally, radiographic views of the spine are performed with an AP projection to place the spine as close to the image receptor as possible. However, the breast tissue in female adolescents is extremely sensitive to the development of radiation-induced breast cancer (with a latent period of 5 to 15 years). When the examination is performed with the PA projection instead of the AP projection, the breast tissue receives the exit dose instead of the entrance dose of radiation. This can reduce the mean glandular dose to the breast tissue by as much as 98%. Shielding of the breast areas with specialized devices also should be used to reduce the dose even further.

8. *Use of gonadal shielding.* Gonadal shielding with at least 0.5-mm lead equivalence should be used whenever the gonads lie within 5 cm of the collimation line and do not interfere with the anatomy of interest. This can reduce the dose to the reproductive organs by as much as 90%. Gonadal shielding may be a flat contact, a shaped contact, or a shadow type of shield.

Fluoroscopic Examinations. Fluoroscopic examinations have the potential to deliver a considerable dose of radiation to the patient. Therefore ALARA protocols including the following should be in place for these examinations:

1. *Keep fluoroscopic milliampere (mA) and time as low as possible when performing fluoroscopy.* The mA is usually kept in a relatively narrow range (0.5 to 3 mA), so reducing the fluoroscopic time is one of the most effective means of reducing patient dose during fluoroscopic procedures.

2. *Use high kilovolt (peak) if possible.* Fluoroscopic examinations should be performed in the 85- to 125-kVp range (depending on the contrast media being used). The use of a higher kilovolt (peak) reduces the fluoroscopic mA required to obtain adequate image brightness, thereby reducing the patient's dose.

3. *Limit field size as much as possible.* This is done with the fluoroscopic collimation shutters and with a smaller size image intensifier. This has the same effect as collimation, which was previously discussed.

4. *Use intermittent fluoroscopy (periodic activation of the fluoroscopic x-ray tube rather than continuous activation).* This can reduce patient dose by as much as 90%. Many departments have incorporated a procedure of recording the total fluoroscopic exposure time of a patient in their medical records or in a department log sheet. This information also should include the name of the radiologist/physician who performed the fluoroscopy, along with the patient case number.

5. *Use the last-image-hold feature.* This feature holds the last image obtained in digital storage and displays it on the monitor. This can reduce total fluoroscopic time by 50% to 80%.

6. *Avoid the magnification mode.* The magnification mode found with multifield image intensifiers can increase patient dose between 2 and 10 times that of the standard mode. This is because the magnification mode reduces the brightness gain of the image intensifier tube, requiring an increase in fluoroscopic milliampere to compensate.

7. *Keep the patient-to-image intensifier distance as short as possible during mobile fluoroscopic studies with a C-arm.* This reduces the source-to-skin distance to the patient.

8. *Reduce the number of spot film images and reduce the spot film size.* Patient dose increases as the number of spot film images increases. In addition, larger spot film size formats require more radiation; therefore, patient dose is increased.

Visitor Protection

"Visitors" to diagnostic imaging departments are persons other than patients or radiology department staff. They may include relatives or friends of patients, hospital volunteers, security personnel, or other hospital employees who do not normally work in radiation areas (e.g., nurses, patient care technicians, respiratory therapists). While these persons are in the diagnostic imaging department or near mobile x-ray equipment in use (e.g., the emergency department or surgical suite), they are entitled to a safe environment with no unnecessary exposure to ionizing radiation. The NCRP lists maximum effective dose equivalent limits for members of the general population in its report, number 116. For members of the general population who may be exposed to frequent or continuous exposure from artificial sources other than medical irradiation (this includes radiography students younger than the age of 18), the NCRP recommends a maximum effective dose equivalent limit of 0.1 rad equivalent, man (rem) (1 mSv) per year. For those who may receive infrequent exposure (e.g., a parent who may be asked to hold a child for an x-ray procedure), a maximum of 0.5 rem (5 mSv) per year is recommended. To help minimize exposure to department visitors, radiographers can make sure that all examination room doors remain closed during radiographic procedures.

During mobile radiographic procedures, visitors should leave the area if possible or move at least 8 feet away from the source of radiation. Visitors who want to accompany patients or observe a radiographic examination (such as a prospective radiography student or a radiology resident) should remain behind a protective barrier or wear protective apparel, or both. In some cases (e.g., pediatric patients), a visitor (nurse, patient care technician, parent or other relative) may be asked to help hold a patient during a radiographic procedure. These persons should be provided with protective apparel (such as lead aprons and gloves) to prevent overexposure to radiation that can occur during the procedure. Avoiding repeat exposure is also important in these instances because repeat exposure increases the patient's and visitor's dose.

Personnel Protection

Personnel who perform diagnostic procedures using ionizing radiation can potentially receive significant amounts of radiation and must therefore follow proper radiation practices. According to NCRP report number 116, maximum total effective dose equivalent is 5 rem (50 mSv) per year for whole body exposure. The limit for the lens of the eye is 15 rem (150 mSv) per year. The limit for all other parts of the body (such as the hands) is 50 rem (500 mSv) per year. Examinations in which mobile equipment, fluoroscopy, cardiac catheterization, and interventional procedures are used pose a higher risk than traditional radiographic procedures. Technologists working with ionizing radiation who become pregnant should be issued a second monitoring device to be worn at the waist to monitor exposure to the embryo or fetus. The embryonic/fetal dose of occupational workers should not exceed 0.05 rem (0.5 mSv) in any 1 month of the 9-month gestation period and 0.5 rem (5 mSv) for the entire gestation period. Medical facilities must have an orientation program on radiation safety for newly employed technologists and a continuing education program to update the skills of all department personnel.

Personnel who work in proximity to radiographic and fluoroscopic procedures (e.g., emergency department, operating room, intensive care unit) also should have the same in-service training. Periodic surveys with properly calibrated instruments such as Geiger Müller (GM) counters and ionization chambers should be performed to assess that radiation in the workplace does not exceed accepted standards. Warning signs marked "Caution: Radiation Area" should be posted for any areas where dosage can exceed 5 milliroentgen (mR)/hr. All personnel must wear a monitoring device such as a film badge dosimeter, optically-stimulated luminescent dosimeter, thermoluminescent dosimeter, or pocket ionization chamber. The cardinal principles of radiation protection (time, distance, and shielding) should be followed by all radiologic technologists to minimize their occupational exposure.

Time. Radiographers should keep the time of exposure to radiation as short as possible because the amount of exposure is directly proportional to the time of exposure, as indicated by the following equation:

$$\text{Total exposure} = \text{Exposure rate} \times \text{time}$$

The exposure rate is the output of radiation from the source per unit time. For example, if a radiation source creates an exposure rate of 225 mR/hr at a position occupied by an occupational worker, and the worker remains at that position for 36 minutes, what is the total exposure?

$$\text{Total exposure} = \frac{(225 \text{ mR/hr})}{(36/60 \text{ hr})} = 135 \text{ mR}$$

The factor of time is especially important during fluoroscopic, angiographic, and interventional procedures.

Distance. Radiographers should always maintain as large a distance as possible between the source of radiation and themselves. The reason is that radiation continually diverges from its source, so as distance is increased, less radiation exists per unit area. Reduction in radiation intensity follows an inverse square relationship and can be determined from the following equation:

$$\frac{\text{New intensity}}{\text{Old intensity}} = \frac{\text{Old distance}^2}{\text{New distance}^2}$$

For example, if the radiation intensity at 90 cm from a radiation source is 1.3 R/min, at 270 cm (3 times the distance as 90 cm), the radiation intensity is reduced to only 0.14 R/min (9 times less than the amount received at 90 cm). Therefore a small increase in the distance from the source causes a large decrease in the amount of

radiation exposure that is received. This factor is especially important in fluoroscopy because it may require the operator of the x-ray equipment to remain in the examination room. As a rule of thumb, the occupational radiation exposure during tableside fluoroscopy is about 1 mrem/min. Moving back away from the side of the examination table (if possible) can significantly reduce this amount according to the inverse square law.

Shielding. Any material that can be placed between you and a source of radiation is considered shielding. Materials with a high atomic number (such as lead) that are not naturally radioactive are best for shielding because the greatest amount of photoelectric absorption occurs in these materials. Shielded booths are required for protecting the area around the control panel of radiographic units. The walls of the examination room are designed to protect personnel, other hospital employees, and the general public from unnecessary exposure. Lead aprons and gloves must be provided to employees when the possibility of exposure rate could exceed 5 mR/hr (e.g., technologists who must be outside the control booth during diagnostic procedures). Lead aprons must have a minimum lead equivalent thickness of at least 0.5 mm and cover 75% to 80% of the active bone marrow of the person wearing it. Protective gloves require a minimum lead equivalent thickness of 0.25 mm, with 0.5 mm preferred. Thyroid shields are available for general fluoroscopic, angiographic, and interventional procedures and must have a minimum lead equivalent thickness of 0.5 mm. Protective eyeglasses with a minimum lead equivalence of 0.35 mm or 0.5 mm are also available.

SUMMARY

Implementing a quality management program requires considerably more than just equipment monitoring and maintenance. A basic knowledge of statistics and data collection, data presentation tools, administrative responsibilities, risk management, and radiation safety practices is essential in order for a quality management technologist to implement a successful quality management program.

Refer to the Evolve website at https://evolve.elsevier. com for Student Experiment 2.1: Attenuation or Transmission of Radiation.

REVIEW QUESTIONS

1. Which of the following terms best describes the entire set or group of items being measured?
   a. Population
   b. Sample
   c. Frequency
   d. Central tendency

2. Which of the following terms best describes the average set of observations?
   a. Mean
   b. Median
   c. Mode
   d. Variance

3. Which of the following terms best describes variables that have only two values or choices?
   a. Continuous variables
   b. Dichotomous variables
   c. Stochastic variables
   d. Statistical variables

4. A cause-and-effect diagram also is known as which of the following?
   a. Fishbone chart
   b. Pareto chart
   c. Trend chart
   d. Scatter plot

5. Which of the following terms best describes a chart that pictorially demonstrates whether key indicators are moving up or down over a given period of time?
   a. Histogram
   b. Pareto chart
   c. Trend chart
   d. Scatter plot

6. The distribution of continuous data can best be demonstrated by the use which of the following?
   a. Histograms
   b. Control charts
   c. Scatter diagrams
   d. Pareto charts

7. Which of the following is not a tool for data presentation?
   a. Control charts
   b. Brainstorming
   c. Pareto charts
   d. Cause-and-effect diagrams

8. The unit of measure used to express the dose equivalent to occupational workers is which of the following?
   a. Roentgen
   b. Rad
   c. Rad equivalent, man
   d. Relative biological effectiveness (RBE)

9. Which of the following terms best describes the square of the standard deviation?
   a. Range
   b. Mode
   c. Variance
   d. Frequency

10. Which of the following does not affect patient dose during diagnostic radiography?
    a. Inherent filtration
    b. Added filtration
    c. Focal spot size
    d. Source-to-image distance (SID)

Film/Screen Image Receptors, Darkrooms, and Viewing Conditions

OBJECTIVES

At the completion of this chapter the reader should be able to do the following:

- State the function and characteristics of a darkroom used for diagnostic imaging
- Explain the importance of proper safelight type and function
- Perform a safelight evaluation test
- Perform an evaluation of white light leakage and processing area condition
- Explain the conditions for proper film and chemical storage
- Discuss the importance of proper viewbox illuminator function on image quality
- Perform a viewbox quality control test
- Explain the evaluation process of image duplicators
- Explain the factors affecting screen speed
- Describe the importance of spectral matching of intensifying screens and film
- Describe the different types of image resolution

Despite the digital revolution that has recently occurred in diagnostic imaging, many radiographic images are still recorded on film. Even with digital imaging, hard copy imaging may be desired, and this necessitates the use of silver-based film. Because all traditional film is light sensitive, it must be handled in a safe area where no light or ionizing radiation is present. Most diagnostic imaging departments use a **darkroom** area for this purpose, whereas other nondigital departments may use some form of a daylight system (discussed in Chapter 5). Even departments with daylight systems usually have a traditional darkroom that can be used for duplicating existing radiographs or used as a backup, in case of a malfunction in the daylight system.

DARKROOM FUNCTION

The function of a radiographic darkroom is to protect the film from white light and ionizing radiation during handling and processing. After a film has been exposed to light or ionizing radiation (such as in a cassette during a radiographic examination), it can be as much as 2 to 8 times more sensitive to subsequent exposure as an unexposed film (depending on the type of emulsion). This increase in sensitivity is formally known as **latensification.** As a result of this phenomenon, any accidental exposure from an unwanted source (such as a darkroom light leak) can destroy a diagnostic image. Film also can be affected by excess heat, humidity, static electricity, pressure, and chemical fumes. All of these variables must be carefully controlled to obtain a diagnostic quality image. The most common result if they are not controlled is the presence of fog on the manifest image. Fog is defined as noninformational density that occurs because silver grains are formed and do not represent any of the anatomic structures within the patient.

DARKROOM ENVIRONMENT

A darkroom is considered a scientific laboratory by common practice standards and the Occupational Safety and Health Administration (OSHA) and should meet all of the requirements and possess all of the equipment of a laboratory. It also should be clean, well ventilated, well organized, and safe. Eating, drinking, and smoking must be prohibited in the darkroom because bits of food or ashes from cigarettes can get into image receptors as they are being loaded and unloaded. These can cause artifacts on the image that can mimic pathologic conditions (especially in mammography cassettes) or otherwise degrade the diagnostic quality of the image. These artifacts are discussed in detail in Chapter 10.

Darkroom Characteristics

Countertops or other work surfaces and rubber floor mats should be grounded to reduce the risk of **static electricity.** Static electricity creates sparks that emit white light (all colors of the visible spectrum). Because all imaging films are sensitive to some portion of the visible light spectrum, this light creates artifacts that appear on the processed image. The types of static artifacts are tree, crown, and smudge (see Chapter 10). In addition to the work surfaces being grounded, static can be minimized by the following:

1. Handle film properly. Proper film handling, placing a film into and out of a cassette or onto a film tray rather than sliding it reduces the risk of static electricity because friction is a primary cause of static electricity.
2. Wear natural-fiber clothing (cotton) versus synthetic-fiber clothing (e.g., nylon, polyester).
3. Maintain a proper **humidity** range (30% to 60% relative humidity). Moisture in the air absorbs the buildup of static charges. This is why static is less of a problem in the summer, when the relative humidity is greater. In some darkrooms, installation of a humidifier or ion generator may be necessary to maintain the recommended level of humidity. A **psychrometer,** which measures humidity, should be available or installed in the darkroom. A psychrometer is a type of hygrometer (a device that measures atmospheric humidity) for calculating relative humidity (Fig. 3-1). It consists of a thermometer with wet and dry bulbs, the readings of which are compared, giving the rate of evaporation of water from which the water vapor saturation of the atmosphere can be calculated. At low relative humidity, moisture evaporates from the wet bulb more rapidly, causing the wet bulb to have a lower reading than the dry bulb. The temperature difference between the two bulbs is used to calculate the relative humidity. Excessive humidity could cause the films to stick together, and the emulsion from the films could be removed when they are pulled apart. Excessive humidity also could cause a condensation problem, and the result could be artifacts (see Chapter 10).
4. *Clean screens regularly with an antistatic nonabrasive cleaner.* Appropriate screen cleaners are available from the manufacturers from whom the screen is

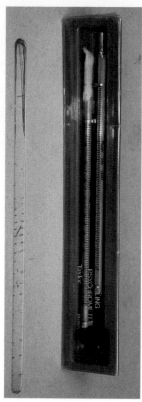

FIGURE 3-1 Psychrometer for measuring relative humidity.

purchased (it is important to match these products to the particular brand of screen). The proper procedure for cleaning intensifying screens is covered in Chapter 7.

The darkroom must be well ventilated to prevent buildup of heat and humidity, which degrade the film. Proper ventilation also removes excessive fumes from the processing solutions that may sensitize film emulsions. The presence of these fumes also can cause condensation of processing chemicals onto work surfaces in the darkroom (e.g., underneath cabinets or shelves). Over time, the residue created by this condensation may fall into open cassettes, causing artifacts to appear in the final images. Removing these fumes, along with periodically wiping these areas with a damp cloth, should minimize the occurrence of these artifacts. **Temperature** should be maintained in a range of 65° to 75° F (18° to 24° C). The fumes from the processing solutions are considered toxic, corrosive, and potentially carcinogenic by OSHA, the Environmental Protection Agency (EPA), and the Department of Transportation. OSHA maintains a listing of Permissible Exposure Limits (PELs), which are the chemical levels to which employees can be exposed in the workplace without risk or harm. An environmental engineer can be consulted to monitor the level of a darkroom area. The following are PELs for some of the components found in processing solutions:

Acetic acid: 10 parts per million (ppm)
Ammonium thiosulfate (as ammonia): 50 ppm
Hydroquinone: 2 mg/m^3 (0.44 ppm)
Phenol: 5 ppm
Sulfur dioxide: 5 ppm
Glutaraldehyde: 0.7 mg/m^3 (0.2 ppm)
Silver: 0.01 mg/m^3

The values just listed were established in 1968, and discussion to revise these figures is taking place. In recent years, many technologists and darkroom technicians have complained of hypersensitivity to darkroom chemicals, a condition sometimes called *darkroom disease,* which manifests in a variety of symptoms ranging from hives to severe fatigue and impairment of the immune system. The Society of Toxicology and the American Society of Radiologic Technologists are currently collecting data on this phenomenon. Proper **ventilation** in a darkroom should keep the levels of chemical vapors well below PELs and should include a source of fresh air, slight positive air pressure (so that chemical fumes are not sucked out of the processor), and ventilation to the outside atmosphere. *This should yield about 8 to 10 room changes of air per hour.* A ventilator duct should be placed near the floor, in either the lower portion of the entrance door or the wall.

Many darkrooms have interior walls that are mistakenly painted black, and these walls can make the room too dark. Instead, darkroom walls should be painted in pastels and light colors to increase the reflectance of the light emitted from the safelight. Enamels or epoxy paints are best because they are easy to clean and more durable. However, a matte finish must be used, because a high-gloss finish could reflect and amplify light leaks. Should any darkroom wall lie adjacent to a radiation area (e.g., radiographic room, nuclear medicine area), proper lead shielding that is appropriate to the type and energy of radiation used must be present in the walls to protect darkroom personnel and prevent fogging of the film.

The processing of most diagnostic images requires a large quantity of clean water. Today, in most automatic film processors, only cold water is used, because the processors have built-in heating systems to regulate solution temperatures (see Chapter 4). Older processors and many cine film processors may require a hot water supply in addition to the cold water and have a mixing valve to regulate the temperature. Adequate drainage must be in place to remove the dirty water and used chemicals after processing is completed. *Adequate drainage* is generally defined as the capacity to handle 2.5 times the maximum outflow of the processor when all drains are open. For most automatic film processors this is about 10 gallons per minute (38 L/min). A floor drain is generally desired for maximum efficiency, with a 3-inch-diameter cast iron or plastic (polyvinylchloride [PVC]) pipe. Local building codes should be referenced before choosing PVC pipe because some municipalities have restrictions on its use. Copper or brass pipes and fittings should be avoided because of the corrosive effect of the processing chemicals. These drains should be dedicated only to film processors and should not share a common line with sinks and toilets, to reduce the chance of blockage. They also must be cleaned on a regular basis with a commercial drain cleaner because buildup forms over time. This is especially important when metallic replacement silver recovery units (see Chapter 6) are used. Flooring around the drain must be easy to clean, moisture resistant, and of a light color to allow identification of objects that may have been dropped in the dark.

Darkrooms should have adequate storage space for film and chemicals. Film must be stored in an upright position (with no heavy objects or other boxes of film stacked on top) to avoid pressure marks. Open boxes of film should be kept in a metal film bin (usually mounted under the work counter) to minimize the chance of being exposed to white light (Fig. 3-2). Passboxes, also known as *film transfer systems,* also should be present to prohibit white light from entering. The darkroom door should be double-interlocked or revolving, or a lightproof maze can be installed if floor space permits.

Darkroom Lighting

A darkroom should have two types of lighting, overhead lights and safelights.

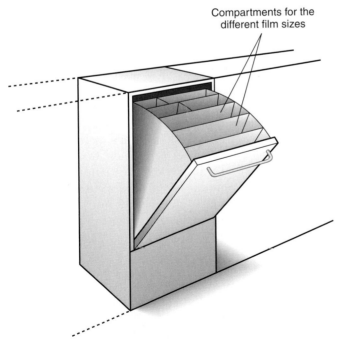

Compartments for the different film sizes

FIGURE 3-2 Standard darkroom film bin.

Overhead Lighting. Overhead lighting is the standard white light that normally illuminates the interior rooms of hospitals and clinics. This standard lighting is necessary for cleaning, maintenance, and possible emergencies (e.g., darkroom personnel becoming ill). Proper overhead lighting normally requires a standard fluorescent fixture (two to four 48-inch fluorescent tubes) per 8 square feet (0.74 m^2) of floor space. The overhead light should be interlocked with the film bin(s) so that if a bin is open, the light cannot be energized. If this is not practical, a cover should be placed over the switch to prevent accidental activation. Film bin alerts also are available (at a minimal cost) that sound a continuous alarm while the film bin is open to prevent accidental exposure to white light.

Safelight. A **safelight** is a light source that emits wavelengths to which particular types of film are not sensitive. Ordinary room light (known as white light) is really a mixture of all of the colors in the visible light spectrum mixed together, as shown in Figure 3-3. Each individual color is determined by the wavelength of the light photon, which is measured in units called angstroms (Å). One angstrom is equal to 10^{-10} m of 10^{-8} cm. Wavelengths range from about 4000 Å for violet light to 8000 Å for red light. In comparison, the wavelengths of diagnostic radiographs generally range from only 0.1 to about 0.5 Å.

Even the best safelight emits some white light (only lasers emit a pure light of one specific wavelength), so it is important not to leave film in safelight indefinitely. Also remember the concept of latensification whereby a film that has been previously exposed is more sensitive than film that has not been exposed. A typical radiographic film (exposed) should be able to remain in safelight for at least 40 seconds without becoming fogged. Mounting safelights at least 3 to 4 feet from feed trays or loading counters also helps minimize safelight fog.

The type of film to be processed in the darkroom determines the type of safelight to be used.

Blue-Violet-Sensitive Film. Blue-violet-sensitive film is a common type of film used in screen cassettes and, as its name implies, is primarily sensitive to the colors blue, indigo, and violet. An amber-colored safelight (a mixture of red, orange, and some yellow) is normally used, with two options available. For the average-size darkroom, a fixture type of safelight containing either a 7.5- or 15-watt (W) light bulb is sufficient (Fig. 3-4). A 7.5-W bulb is recommended for single emulsion film. The light bulb is covered by a colored piece of plastic or glass called a *filter*. The most common types of filters for blue-violet-sensitive film are the Kodak Wratten 6B or the Kodak Mor-Lite (which is slightly brighter). Both

Red	Orange	Yellow	Green	Blue	Indigo	Violet

FIGURE 3-3 Visible light spectrum.

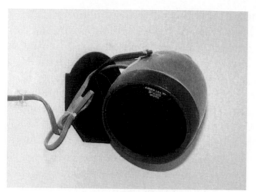

FIGURE 3-4 Fixture type of darkroom safelight.

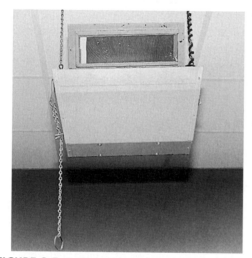

FIGURE 3-5 Sodium vapor lamp darkroom safelight.

of these filters emit an amber- or brownish-colored light. The other option, called a *sodium vapor lamp* (Fig. 3-5), is used in a large darkroom or when bright safelight conditions are desired. This works on the same principle as mercury streetlights; however, sodium yields a bright amber color when energized, instead of the bright white color of the mercury lamps. These lights are large, expensive, and require a long warm-up time to reach maximum brightness. They must be mounted on the darkroom ceiling (at least 6 feet above counters and film bins) because of their brightness level and to provide indirect lighting. Shutter or door openings on top are adjusted with a pull-chain to regulate the level of brightness.

Orthochromatic Film. Orthochromatic film is mainly sensitive to the green portion of the visible spectrum, in addition to the blue-violet portion. A red or magenta dye is added to the film emulsion to increase the absorption of green light by the silver halide crystals. Amber is a mixture of red, orange, and yellow; therefore, the safelights discussed previously are not compatible with this type of film because orange and yellow are too close to green in the spectrum. It is therefore necessary to use a safelight

with the same fixture and light bulb combination mentioned previously, but to use a safelight filter that emits light that is pure red. The most common of this type is the Kodak GBX Series of all-purpose filters (*GBX* stands for green/blue/x-ray). In addition, all Kodak duplicating film requires a GBX-2 filter. An older type of safelight filter that is still acceptable for **orthochromatic** film is the Kodak 2 filter, which is dark red. Another option is an LED safelight, which uses a light-emitting diode that consumes low power and can last up to 15 years. These safelights are perfectly compatible for use with blue-violet-sensitive film but are not as bright as safelights with amber filters. Facilities should avoid the use of red-colored light bulbs such as those found in Christmas decorations. Although considerably less expensive than actual safelight fixtures, they can emit too much white light, resulting in safelight fog.

New Modality Film. New modality film is designed to obtain images from either a cathode-ray tube (multiformat camera) or a laser camera (often used in computed tomography [CT], sonography, nuclear medicine, magnetic resonance imaging [MRI], and digital radiography [hence the name]). The light source for many of these devices usually emits light that is red or amber colored, so the film emulsion is designed accordingly (it is also sensitive to infrared). A fixture and light bulb combination safelight with a dark green filter (Kodak Number 7) can be used with these emulsions. This filter is dark, and some time is necessary for the eyes of technologists or darkroom personnel to adapt. Some types of new modality film are **panchromatic** (sensitive to all colors of the visible spectrum) and therefore cannot be exposed to any safelight. It is best to consult the literature accompanying the box of film or the manufacturer's technical representative before dark green safelight is used.

Other Film Types. Most other types of film (e.g., duplicating, subtraction, spot, industrial) can be processed in darkrooms with the safelights just discussed. It is best to consult the film manufacturer to determine the correct type of safelight for these films. Cine film used in cardiac catheterization studies is black-and-white motion picture film (**panchromatic**) and cannot be exposed to safelights. It normally requires its own dedicated processor (see Chapter 9).

Light and Leakage Testing

Safelight Testing. Safelights may become unsafe over time as a result of cracks or pinholes in the filter (resulting from expansion and contraction with heat), the wrong wattage of the bulb being installed, or the doors on a sodium vapor lamp being open too far; therefore a safelight test should be performed at least semiannually or more frequently if problems are discovered. Testing also should be performed when the safelight bulb or filter is changed. Safelights that are turned on for 24 hours a day, 7 days a week, should have their filters changed annually.

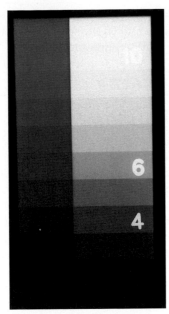

FIGURE 3-6 Image of penetrometer showing safelight fog. *(Courtesy Nuclear Associates, Carle Place, N.Y.)*

6. Expose the film to normal safelight conditions for 2 minutes and then process the film.
7. Place the film on a viewbox illuminator and observe if there is a defined line or break between the halves (see Fig. 3-6). If there is no defined line between the halves, then there is no safelight fog because the human eye can observe differences of as little as 0.01 optical density units. If a discernible line is present, use a **densitometer** to measure the optical density on each side of the line. The difference between the two sides is a measure of darkroom fog. Because the difference in optical density measurements varies for each step, the step with the maximum density difference must be found. Record the density difference value and the step on which it was measured. This same step should be used for all future safelight tests. The maximum density difference (or darkroom fog level) should be less than 0.05 optical density units. Levels in excess of this value indicate serious safelight fog, which can reduce the image contrast of any films that are exposed to these conditions. If the fog levels are greater than 0.05, readjusting the position of the safelight, replacing the safelight filter, checking to see that the proper wattage bulb has been installed into the safelight, or closing the shutters on a sodium vapor lamp can usually correct the situation.

If safelights are turned on an average of 12 hours a day, 7 days a week, the filter should be changed every 2 years. Testing requires a sensitized film (pre-exposed) because this makes it more sensitive to safelight fog.

Safelight testing (Fig. 3-6) can be accomplished by either of the procedures discussed in the following paragraph.

PROCEDURE

This procedure is performed with a penetrometer on dual emulsion films only.

1. Use a tape measure to verify the proper distance from the safelight to the work counters or feed trays. Also check the wattage of light bulbs and inspect the filter for cracks or pinholes. Make sure that the filter type matches the film type.
2. Load an 8 ×10 inch (20 × 25 cm) cassette with film from a fresh box of film. If more than one type of film is used by the facility, a separate test should be performed for each type of film.
3. Take the loaded cassette to a radiographic room and center the cassette on a radiographic table at a source-to-image distance (SID) of 40 inches (100 cm). Place a penetrometer (step wedge) in the center of the cassette, aligning the long dimension of the wedge with the long axis of the cassette. Collimate the light field to the edges of the step wedge.
4. Expose the cassette at approximately 70 kilovolts (peak) (kVp) and 5 milliamperes-second (mAs). Ideally, the image of the step wedge on the film should have an optical density of approximately 1 when measured with a densitometer. The kilovolt (peak) and milliampere-second can be adjusted depending on the speed of the image receptors that are used.
5. Bring the cassette back into the darkroom, lay the exposed film on the counter, and cover one half of the film with an opaque material such as cardboard. Be sure to bisect the latent image of the penetrometer into right and left halves and not top and bottom.

PROCEDURE

This procedure is performed with a sensitometer and is acceptable for both single emulsion (which is usually slower speed) and dual emulsion film, if one does not want to use the previous procedure.

1. In the darkroom (in complete darkness with the safelights turned off), remove a sheet of film from a fresh box of film.
2. Expose this sheet of film with a **sensitometer** and place it on the counter in the darkroom. Place an opaque card over one half of the exposed wedge pattern on the film, just as in the first procedure.
3. Expose the film to normal safelight conditions for 2 minutes and then process the film.
4. Use a densitometer to determine the step that will have an optical density closest to 1.4 optical density units (using the side that was covered with the opaque card).
5. Determine the maximum density difference (the difference in optical density between the covered side and the uncovered side) for this step and record for future use. For dual emulsion films, the maximum density difference should not exceed 0.05 optical density units (as in the first procedure). For single emulsion films, the maximum density difference between the halves cannot exceed 0.02 optical density units. Since single emulsion film generally has a lower inherent contrast, it is vitally important to keep any additional fogging (which reduces contrast even further) to a minimum.

Leakage Testing and Processing Area Condition. While safelights are tested, a check for light leaks, other extraneous light sources (e.g., indicator lights on processors, duplicators, luminous dials on a clock), and processing area conditions usually also can be performed.

PROCEDURE

1. Turn on all white lights in the area surrounding the darkroom. Enter the darkroom and shut off all safelights and overhead lights.
2. After eyes adapt to the dark (about 5 minutes), check for white light leaks, especially near the processor, darkroom doors, water pipes, ventilation ducts, and suspended ceiling tiles. Light leaks can cause artifacts and reduce image contrast.
3. Turn on the overhead lighting and inspect the counter tops and processor feed tray for foreign objects, dampness, cleanliness, and sharp edges. These conditions can cause artifacts if not corrected.
4. Locate the reserve fixer and developer tanks. Check to ensure that they are properly ventilated and that the temperature of the area is within accepted limits. Excessive temperature can cause a deterioration of the processing solutions.
5. Locate the film storage area and verify that the boxes of film are being stored vertically and under the proper temperature conditions. Also check the age of the film and the visibility of the expiration date. The oldest boxes of film should be positioned so that they will be used first. Artifacts can result if these conditions are not within proper parameters.
6. Correct any problems or deficiencies.

Film and Chemical Storage

Film should be stored at a temperature range between 55° and 75° F (14° to 24° C), whether in the darkroom (only open boxes of film, kept in the film bin); storage closet; or warehouse. Excessive heat can cause age fog, and too low of a temperature can lead to moisture condensation on the film, resulting in artifacts. Humidity also must be controlled (30% to 60% relative humidity), especially with film in which the moisture-proof inner seal has been opened. As previously mentioned, static artifacts can appear if the air is too dry. Premature aging of the film, condensation, and films sticking together could be a problem in high-humidity conditions. Film can be stored in a refrigerator or freezer to prolong the shelf life, provided the inner seal is unopened. If kept in a freezer at 0° F or below, the deterioration or aging process stops and the expiration date can be extended for any time that the film was in the freezer. After removal, a 24-hour warm-up period is required before the inner seal can be opened and the film used. This is to prevent condensation and the associated artifacts from appearing on the film.

Chemicals should be stored in a well-ventilated area with a temperature range between 40° and 85° F (5° and 30° C). The temperature should not exceed 70° F (21° C) for a prolonged period. The area should be darkened or have minimal lighting because the developer solution can degrade if exposed to bright light. It is best not to store film and chemicals near each other because film chemistry contains quantities of potassium, a percentage of which is in the form of potassium-40, which is a naturally occurring radioactive isotope that can fog film over time. Most film manufacturers recommend that background radiation not exceed 7 microroentgens (μR)/hr. Levels near large quantities of processing chemicals can reach 12 μR/hr. Most manufacturers of film and processing chemicals give a 12-month expiration date on the basis of an ambient temperature of 68° F (20° C).

VIEWBOX QUALITY CONTROL

Viewbox Illuminators

Most diagnostic images are transparencies and therefore require an illuminator to view the final image. Proper functioning of the **viewbox illuminator** is essential in maintaining image quality because it has a direct effect on the contrast. Over time, heat from the fluorescent bulb inside can discolor the plastic front of the viewbox. Dirt and dust can form on both the inside and outside of the plastic viewing surface, as well as the outside surface of the fluorescent bulb. This can reduce light output by as much as 10% per year, and the image contrast is decreased. For this reason, the bulbs should be changed every 2 years (especially viewboxes used in mammography), even though the typical fluorescent bulb has a rated life of 7500 to 9000 hours. With multiple viewboxes, replace all lamps at the same time and replace them with bulbs of the same manufacturer, production lot, and color temperature to maintain consistency. All viewboxes should be cleaned weekly with an antistatic, non-abrasive cleaner, and the intensity of all viewboxes within the department should be checked for consistency. A viewbox quality control test should be performed on acceptance and then at least once a year (weekly for those used in mammography).

Viewbox Quality Control Test

The viewbox quality control test requires a screwdriver and either a photographic light meter or a 35-mm camera with a built-in light meter (Box 3-1, Fig. 3-7).

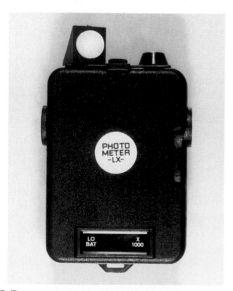

FIGURE 3-7 Photographic light meter (photometer) for viewbox evaluation. *(Courtesy Nuclear Associates, Carle Place, N.Y.)*

The radiant energy that strikes or crosses a surface per unit of time or radiant energy emitted by a source per unit time is called *radiant flux* and is measured in watts (W). The watt is defined as the number of joules (J) of energy per second or 1 W = 1 J/sec. Radiant flux, evaluated with respect to its capacity to evoke the sensation of brightness, is called *luminous flux*. The unit of luminous flux is the lumen and is affected by the radiant flux and the wavelength of the light. One standard candle radiates about 12.5 lumens. The luminous intensity of a light source is the amount of luminous flux per solid angle and is represented by the equation:

$$I = \frac{dF}{d\omega}$$

where I = Luminous intensity, dF = Luminous flux in lumens, and dω = Solid angle in steradians and where ω is equal to the area on the surface of a sphere divided by the square of the radius of that sphere. This value of lumens per steradian is also called the *candle*, or *candela* (cd), and is the official unit of luminous intensity. One candle or candela corresponds to 3.8×10^{15} photons per second being emitted from a light source through a conelike field of view.

The actual brightness of a particular area or source can be evaluated by one of two values, illuminance and luminance.

Illuminance

Illuminance is the amount of luminous flux incident per unit area, or the amount of light that falls on a given surface. It is not the amount of brightness of a light source, but rather the result of that light source in illuminating a particular area. For example, we are often more interested in the intensity of light falling on a surface than we are in the brightness of a light source. If you are reading, you are more concerned with the brightness of the page than in the brightness of a particular light bulb. The brightness of the page that you are reading is the illumination; the brightness of a particular light bulb is the luminance. The illumination that you obtain depends not only on how bright the bulb is (the luminance) but also on how far away it is (light intensity follows the inverse square law). Illuminance can be measured in units of lux (lumens per square millimeter) or **foot-candles** (ft-cd) (lumens per square foot). Conversion of foot-candles to lux can be accomplished by the following equation:

$$\text{Lux} = \text{Foot-candles} \times 10.8 \text{ (because 1 ft-cd} = 10.8 \text{ lux)}$$

The illuminance of the interior of a typical home or office building from artificial light is approximately 1000 lux or 100 ft-cd. The light-localizing variable-aperture collimator must be able to illuminate a minimum of 15 ft-cd or 160 lux according to Food and Drug Administration guidelines (discussed in Chapter 7). Viewbox brightness can be measured with illuminance (because the light bulb is illuminating the acrylic plastic [Plexiglass] front), but luminance is more accepted. If illuminance is used, standard viewboxes will have a value of about 5000 lux, 500 ft-cd, or 13 EV. A photodetector that is covered with both a photometric filter and a cosine diffuser is required for the measurement of illuminance (see Fig. 3-7).

Luminance

Luminance is the luminous intensity per unit of projected area of source, or the amount of light that is emitted or scattered from a particular surface. In other words, luminance measures the brightness or intensity from a particular light source. Luminance is the preferred method of measuring viewbox brightness and is required for inspections according to the Mammography Quality Standards Act. Units that can measure luminance include candles or candela per square meter (also known as **nit**), candles per square centimeter, or candles per square foot. The range of human vision is from 6×10^{-6} nit to $10 \times 10 = 6$ nit. The optimum range is from about 1000 to 10,000 nit. The average viewbox for viewing film images has an average brightness level of 2000 nit, while a 36 W fluorescent tube has a brightness level of 8000 nit. Another set of units also can be used for measurement of luminance and is 1/π as great as those mentioned earlier. These units are the lambert, foot-lambert (often used to measure television and computer monitor brightness), and meter-lambert.

$$1 \text{ lambert} = 1/\pi \text{ cd/cm}^2$$
$$1 \text{ foot-lambert} = 1/\pi \text{ cd/ft}^2$$
$$1 \text{ meter-lambert} = 1/\pi \text{ cd/m}^2$$

For conversion of nit to foot-lamberts, the following equation can be used:

$$1 \text{ cd/m}^2 (\text{nit}) = \text{foot-lambert} \times 3.43$$
$$(\text{because 1 foot-lambert} = 3.43 \text{ nit})$$

For the luminance and illuminance units to be equated (because both can be used to measure viewbox brightness), 1 lux of illuminance may be thought of as the reflectance of a perfectly diffusing surface to 1 cd/m^2 (nit) of luminance (or 1 lux = 1 nit).

IMAGE DUPLICATING UNITS

Film duplicating units, or copiers, are standard pieces of equipment in diagnostic imaging darkrooms (Fig. 3-8). Because legal considerations make hospitals reluctant to release original images, copies are made so that patients can consult with specialty physicians without having to repeat the examinations. Most units emit **ultraviolet (UV)** light using special black light bulbs (BLBs). UV light is more penetrating than visible light; thus, it can penetrate the darker areas of a processed image so that the image can be duplicated. The copy film is single-emulsion film sensitive to UV light, so a standard safelight can be used. The emulsion side of the film should be placed against the original image during the duplication process. The emulsion of duplicating film is more unstable than conventional film because of

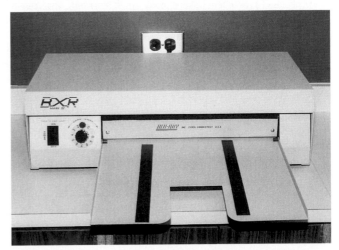

FIGURE 3-8 Duplicating unit for copying diagnostic images.

PROCEDURE

1. Inspect the acrylic plastic (Plexiglas) front of the viewbox for discoloration, dust, and other artifacts. Clean or replace the acrylic plastic if necessary.
2. Unplug the viewbox and remove the acrylic plastic front with the screwdriver. Inspect the fluorescent light bulb for proper wattage, cleanliness, and discoloration; clean or replace if necessary. When finished, replace the acrylic plastic front and screws.
3. Determine the brightness level. This procedure requires a basic understanding of the concepts of photometry, which is the study and measurement of light (see Box 3-1).

   To measure the brightness level of viewbox illuminators, use a photographic light meter (photometer) (see Fig. 3-7), which ideally can measure both luminance and illuminance. The American College of Radiology (ACR) recommends measuring the luminance in nit. The aperture of the photometer should be 9 inches away from the viewbox front when brightness is measured. This can vary slightly, depending on the manufacturer of the photometer (follow the manufacturer's instructions for your particular model). Make the first reading in the center viewbox. Conventional viewbox luminance should be at least 1500 nit, with 1700 nit being standard. Viewboxes used for viewing mammograms should have a luminance of about 3500 nit. If illuminance is used to measure brightness, the minimum illuminance should be 5000 lux or 500 foot-candles (ft-cd). The greater the brightness level of the viewbox, the greater the contrast observed in the viewed diagnostic image.
4. Determine viewbox uniformity. Once it has been determined that the viewbox has sufficient luminance (brightness level), then the uniformity of the brightness for each viewbox panel, each bank of viewboxes, and all viewbox banks within the entire radiology department must be determined. For an individual viewbox or a single-viewing panel (usually 14 × 17 inches) within a bank, mentally divide the viewing panel into quadrants. Hold the photometer 9 inches away (or per manufacturer's instructions) from the center of each quadrant and record the luminance. Compare this value with the center reading obtained in Step 3. These readings should not deviate by more than ±10% of each other.

   To determine the uniformity of a single bank of viewboxes, hold a photometer 9 inches away from the center of each individual viewbox within the bank, record the readings, and compare with each other. These readings should not vary by more than ±15% of each other.

   The uniformity of each bank of viewboxes found in the entire radiology department also should be determined. This can be accomplished by taking the average of the center readings from each bank of viewboxes in the radiology department and comparing them with each other. These values should be within ±20% of each other.

   If a photometer is unavailable, a photographic light meter or a 35-mm camera with a built-in light meter can be substituted (this cannot be accepted during Mammography Quality Standards Act inspections). A photometer can only measure illumination and not luminance. If the camera uses an exposure value (EV) scale to measure light intensity, set the film speed indicator to ASA 100. Place the camera lens in contact with the center of the viewbox front, look into the viewfinder, and record the reading. Repeat this procedure for each quadrant to verify viewbox uniformity. An EV of 13 indicates 500 ft-cd of illumination (the minimum acceptable value for a standard viewbox). An EV of 14 indicates twice as much light (or 1000 ft-cd), and an EV of 12 is one half as much (250 ft-cd). If the light intensity is doubled, the maximum optical density that can be viewed is also doubled. For example, if 500 ft-cd can illuminate a maximum optical density of 2.5 on the image, then 1000 ft-cd can illuminate a maximum optical density of 2.8. Some cameras have a light meter that does not use an EV scale but instead indicates the shutter speed to use when taking the photograph and looking into the viewfinder. In this case, set the film speed indicator to ASA 64 and the shutter to f8. The denominator of the shutter speed indicated is the light intensity in foot-candles. For example, if the indicated shutter speed is 1/400 seconds, the light intensity is 400 ft-cd.
5. Measure the color temperature. The quality or spectrum of light that is emitted from a light source can be defined by its color temperature. This is the temperature at which a black body radiator emits light of a comparable color. A surface that absorbs all of the radiant energy that is incident on it would appear black and is called a black body. The color temperature is measured in degrees Kelvin (°K) and measured with a color temperature meter (available from scientific supply companies). Standard viewboxes should have color temperatures ranging from 5400° K to 10,000° K. Most viewbox manufacturers prefer a rating of 6250° K.
6. Measure the ambient light conditions. The ambient light is the light level of the viewing room and the radiologist viewing area separate from the viewbox. This light must be less than that of the viewbox, or a decrease in contrast level is observed in the image. To survey this level, turn the illuminators off and place the meter or camera 1 foot away from the viewbox to record the reading. The maximum ambient room light should be 30 ft-cd (320 lux) or 8 EV. For mammographic viewing areas, the maximum ambient light should be 4.5 ft-cd (50 lux) or less (equivalent to a moonlit night). Ambient light can vary considerably in various areas of a hospital. Operating rooms typically have a range of 300 to 400 lux, emergency department rooms about 150 to 300 lux, and staff offices about 50 to 180 lux.

latensification. This is because it has been pre-exposed by the manufacturer to the point of **solarization**, or image reversal. For this reason, large quantities should not be stockpiled. More information on solarization or image reversal can be found in Appendix A.

Most units have an exposure level switch to regulate the quality of the copy image. Film duplicators should faithfully copy optical densities of up to 2.5 from the original image. To verify this, make a copy of a sensitometer film, use a densitometer to measure each step, and compare with the original image. They should be the same or within an optical density of 0.02 and should be evaluated on a weekly basis. To check the contact between the copy film and the original during duplication, use a radiograph of a wire mesh screen (used to evaluate film/screen contact) and make a copy. The copy should demonstrate the same sharpness level of the mesh pattern throughout the image. This should be performed monthly.

Images obtained with a multiformat camera or a laser camera can be particularly difficult to duplicate because of its single emulsion. An image from a Society of Motion Picture and Television Engineers test pattern or AAPM TG 18-QC test pattern (see Chapter 9) should be produced from the camera and then duplicated with the copier. Optical density readings from the same areas of the copy and the original should be taken with a densitometer and compared. Again, they should be the same or within a value of 0.02.

FILM/SCREEN IMAGE RECEPTORS

Most of the images recorded during conventional analog radiography are obtained with film/screen combination image receptors. Thomas Edison developed intensifying screens in 1896, and Michael Pupin first used a film/screen combination in radiography later that same year. The x-rays exiting the patient energize the phosphor crystals, and the result is the emission of light called **luminescence.** Luminescence can occur by one of two different processes, **fluorescence** or **phosphorescence.**

1. **Fluorescence** is the light of certain crystals emitted within 10^{-8} seconds after the crystals are exposed to radiation. This means that light is emitted promptly. This is the type of luminescence that is desired for use in intensifying screens.
2. **Phosphorescence** is the light of certain crystals emitted sometime after 10^{-8} seconds after the crystals' exposure to radiation, resulting in a delayed emission of light. This delayed emission of light is often called *afterglow* or *lag.* This is not desired for use in intensifying screens because the delayed emission of light fogs the film in the cassette before the radiographer can get it to the processor or daylight system. This type of luminescence is desired for the output phosphor of fluoroscopic image intensifiers and cathoderay tube (CRT) displays such as television and computer monitor screens.

The fluorescent light from the crystals in the intensifying screen is used to expose the film (rather than for x-ray interaction) and creates 95% to 98% of the optical density. This results in lower patient exposure (compared with a nonscreen exposure) because only a relatively small number of x-rays are necessary for the screens to emit a relatively large quantity of light. Proper application of intensifying screens is necessary to create adequate images. Because considerable variation can occur with the use of screens, proper quality control protocols should be in place. Several intensifying screen variables are discussed.

Intensifying Screen Speed

Intensifying **screen speed** refers to the amount of light emitted by the screen for a given amount of x-ray exposure. A screen that is designated as fast creates an increased amount of light compared with a screen designated as slow when both are exposed to identical kVp and mAs factors. Screen speed can be measured by intensification factor, relative name, or speed value.

Intensification Factor. The exposure required to create a certain optical density without a screen (direct exposure) is divided by the exposure required with a screen to create the same optical density, which determines the **intensification factor.**

$$\text{Intensification factor} = \frac{\text{Exposure without screens}}{\text{Exposure with screens}}$$

For example, if 100 mAs creates an optical density of 1.0 on a direct exposure film and 5 mAs creates the same optical density value with a film/screen combination, then that screen has an intensification factor of 20. The larger this value, the faster the speed of the screen.

Relative Speed Value. Relative speed is the most common method of designating screen speed and is used for all screens with rare earth phosphors. A mathematic number that is a multiple of 100 is used, with a larger number designating a faster speed. When one speed is changed to another, a change in mAs is required to maintain optical density. This can be calculated with the following equation:

$$\text{New mAs} = \frac{\text{Old mAs} \times \text{Old relative speed value}}{\text{New relative speed value}}$$

For example, if 10 mAs were used with a 100-speed screen, then 5 mAs would be used with a 200-speed screen.

Name of Screen. Older, non-rare earth screens use specific names such as *fast* or *slow* to designate screen speed. A listing of these older names, along with their relative speed values, is presented in Table 3-1.

TABLE 3-1	Older Names for Screen Speed
Name of Screen	**Relative Speed Value**
Ultra high or hi-plus	300
High or fast	200
Medium, par, or standard	100
Detail, slow, or high resolution	50
Ultra-detail	25

Factors Affecting Screen Speed.

Type of Phosphor Material. Many different phosphor materials have been used in screens since 1896. They are generally divided into two categories, rare earth and non-rare earth phosphors. The non-rare earth phosphors are the original type of screen material and emit light in the blue-violet portion of the color spectrum. Examples include calcium tungstate, barium strontium sulfite, and barium fluorochloride. The rare earth phosphors were developed in the early 1970s and are currently the most common type of intensifying screen material. The name *rare earth* is used because these materials have atomic numbers ranging from 57 through 71 and are known as the *lanthanide*, or *rare earth*, series from the periodic table of elements. These materials possess a greater detective quantum efficiency (DQE) (the ability to interact with x-rays) and a greater conversion efficiency (the ability of screens to convert x-ray energy into light energy). The older calcium tungstate screens have a conversion efficiency of 4% to 5%, whereas the newer rare earth screens have values ranging from 15% to 25%. Thus the rare earth phosphors are faster than the non-rare earth phosphors. Table 3-2 presents the more common rare earth phosphors and the color of light emitted.

The rare earth phosphors are mixed with materials called *activators* (the elements terbium, niobium, or thulium) that help determine the intensity and color of the emitted light.

Thickness of Phosphor Layer. A thicker layer of phosphor material causes the screen to emit more light because the extra material can absorb more x-rays. This decreases the resolution of the resulting image because of increased light diffraction or diffusion (Fig. 3-9). Rare earth screens generally demonstrate better resolution than non-rare earth screens because they have greater conversion efficiencies and therefore do not have to be placed in as thick a layer. The average range of phosphor thickness is from 150 to 300 μm.

Size of Phosphor Crystals. Using larger-sized phosphor crystals increases the speed of the screen but decreases image resolution because of light diffusion.

Reflective Layer. When x-rays interact with the phosphor material of a screen, light is emitted isotropically (in all directions). Because the film is only on one side of the screen, light traveling away from the film is

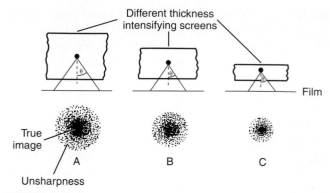

FIGURE 3-9 Effect of screen active layer on light diffusion and image sharpness.

normally lost to the imaging process. Faster speed screens add a layer of titanium dioxide to reflect light back toward the film. This increases the speed but decreases the resolution because of the angle of the reflected light.

Light-Absorbing Dyes. Slower speed screens have light-absorbing dyes added to the phosphor layer to control reflected light (Fig. 3-10). This dye decreases speed but increases image resolution.

Ambient Temperature. When the ambient temperature of an intensifying screen increases significantly above room temperature (above 85° F [30° C]), the screen may function slower than usual. The higher temperature gives the phosphor crystal more kinetic energy. This additional energy does not cause more light to be emitted, but rather, increases the energy (and therefore the color) of the light emitted. Because the film may not be sensitive to this new color, the resulting radiograph appears underexposed.

Kilovolt (Peak) Selection. The phosphor material in a screen must interact with the x-ray photon for luminescence to occur. The greatest absorption of x-rays occurs when the x-ray photon energy and the binding energy of the K-shell electron are almost the same. This is called the *K-edge effect*. Because the kVp setting on the control panel regulates the x-ray photon energy and the phosphor material used controls the K-shell binding energy, care must be taken to match the kVp used in technique selection. For example, a dedicated mammography cassette usually has a lower K-edge value (15 to 20 kiloelectron

TABLE 3-2	Emission Color of Common Rare Earth Phosphors
Rare Earth Phosphor	**Color of Emission**
Gadolinium oxysulfide	Green
Lanthanum oxysulfide	Green
Yttrium oxysulfide	Blue-green
Yttrium tantalate	Blue-green
Lanthanum oxybromide	Blue
Lutetium tantalate	Blue

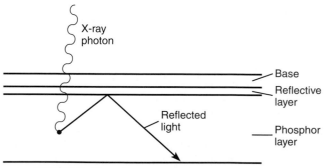

FIGURE 3-10 Reflected light within phosphor layer.

TABLE 3-3	K-Shell Binding Energies for Some Phosphor Materials	
Element	Atomic Number	K-Shell Binding Energy (keV)
Yttrium	39	17.05
Barium	56	37.4
Lanthanum	57	38.9
Gadolinium	64	50.2
Tungsten	74	69.5

keV, Kiloelectron volt.

volts [keV]), because lower kVp techniques are used. If one of these cassettes is used at 100 kVp instead, it functions much more slowly than if used at its proper kVp. Table 3-3 indicates the K-shell binding energies for different phosphor materials.

PROCEDURE

1. Make an exposure of a step wedge or homogenous phantom onto an image receptor so that the center of the image has an optical density of about 1.5.
2. Expose each image receptor to the same technical factors.
3. Process each radiograph and take optical density readings of the same center area in each. If the image receptors are all the same relative speed, the optical density readings should not vary by more than a value of ± 0.05.

Quality Control Testing of Screen Speed

Quality control testing of screen speed should occur on acceptance and then yearly. First, one should evaluate whether similar cassettes marked with the same relative speed are the same using the following procedure.

Cassettes also should be evaluated to ensure that the screen speed is uniform throughout the entire surface. Intensifying screens should be uniform in speed throughout the entire surface of the screen itself. In other words, the speed in the center should be the same as the speed at the outer edges or anywhere else on the screen. During manufacturing processes, inconsistencies may occur in which the phosphor layer is applied more thickly at one portion of the screen than at another. Also, during screen cleaning, excessive rubbing may remove more of the phosphor layer at one point than at another; therefore, a test of screen uniformity should be performed on acceptance and then yearly.

PROCEDURE

1. Make an exposure of a homogenous phantom onto an image receptor that yields an optical density of approximately 1.5.
2. Process the radiograph and take optical density readings in the center and in each of the four quadrants of the image. These values should not vary by an optical density value of more than ± 0.05. Any film/screen image receptors that exceed this limit should be removed from service.

Spectral Matching

Previously in this chapter, it is mentioned that various films are sensitive to specific colors of light and therefore require special colored safelights to illuminate the darkroom. Because intensifying screen phosphors emit blue, blue-green, or green light, the film used inside the cassette should be sensitive to the corresponding color. This is known as **spectral matching.** Any blue-violet-emitting screen phosphor should be used with monochromatic blue-violet film, and green-emitting phosphors must be used with **orthochromatic** film. The non-rare earth screen phosphors tend to emit a broadband of light (Fig. 3-11), whereas rare earth phosphors emit specific colors of light, also known as *line emission* (Fig. 3-12).

Screen Resolution

Intensifying screens should be able to demonstrate clear images of patient anatomy so that the proper diagnosis can be obtained. The ability of an imaging system to accurately display these images is known as *resolution,* of which there are two types, contrast resolution and spatial resolution.

Contrast Resolution. **Contrast resolution** is the ability of an imaging system to distinguish structures with similar x-ray transmission as separate entities (the term not only applies to intensifying screens, but all imaging systems including computed radiography (CR), digital

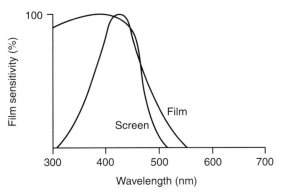

FIGURE 3-11 Broadband spectrum from non-rare earth phosphor.

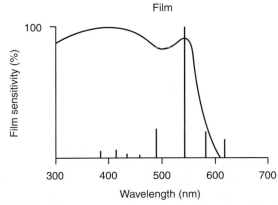

FIGURE 3-12 Line spectrum from rare earth screen phosphor.

radiography (DR), conventional and digital fluoroscopy, computed tomography, magnetic resonance imaging, and sonography). In other words, separate shades of gray (contrast) should appear so that one structure stands out from the other. Contrast resolution is affected by the sensitivity of the image receptor (speed) and the amount of radiographic mottle (also called *noise*). If the radiographic mottle is increased, the contrast resolution decreases. The radiographic mottle is determined by film graininess (also called *random* or *stochastic noise*), the uniformity of the screen phosphor layer (also called *structured* or *nonstochastic noise*), and **quantum mottle** (also called *quantum noise*), which is the statistical fluctuation in the number of photons per unit area that contribute to image formation. The quantum noise that is perceived in the image is normally stated as a percentage and determined by the following equation:

$$\text{Quantum noise} = 100 \times \frac{\sigma}{N}$$

N is the mean number of photons per unit area, and σ is the standard deviation that measures the width of the distribution about that mean and is equal to the square root of N. For example, if a mean of 100 photons exposes a film, the σ is 10 and the quantum noise is 10%. If a mean of 100,000 photons exposes a film, the σ is 316, but the quantum noise is only 0.3%; therefore, as the total number of photons increases, the quantum noise perceived in the image decreases. The number of x-ray photons used to create a radiographic image is approximately $10^5/\text{mm}^2$ of image receptor. Care must be taken with very fast speed screens because lower mAs values are required. This decrease in the number of photons increases the quantum noise, which manifests as a blotchy appearance to the image and decreased contrast resolution. Contrast resolution is often measured with a value known as the **signal-to-noise ratio (SNR)**.

$$\text{SNR} = \text{Signal}/\text{Noise}$$

The signal in diagnostic imaging is the contrast, or gray scale, of the image. Because this value should be relatively large and the noise should be relatively small, a large SNR indicates high-contrast resolution. Increasing the SNR in film screen imaging can be accomplished by increasing the mAs (which can increase patient exposure and heat created in the x-ray tube), increasing the kVp (which can decrease radiographic contrast), increase phosphor layer thickness (which may degrade spatial resolution), or increase the x-ray attenuation capability of the phosphor material used in the screen. The SNR value is more commonly used when television and computerized images are described.

Contrast resolution also can be described using a value known as **contrast-to-noise ratio (CNR)**. As with the SNR, the CNR is defined as the contrast seen in the image, divided by the amount of noise existing in the image. Increasing the contrast and reducing image noise will increase the CNR and therefore improve image quality

and increase the ability to detect a lesion (especially in mammographic images). Contrast can be improved by reducing the amount of scattered radiation, reducing all causes of fogging, or the use of a contrast agent. Reducing image noise can be obtained by reducing quantum mottle (accomplished by increasing the number of photons used to make the radiographic image) or by image postprocessing in digital imaging.

Digital imaging systems generally have superior contrast resolution to film/screen systems. Magnetic resonance imaging possesses the greatest contrast resolution capability of all current imaging modalities.

Spatial Resolution. Spatial resolution (also known as high-contrast resolution) is the ability of an imaging system to create separate images of closely spaced high-contrast (black and white) objects (as with contrast resolution, spatial resolution also applies to all imaging modalities). In other words, do the two objects appear sharp and clear, or do they blur together? This is determined by the amount of light diffusion that occurs between the screen and film, which is in turn affected by the screen thickness, phosphor crystal size, and film/screen contact. The most common method of measuring spatial resolution is to use a value known as *spatial frequency*. The unit of spatial frequency is the line pairs per millimeter (lp/mm) and is obtained with a resolution chart (Fig. 3-13). A line pair includes an opaque line and a radiolucent space. In the resolution chart, one lp/mm would have a 0.5 mm lead bar separated by 0.5 mm of radiolucent material. Two lp/mm would have 0.25 mm lead bars separated by 0.25 mm of radiolucent material and so on (see Table 3-4). The greater the lp/mm value, the smaller the object that can be imaged and the better the spatial resolution. The *limiting spatial resolution* (also known as the **Nyquist frequency**) is the maximum number of lp/mm that can be recorded by the imaging system. The resolving power of the unaided human eye is approximately 30 lp/mm when

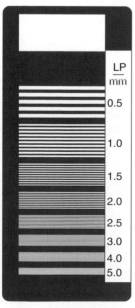

FIGURE 3-13 Line pairs per millimeter resolution chart.

TABLE 3-4	Comparison of Spatial Resolution and Line Size
Spatial Resolution	**Line or Space Width in mm**
1 lp/mm	0.5
2 lp/mm	0.25
3 lp/mm	0.167
4 lp/mm	0.125
5 lp/mm	0.10
6 lp/mm	0.083
7 lp/mm	0.071
8 lp/mm	0.063
9 lp/mm	0.056
10 lp/mm	0.050

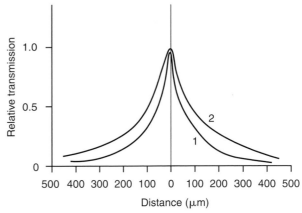

FIGURE 3-15 Line spread function (LSF) graph.

inspecting an image up close, and at normal reading distance (about 25 cm), it is about 5 lp/mm. Most film/screen systems cannot provide this level of spatial resolution. Non-screen film holders that were once used in radiography could yield up to 100 lp/mm (but at a price of extremely high radiation dose to the patient). Other methods of measuring spatial resolution include point spread function (PSF), line spread function (LSF), edge spread function (ESF), and **modulation transfer function** (MTF).

Point Spread Function. **Point spread function** is a graph that is obtained with a pinhole camera and a microdensitometer. The pinhole camera creates a black dot in the center of a film, and a microdensitometer is used to take readings of this point. These values are plotted on a graph versus the distance from the center of the point, as shown in Figure 3-14. The narrower the peak on the graph, the better the spatial resolution and quality of the image. The width of the peak (in millimeters) of the PSF graph can be measured to yield a numerical value to indicate spatial resolution (the smaller the number, the better the spatial resolution and vice versa). The width is usually measured at half the maximum value and is termed **full width-half maximum** (FWHM). The limiting spatial resolution in lp/mm may be estimated by using the following equation:

$$1/(2 \times FWHM)$$

For example, if the PSF has an FWHM value of 0.1 mm, the limiting resolution would be 1/(2 × 0.1 mm) or 5 lp/mm.

Line Spread Function. **Line spread function** is a graph that is more accurate and easier to obtain than the PSF graph. It requires an aperture with a slit that is 10 μm wide instead of the pinhole camera. Density readings of the centerline are taken and plotted (Fig. 3-15). FWHM values also can be obtained from this graph and interpreted much the same way as discussed with point spread function.

Edge Spread Function. **Edge spread function** requires a sheet of lead to be placed on a cassette and exposed. Density readings are taken at the border between the black-and-white areas and plotted on a graph (Fig. 3-16).

Modulation Transfer Function. **Modulation transfer function** is a numeric value that is used to measure the spatial resolution and is obtained from the LSF graph with a mathematic process known as *Fourier transformation*. Just as a mathematic number (slope) can be obtained from a linear graph, Fourier transformation can obtain a number from a curve. This number ranges from 0 to 1 (0% to 100%), with 1 being the

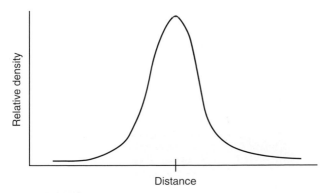

FIGURE 3-14 Point spread function (PSF) graph.

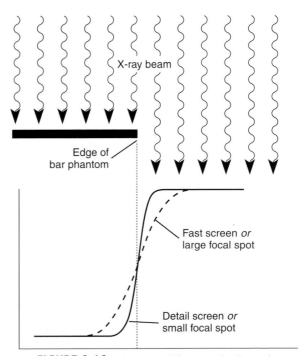

FIGURE 3-16 Edge spread function (ESF) graph.

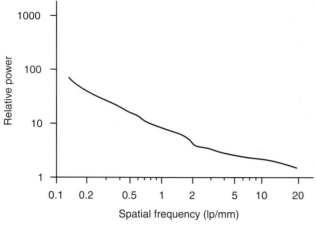

FIGURE 3-17 Weiner spectrum indicating the modulation transfer function (MTF).

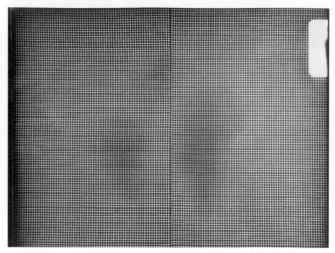

FIGURE 3-19 Wire mesh image.

maximum spatial frequency. An easier way to think of MTF is demonstrated by the following equation:

$$MTF = \frac{Information\ recorded\ in\ an\ image}{Information\ available\ in\ the\ part}$$

If all of the patient information is recorded in the image, a value of 1 is obtained. For example, an MTF value of 0.5 indicates that 50% of the patient's anatomy is recorded. The total MTF of an imaging system is obtained by combining all of the component MTF values.

$$MTF_{total} = MTF_1 \times MTF_2 \times MTF_3, \text{ and so on}$$

For example, if a film can demonstrate 80% of the patient anatomy on an image (MTF = 0.8) and a screen can demonstrate 70% (MTF = 0.7), the total system MTF equals 0.8 × 0.7, or 0.56. A Weiner spectrum graph is sometimes used to demonstrate the relationship of MTF and spatial frequency (Fig. 3-17).

The resolution test tool (see Fig. 3-13) can be imaged with a cassette on acceptance and then yearly to evaluate any variation. One variable that can affect resolution is the film/screen contact. Because poor film/screen contact increases light diffusion, (Fig. 3-18) and therefore

decreases resolution, a wire mesh test should be performed at least annually (more often with larger cassette sizes because they are more prone to develop poor contact) (Fig. 3-19).

PROCEDURE

1. Expose the wire mesh test tool that is placed on the cassette front, using exposure factors of 50 kVp and 5 mAs tabletop.
2. Process the film and evaluate the resulting image. Areas of poor contact appear as localized blurring (see Fig. 3-19). Bent or warped cassettes, warped screens, and foreign objects inside the cassette are the most common causes of poor film/screen contact.

Screen Condition

Cassettes containing intensifying screens must function as designed in order to create optimum radiographic images. Errors to avoid include improper film position

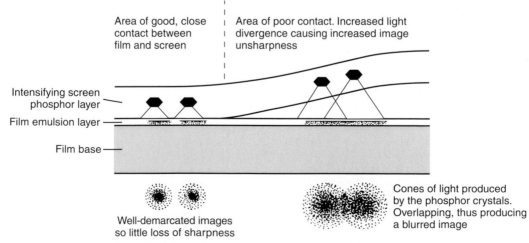

FIGURE 3-18 Effect of film/screen contact on light diffusion.

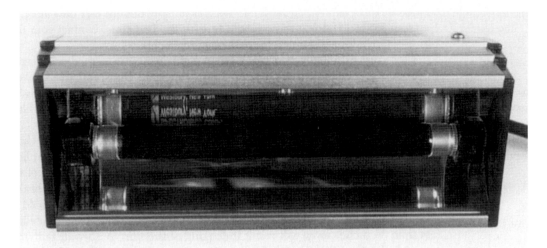

FIGURE 3-20 Ultraviolet (UV) lamp for inspecting intensifying screens. *(Courtesy Nuclear Associates, Carle Place, N.Y.)*

within the cassette, poor film/screen contact, and uneven closure of the cassette. Intensifying screens also must be free of dirt, stains, and defects to properly image anatomic structures. A regular schedule (at least every 6 months) of screen cleaning with an antistatic solution should be standard department policy because artifacts can mimic certain pathologic conditions. The end of the day is usually the best time to clean cassettes because of decreased demand for their use. An ultraviolet (UV) lamp can be used in the darkroom to examine the surface condition of the screens (Fig. 3-20). Be sure to remove the film from the cassette before turning on the UV lamp. The following is an accepted procedure for cleaning intensifying screens.

PROCEDURE

1. Choose a clean location to clean screens and cassettes. Wipe the outside of cassettes and clean the countertop before cleaning screens.
2. Moisten a lint-free wipe with a small amount of commercially available screen cleaner and antistatic solution. A mild soap and water solution or a 70% solution of isopropyl alcohol may be used as an alternative (check with your screen manufacturer to see if this is acceptable), but a screen cleaner and antistatic solution must be used afterwards.
3. Clean and dry the screen. Be sure to avoid excessive pressure or rubbing on the screen surface.
4. Use a second lint-free wipe to clean the frame and inside cover (for single-screen cassettes).
5. Stand the cassettes on edge to dry.
6. Once the screen and cassette cover are dry, inspect them for any particles of dust. Use a UV light if necessary. If they are clean, reload with fresh film. For mammography cassettes, the screen surface should be carefully brushed with an antistatic brush and then inspected before loading with fresh film. This is discussed more completely in Chapter 11.

SUMMARY

Maintaining proper darkroom conditions and procedures is essential to achieving the desired film-based radiographic image. These images also must be displayed with the use of proper viewing conditions for optimum diagnostic capability. Quality control procedures must also be performed for film/screen image receptors and film-based image duplicator units. All radiographers also should have knowledge of image receptor factors such as spatial resolution, contrast resolution, signal-to-noise ratio, etc, as these factors are also important in discussing image quality with digital image receptors.

Refer to the Evolve website at https://evolve.elsevier. com for Student Experiments 3.1: Darkroom Fog Check and Viewbox Illuminations and 3.2: Measurement of Spatial Frequency.

REVIEW QUESTIONS

1. Which of the following is the main reason to prohibit food and drink in a film darkroom?
   a. Avoid contamination of processor solutions
   b. Prevent artifacts
   c. Prevent pressure marks on the film
   d. Prevent static artifacts
2. Which of the following terms best describes the amount of light that is emitted from or scattered by a surface?
   a. **Photometry**
   b. Luminance
   c. Illuminance
   d. Optical density

3. Which of the following names a device that can be used to measure darkroom humidity levels?
   a. Sensitometer
   b. Densitometer
   c. Hydrometer
   d. Psychrometer

4. Proper darkroom ventilation should include _____ room changes of air per hour.
   a. 3 to 5
   b. 6 to 8
   c. 8 to 10
   d. 10 to 12

5. Which of the following terms refers to the amount of light emitted by a screen for a given amount of x-ray exposure?
   a. Speed
   b. Sensitivity
   c. Lag
   d. Resolution

6. Which of the following terms best describes the ability of a screen material to convert x-ray energy into light energy?
   a. Screen speed
   b. Quantum Detection Efficiency (QDE)
   c. Conversion
   d. Resolution

7. Why should boxes of film and containers of developer solution not be stored near each other?
   a. Developer contains naturally occurring radioactive material.
   b. Pressure marks can occur on the film.
   c. Static electricity is more common.
   d. None of the above are correct.

8. Photometric readings from each quadrant of a single view box panel should not vary by more than ± _____ %.
   a. 2
   b. 5
   c. 10
   d. 20

9. Which of the following terms is the unit most commonly used to measure luminance?
   a. Lux
   b. **Nit**
   c. Foot-candle
   d. Lumen

10. Which of the following terms best describes the ability of an imaging system to create separate images of closely spaced high-contrast objects?
    a. Screen speed
    b. Spatial resolution
    c. Contrast resolution
    d. Quantum mottle

Film Processing

KEY TERMS

agitation	flood replenishment	oxidation/reduction reaction
archival quality	hyporetention	synergism
developer	latent image	volume replenishment
fixer	manifest image	

OBJECTIVES

At the completion of this chapter the reader should be able to do the following:

- Describe the main differences between manual and automatic film processing
- List the main components of the developer and fixer solutions and state the function of each component
- Explain the proper mixing procedure for developer and fixer concentrate solutions
- State the chemical safety procedures for the safe handling of processing chemicals as described by the
- Occupational Safety and Health Administration (OSHA)
- Describe the basic tests for determining the archival quality of processed images
- List the six main systems of automatic film processors and state the function of each system
- Describe the methods of installing film processors in a darkroom

After a film has been exposed to radiation, the image that it contains is still invisible to the human eye and is called a **latent image.** For the film to be converted into a visible image, or **manifest image,** the silver contained in the film must be changed from an ionized state (Ag^+) into a neutral, or reduced, state ($Ag°$), in which the silver turns black. This requires the film to be processed by various solutions that convert the latent image into a visible one and also preserve the image for permanent storage. The two basic methods of film processing are manual and automatic.

MANUAL AND AUTOMATIC FILM PROCESSING

Manual Processing

In the manual processing method, film is moved from one solution to the next manually until processing is complete. This method requires more labor and time and is more prone to variations than automatic processing. For this reason, manual processing is seldom used in diagnostic imaging today. For film to be processed manually, several steps are required after the films are hung on special hangers.

Procedure

1. *Wetting agent.* The wetting agent is a chemical that loosens the emulsion so that subsequent solutions can reach all parts of the emulsion uniformly, which reduces development time. This step is optional because developer ingredients also soften the emulsion. If a wetting agent is used, the film should remain in the solution for about 15 seconds.
2. *Developer.* The developer solution converts the latent image into the visible image; therefore, this is the most important processing chemical. The film remains in the developer for 3 to 5 minutes depending on the temperature of the solution.
3. *Stop bath or water rinse.* The stop bath or water rinse step stops the development process and removes excess developer from the film. A stop bath is a 1% solution of acetic acid that chemically neutralizes the developer (because it is an alkaline solution) and requires only 5 to 10 seconds of film immersion time. A water rinse relies on water to remove the excess developer and requires about 30 seconds of film immersion.
4. *Fixer.* The fixer solution removes the unexposed and undeveloped silver halide crystals from the film emulsion and also hardens the emulsion so that the film can be permanently stored. The time of fixation varies with solution temperature, but the general rule for manual fixation is use of the following equation

   Fixing time = Clearing time + Hardening time

   The clearing time is the time necessary for the fixer to clear away the unexposed and undeveloped silver halide crystals, which should be accomplished within 5 minutes. The hardening time is the time it takes the emulsion to properly harden and is usually equal to the clearing time; therefore, a film that requires 5 minutes to clear requires another 5 minutes to harden, leaving a total fixing time of 10 minutes.
5. *Washing.* Excess fixer must be removed from film before it is allowed to dry, or the fixer components crystallize onto the film surface, a process known as **hyporetention**. This white, powdery residue can impair the diagnostic quality of the final image and must therefore be avoided. An example of an image

with hyporetention can be found in Chapter 10. This step may take up to 20 minutes.
6. *Drying.* Drying prepares the film for viewing and storage and can be accomplished either by an electric dryer, which works in less than a minute, or by exposure to room air while the film is mounted on a special hanger, which may require an hour or more.

Automatic Processing

Automatic processing requires an electromechanical device called an *automatic film processor,* which transports the film from one solution to the next without any manual labor except for placing the film into the device. This shortens the overall processing time, increases the number of films that can be processed in a given period, and ensures less variability of overall film quality than manually processed films because the processing time, solution temperature, and chemical replenishment are automatically controlled. The disadvantages of automatic processing include higher capital and maintenance costs, increased chemical fog due to higher processing temperatures, and transport problems that can damage or destroy images during processing. In a diagnostic imaging department that has not converted to digital imaging, the advantages far outweigh the disadvantages and automatic film processing is virtually exclusive.

PROCESSING CHEMICALS

Developer

As previously mentioned, the **developer** is the most important processing solution; it converts the latent image into a manifest image. This is accomplished by the developer solution carrying out an **oxidation/reduction reaction,** or *redox.* When a chemical is oxidized (broken down), it releases electrons. These electrons are then available to convert another compound into a more simplified, or reduced, state (hence the term *oxidation/reduction reaction*). During film processing, the developer solution ingredients are oxidized and the silver halide crystal is reduced to black metallic silver. This chemical reaction can be summarized by the following equations:

During exposure to radiation:

$$Ag^+ Br^- + radiation \rightarrow Ag^\circ + Br^- + Ag^\circ$$
$$\text{(5 atoms latent image)}$$

During immersion in developer:

$$Ag^+ + developer + Ag^\circ (5 \text{ atoms latent image}) \rightarrow$$
$$Ag^\circ (10^8 \text{ atoms visible image}) + oxidized \ developer$$

Developer Components. Developer is composed of developing or reducing agents, preservatives, accelerators or activators, restrainers, regulators, antifoggants or starters, hardeners, solvents, and sequestering agents; all act on the film.

Developing or Reducing Agents. Developing or reducing agents carry out the oxidation/reduction reaction that converts the latent image into a manifest image. Two different reducing agents are used in standard developer solutions: phenidone and hydroquinone.

Phenidone (Elon or Metol in Manual Developer). Phenidone is fast acting and produces the image optical densities of up to about 1.2. It is responsible for the minimum diameter (D_{min}) and speed indicators used in sensitometric testing (described in Chapter 5).

Hydroquinone. Because hydroquinone acts more slowly than phenidone, the developmental process is completed so that the image optical densities that are greater than 1.2 are visualized. Hydroquinone is responsible for the maximum diameter (D_{max}) and contrast indicators used in sensitometric testing. These indicators are the first variables to show an indication of developer failure because hydroquinone is the processing chemical most sensitive to changes in temperature, concentration, and pH and to exposure to light and heavy metals. Hydroquinone levels should be maintained in the range of 20 to 25 g/L.

The overall optical density is created by the synergistic action of the two reducing agents. *Synergism* means that the action of the two agents working together is greater than the sum of each agent working independently. **Synergism** is also known as *superadditivity* (Fig. 4-1).

Preservative. The preservative, or antioxidant, protects the hydroquinone from both aerial oxidation (chemical reaction with air) and internal oxidation (chemical reaction with other developer ingredients). If the hydroquinone is oxidized, there is a decrease in the D_{max} and contrast indicators during a sensitometric test, along with a loss of the shoulder on the H and D curve. Oxidized developer causes the developer solution to turn from a clear, brown liquid into one that is dark and muddy. If strongly oxidized, the solution also has the odor of ammonia because this is a byproduct of the oxidation chemical reaction. Most developer replenishment tanks have a floating lid inside the tank in addition to the main lid on the outside, to minimize contact with the outside air. The chemicals sodium sulfite, potassium sulfite, and cycon can be used as developer solution preservatives.

Accelerator, Activator, or Buffering Agent. The accelerator, activator, or buffering agent has two functions: to soften and swell the emulsion so that reducing agents can work on all of the emulsion and to provide an alkaline medium for the reducing agents. The developing agents must exist in an alkaline medium to have the free electrons available to reduce the silver to Ag°.

An indicator known as *pH* is used to measure the alkalinity of a solution. Potential hydrogen (pH) refers to the exponential (p) value of hydrogen ions (H^+) available for a reaction. Those chemicals having a high hydrogen potential (H^+) are called *acids,* and those having a high alkaline or hydroxide potential (OH^-) (and therefore, a low hydrogen potential) are called *bases.* The pH scale ranges from 0 to 7 (acids) and 7 to 14 (bases) (Fig. 4-2). This scale is based on the concentration of positively charged hydrogen ions (H^+) in moles per liter. For example, a pH of 4 would mean that a particular solution contains one ten-thousandth (10^{-4}) of a mole of hydrogen ions per liter. For this value to be converted to pH, the negative exponent (-4) is changed to a positive number (4). A solution with a H^+ concentration of one ten-millionth (10^{-7}) moles per liter would then have a pH of 7, and so on. Because the pH scale is logarithmic in nature, a change of one whole number on the pH scale can represent a tenfold change from the previous concentration. A pH of 1 denotes 10 times more H^+ ions than a pH of 2; a pH of 3 has 10 times fewer H^+ ions than a pH of 2, and so on. Pure water is neutral and has a pH of 7. Fixer is an acid solution; therefore, care must be taken not to introduce it into developer solutions because only 0.1% contamination deteriorates the developer activity enough to compromise image quality. Chemicals that can be used as accelerators include sodium carbonate, sodium hydroxide, potassium carbonate, and potassium hydroxide.

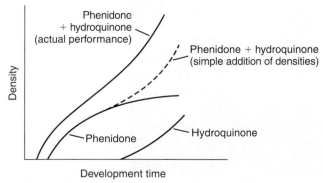

FIGURE 4-1 Graph demonstrating superadditivity effect of phenidone and hydroquinone.

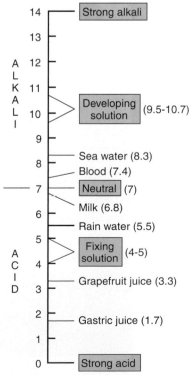

FIGURE 4-2 Potential hydrogen (pH) scale.

Restrainer, Regulator, Antifoggant, or Starter.
The restrainer (regulator, antifoggant, or starter) holds back, or restrains, the action of the developing agents so that they reduce only the silver halide crystals that have been exposed to radiation. The chemical used in most brands of developer is potassium bromide in the form of K^+Br^-, which is chemically similar to Ag^+Br^-. If the reducing agents become too active, they attack the potassium bromide instead of the silver halide. Potassium iodide also can be used as the restrainer. Overdiluting or underreplenishing water can reduce the levels of restrainer and increase the speed indicator during a sensitometric test.

Hardener. When a film enters the warm developer solution, the gelatin emulsion begins to soften and swell, which can cause the film to stick to the rollers of an automatic film processor; therefore, developer manufacturers add a weak hardener (a stronger one is present in fixer solutions) to control emulsion swelling and stickiness. If the amount of hardener is depleted because of underreplenishment, wet films, transport problems, and uncleared films may result. The chemical agent used as a hardener is glutaraldehyde.

Solvent. The previously mentioned ingredients are mixed with a solvent to form developer solution. The most common and readily available solvent is water.

This water should be drinkable and have the following characteristics: filtration to particles under 40 μm, dissolved solids less than 250 parts per million (ppm), pH of 6.5 to 8.5, hardness of 40 to 150 ppm, heavy metals less than 0.1 ppm, chloride less than 25 ppm, and sulfate less than 200 ppm.

Sequestering Agent. Much of the developer used in hospital darkrooms is shipped in concentrate form and then mixed with tap water at the clinical site. Because impurities (e.g., calcium ions, metals such as iron and copper) can be found in tap water, many manufacturers add a sequestering agent called *ethylenediamine tetraacetic acid (EDTA)* or *edetate* to prevent impurities from interfering with the developer chemicals. EDTA is an oily substance that causes calcium and other mineral contaminants to stick together and dissipate to the bottom of processing tanks. EDTA also helps form stable chemical complexes with metallic ions.

Developer Activity. How well a developer functions is called the *developer activity* and is governed by the following five factors: solution temperature, immersion time, solution concentration, type of chemicals used, and solution pH.

Solution Temperature (Fig. 4-3). The greater the solution temperature, the more active the developing

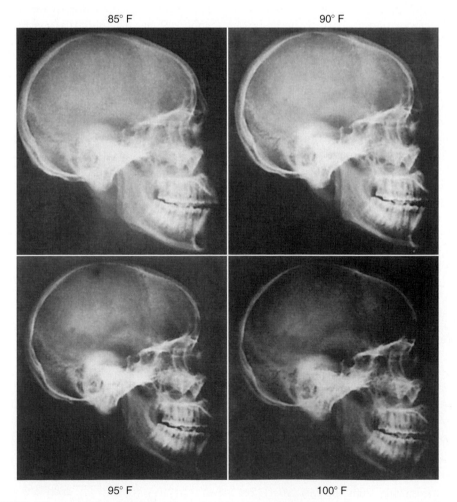

85° F   90° F

95° F   100° F

FIGURE 4-3 Radiographs showing effect of solution temperature on optical density and contrast.

agents become, especially hydroquinone. This increases the optical density of the resultant image. If the temperature drops below 60° F (15.5° C), the hydroquinone stops working, which causes the resulting images to decrease in optical density and contrast. At temperatures above 75° F (24° C), the developing agents become increasingly active, which increases the optical density of subsequent images. The optimum temperature range for developer solution is 68° to 72° F (20° to 22.2° C). However, automatic processing solutions may range from 85° to 105° F (29.4° to 40.5° C) to process images more rapidly.

Immersion Time (Fig. 4-4). The greater the length of time in the solution, the greater the optical densities recorded on the processed image (and vice versa). The reason for this is that the developing agents are in contact with the silver ions for a longer period and can therefore reduce more silver ions to metallic silver.

Solution Concentration. *Solution concentration* refers to the percentage of water versus other chemicals in the solution and can be measured by specific gravity (the density of a liquid compared with water). An instrument called a *hydrometer* measures specific gravity,

which ranges from 1.07 to 1.10 in typical developer solutions. The specific gravity should not vary by 14 ± 0.004 from the manufacturer's specifications. This is discussed further in the next chapter.

Type of Chemicals Used. Developer solutions that contain elon or metol behave differently from those that contain phenidone. The DuPont Cronex HSD system uses an acid developer solution to process the film and therefore behaves quite differently from conventional developer solutions.

Solution pH. The developer solution should maintain a pH between 10 and 11.5 and should not vary by more than ± 0.1 from the manufacturer's specifications. Excessive pH increases the optical density of a processed image or causes increased oxidation, whereas too low of a pH value decreases the optical density of any resultant image.

Over time, the developer becomes exhausted and requires replenishment. Reasons for this replenishment include the following:

- Significant quantities of developer are consumed during the development process.

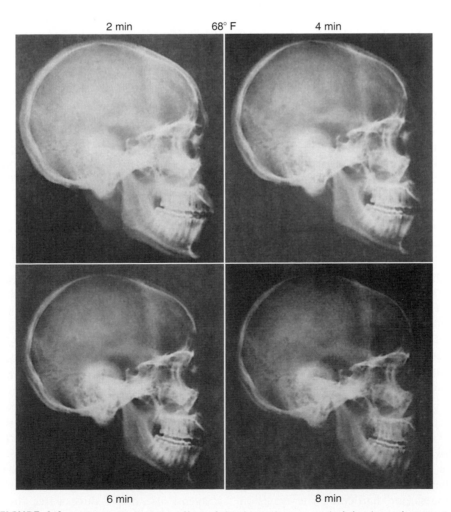

FIGURE 4-4 Radiographs showing effect of developer time on optical density and contrast.

- The liberating of bromide and hydrogen bromide acid into the developer during development can lower the pH and cause a decrease in activity. These bromide levels should be maintained in a range of 4 to 8 g/L to maintain proper pH.
- Aerial and internal oxidation begins as soon as the solution is mixed, and developing agents are consumed.
- A certain volume of developer solution is removed by the film's emulsion each time a film is fed into the processor. The squeegee action of the crossover rack helps minimize this effect.

Developer Mixing Procedure. Developer solution is generally available in two options, as a premix or a concentrate.

Premix or Ready-Mix. As the name implies, this solution has all of the ingredients combined with the solvent so that no mixing is required at the clinical site. The solutions usually are delivered in 5- or 10-gallon containers and should be poured directly into the replenishment tanks. The disadvantages of this method include a relatively short shelf life (from 2 weeks to 3 months) and higher cost (about 40% more than concentrate); therefore, large quantities should not be stockpiled, and frequent deliveries must be made.

Concentrate. The main ingredients are shipped to the clinical site in a concentrate form and must be mixed with water at the clinical site. This is less convenient but greatly reduces the cost of the solutions. The concentrate kit usually comes in three parts. Part 1 contains the hydroquinone, preservative, and accelerator and has a pH between 11 and 12. Part 2 contains the phenidone and restrainer and has a pH of 3. Part 3 contains the hardener and has a pH of 3.

When solution from concentrate is mixed, the proper amount of water should be present in the tank and then each solution added in the proper order. Large quantities of chemicals should be mixed electrically with a commercially available system. These systems use a propeller type of variable-speed mixer. The speed must be regulated because excessive speed introduces unwanted air into the chemicals, which can oxidize the developer. These systems are not useful in facilities that use only a small volume of developer each week. Fresh chemistry should last 2 weeks and then be discarded. Concentrate lasts 1 year when stored at room temperature and away from direct sunlight. Excessive agitation (shaking of the bottles) during mixture and storage should be avoided because this may cause a decomposition of the chemicals, resulting in reduced activity of the solution.

Fixer

Fixer solutions remove all of the unexposed and undeveloped silver halide crystals from the film; thus, the image is cleared. They are also responsible for halting the development process and hardening the emulsion for permanent storage.

Fixer Ingredients. Fixers are composed of the following six components: fixing agent, preservative, hardener or tanning agent, acidifier, sequestering agent, and solvent.

Fixing Agent, Clearing Agent, or Hypo. The fixing agent (clearing agent or hypo) removes the unexposed and undeveloped silver halide crystals from the film. The chemical ammonium thiosulfate is used in most modern fixing solutions (sodium thiosulfate has been used in manual solutions). *Hypo* is a common name for thiosulfate compounds. It picks up unexposed silver atoms from the silver halide crystal to form ammonium thio-silver-sulfate. The fixing process can be summarized by the following equation

$$2AgX + Na_2S_2O_3 \rightarrow Ag_2S_2O_3 + 2\,NaX$$

where X designates the halide used in the film emulsion (either bromide or iodide).

The action of this agent is controlled by dilution, replenishment, and the use of a recirculating electrolytic silver recovery unit (discussed in Chapter 6).

The effectiveness of the fixing agent can be evaluated by a clearing time test.

PROCEDURE

1. Take a strip of undeveloped green film and dip it into the fixer solution. Use a stopwatch to measure the clearing time.
2. Film should clear in 10 seconds at room temperature and in less than 7 seconds at 90° F (32° C). If it does not, the fixing agents are not working properly and the problem may be due to improper mixing (usually too much water), too high of a pH, or expired solution. To correct this problem, dispose of the fixer, clean out the replenishment tank, and fill with fresh solution. It is then recommended that the clearing time test again be performed on the new solution to be sure that it is functioning according to accepted levels.

Preservative. The chemical sodium sulfite dissolves the silver out of the ammonium thio-silver-sulfate, and it is returned or recycled back to ammonium thiosulfate. In this way, sulfite is available to clear more of the undeveloped silver from the film. It can be depleted by excess developer carry-in, underreplenishment, and the use of recirculating electrolytic silver recovery units, which deplete sodium sulfite. The concentration of this chemical should be maintained in the range of 15 to 50 g/L.

Hardener or Tanning Agent. For the film to be stored permanently, the emulsion must be hardened to keep the image from fading or being scratched during handling. This is called *tanning*. Potassium alum, chrome alum, and aluminum chloride are the more common chemicals used as fixer hardeners. These materials' combining with the gelatin proteins to form complex molecules results in a "hardened" emulsion. These agents also help reduce water absorption during washing, and drying time is reduced.

Acidifier, Activator, or Buffer. The acidifier, or activator or buffer, has two functions: neutralizing any developer remaining in the emulsion and providing an acid medium for the fixing agent.

Just as the developing agents need an alkaline medium in which to function, the fixing agent can dissolve undeveloped silver only in an acid solution. The acid allows the fixing agent to diffuse into the emulsion, and thereby the necessary contact with the undeveloped silver ions is made. Fixer pH should be maintained at a level between 4 and 4.5 and should not vary more than ±0.1 from the manufacturer's specifications. Chemicals that help maintain the pH are commonly known as *buffers*. Both acetic acid and sulfuric acid can be used as the acidifier.

Sequestering Agent. These agents help prevent the development of aluminum hydroxide, which forms as the developer solution is carried into the fixer. Because aluminum hydroxide is an alkaline compound, its formation results in an increase in fixer pH. Carboxylic acids, boric acids, or borate salts may be used as the sequestering agents in fixer solutions.

Solvent. Water is used as the solvent in which to suspend the other chemicals. The same standards listed for the developer solvent water also apply to the fixer. The concentration of fixer can be measured by specific gravity and may range from 1.077 to 1.11. The specific gravity should not vary by more than ± 0.004 from the manufacturer's specifications.

Fixer Mixing Procedure. The fixer solution may be purchased in either ready-mix or concentrate form. The ready-mix may cost as much as 20% more but has the same convenience as ready-mix developer. The concentrate must be mixed with water and usually comes in two parts. Part 1 contains the ammonium thiosulfate, preservative, and acidifier. Part 2 contains the hardener in a strong acid solution.

As with developer, one may start with water in the tank and mix large quantities with a commercial mixing unit. It is recommended that the fixer be mixed before the developer because inadvertent splashing of fixer could contaminate the developer.

Washing

Washing is important for the **archival quality** of the film because it removes the fixer from the film emulsion before drying. If hyporetention is allowed to take place, the reaction of the thiosulfate with the silver in the emulsion produces Ag_2S, or silver sulfide, which can stain the image from pale yellow to dark brown. By law, films must be archived 5 years; groups such as the military require 40 years after death, separation, or retirement. Commercial test kits are available to measure the amount of hyporetention (Fig. 4-5). One type of test kit involves the use of a specialized test strip that is placed in contact with a processed film after a drop of solution is applied to its surface, and the test strip

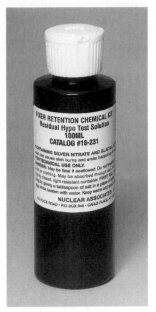

FIGURE 4-5 Hyporetention kit for evaluating residual fixer in processed films. *(Courtesy Nuclear Associates, Carle Place, N.Y.)*

changes color. An accompanying color guide then allows the matching of the color on the strip to the appropriate value on the guide, which then indicates the amount of hyporetention.

Another type of hyporetention test kit involves placing a drop of hypo test solution on a film and then judging the color of the resulting stain. The hypo test solution is a mixture of silver nitrate, acetic acid, and water and must remain in a dark container because it is light sensitive. When a drop of this solution is applied to a processed film, it causes a chemical reaction with any fixer that may still remain; the result is a brown stain. The more fixer that remains on the film, the darker this stain becomes. A test strip containing different color stains is supplied with the solution test kit and then is used to indicate the exact level of hyporetention. The solution is applied to a processed film in the darkroom and is allowed to stand for 2 minutes. After the 2 minutes has elapsed, the excess solution is blotted off (do not wipe) and the film is taken to the lightroom area for comparison with the test strip. The American National Standards Institute (ANSI) suggests that the amount of hyporetention not exceed 2 $\mu g/cm^2$ for radiographic film images and .5 $\mu g/cm^2$ for mammographic film images. These ANSI tests should be performed at least semiannually (every 6 months) for radiographic images (preferably every 3 months) and must be performed quarterly (every 3 months) for mammographic images. If the level of hyporetention exceeds these values, check to see if the wash tank has the correct amount of water present (there should be a level mark on the side of the tank). If this is sufficient, then check the water flow rate to ensure that it is set to the processor manufacturer's standard.

The water used in washing should have the following characteristics: hardness of 40 to 150 ppm, pH of 6.5 to 8.5, dissolved solids less than 250 ppm, and a specific gravity of 1. Washing time should be at least 50% to 100% of the developer time, and the temperature should be about 5° F (3° C) below the developer temperature to help trigger the heater thermostat in the automatic processor. The water flow rate should be at a rate of 1 to 3 gal/min for removal of hyporetention, proper agitation, and prevention of algae and bioslime. If this is a problem, a few milliliters of laundry bleach (5% sodium hypochlorite) may be added to the wash tank at shutdown.

Chemical Safety

Because OSHA considers the darkroom a scientific laboratory, it has several safety requirements in place, including the implementation of hazard communication standards and the use of personal protective equipment (PPE).

- Hazard communication standards were established by OSHA to ensure that both employers and employees have knowledge of all workplace chemical hazards, in addition to the appropriate protection procedures from these hazards. One important tool to help diagnostic imaging departments comply with these standards is the Material Safety Data Sheet (MSDS), which should be displayed for all chemicals used by employees. These forms must be kept on file for each hazardous chemical and must be readily accessible to all employees. They also must contain the potentially toxic chemical agents to which a worker may be exposed, the chemical and physical characteristics, precautionary and control measures for the chemical, primary routes of chemical entry, and limits of exposure to the chemical. They also should contain basic warnings concerning the product such as any possible health effects from exposure and any emergency treatment information. The MSDS also must contain the preparation date of the chemical and the name and address of the manufacturer. Each MSDS uses a rating scale to indicate the hazard level of various chemicals. A level 1 rating indicates a slight hazard, level 2 is a moderate hazard, level 3 is a serious hazard, and level 4 is a severe hazard. The MSDS also must indicate the category of chemical hazard. OSHA categorizes hazardous chemicals as being either a physical hazard or a health hazard. Chemicals that are a physical hazard are those that can cause either a physical injury or a burn. Examples include compressed gases (such as oxygen), oxidizers (such as chlorine bleach), combustible liquids (such as gasoline or kerosene), and flammable materials (such as cleaning solvents). Chemicals that can cause acute or chronic health effects such as irritants, corrosives, sensitizers, and carcinogens are categorized as health hazards. Processing solutions are considered health hazards. An MSDS should be included with each shipment of processing solution. If not, one can be obtained by contacting the manufacturer. OSHA's hazard communication standards also include information on hazard evaluation, the proper labeling of containers, the maintaining of lists of chemicals used by the facility, and employee training. These have been discussed already in Chapter 1.

- OSHA developed PPE standards to ensure that employees have proper protection from workplace hazards. These standards include selecting the appropriate PPE, training employees in the proper use of the PPE, maintaining the PPE in a safe and sanitary condition, and replacing the PPE when it becomes damaged or defective. Safety equipment such as eye protection (preferably full-face or non-vented goggles) must be available to personnel who handle, mix, transport, or use processing chemicals. The equipment must meet or exceed the requirements of ANSI Standard Z87.1-1989, "American National Standard Practice for Occupational and Educational Eye and Face Protection." In case of failure or nonuse of the PPE, an eyewash station should be prominently located in the area where chemicals are in use. Should any amount of processing solution come in contact with the eye, the employee should wash copiously and immediately contact a physician. For protection of the rest of the body, chemically resistant aprons composed of neoprene (chemically resistant) or similar material should be provided. In addition, shower facilities should be available to remove any chemical that has come in contact with the skin. For hand protection, gloves made of neoprene or similar material should be available for employees who handle processing solutions. OSHA's PPE standards require gloves whenever employees' hands are exposed to potential absorption of harmful substances (such as processing solutions). Training programs for personnel also must be established and attendance of participants documented. Only trained personnel should perform mixing, cleaning, or maintenance work.

The Environmental Protection Agency (EPA) also has regulations concerning the use and disposal of processing chemicals. The EPA-SARA Title III (Superfund Amendments and Reauthorization Act of 1986) requires all users of developer solution to report the quantity used. The Resource Conservation and Recovery Act of 1987 governs waste management practices and limits liquid waste containing silver to a level of no more than 5 mg/L, or 5 ppm. This can limit the amount of used processing chemicals and wash tank water that can be placed into public sewers and private septic systems before a special permit is required. This also may come under the jurisdiction of the Clean Water Act of 1977. This is a 1977 amendment to the federal Water Pollution

Control Act of 1972, which set the basic structure for regulating discharges of pollutants to water in the United States. It prohibits the discharge of pollutants into any surface water unless strict standards are in place and a special National Pollution Discharge Elimination System (NPDES) permit has been filed with the EPA. Any medical facility that discharges directly to any surface water must have an NPDES permit. The EPA describes one's local wastewater treatment facility as a publicly owned treatment works (POTW), which also must have NPDES permits. If the wastewater from the diagnostic imaging department is discharged to the local POTW and it has a silver concentration of 5 ppm or greater and more than 15 kg/mo is being discharged, the facility must submit a one-time written notification to the local POTW, the EPA, and the state hazardous waste authority. The discarding or recovery of silver is discussed further in Chapter 6. Material with a pH between 5.5 and 10 can safely be disposed of down the drain; all three parts of the concentrated developer and both parts of concentrated fixer are disqualified. A shipment of scrap film, a silver-laden fixer, and silver recovery cartridges from the clinical site to a refiner or treatment plant also require a special permit from the EPA or the Department of Transportation, or both.

The developer solution is considered the most dangerous processing chemical because of its high alkalinity. This makes it especially dangerous to the eyes (hence OSHA's requirement of eye protection) and skin. A main component of film emulsion is gelatin (a form of collagen), which is an organic form of protein that is broken down by chemicals with a high pH. Because human soft tissue contains collagen, the skin and eyes are at risk if contact is made with developer. Hydroquinone can be absorbed through the skin and is corrosive to the eyes and nasal membranes. Glutaraldehyde is a tanning agent (made to harden collagen-based material) and therefore a skin irritant. Wearing eye protection, rubber gloves, and an apron should always be standard operating procedure when pouring or mixing developer. Fixer is a strong acid that can burn the eyes and irritate the skin. As with developer, proper safety apparel should be worn when pouring and mixing fixer. Wash immediately any skin that has been in contact with processing solutions.

AUTOMATIC PROCESSOR MAIN SYSTEMS

All automatic film processors have six main systems: transport, temperature, circulation, replenishment, drying, and electrical.

Transport System

The transport system is responsible for transporting the film through the various steps in processing and for controlling the development and total processing times.

It also plays a minor role in solution agitation and concentration. This is the largest and most complex system in an automatic processor. Because it has many moving parts, it is also the system most likely to break down. The transport system is made up of three smaller subsystems.

Roller Subsystem. The rollers are responsible for "grabbing" the film and transporting it through the various stages of processing. They also provide a squeegee action that helps prevent too much solution carryover. There are three main types of rollers:

- *Entrance rollers* usually are serrated rollers made of rubberized plastic. This better enables these rollers to grip the film as it enters the processor (Fig. 4-6).
- *Transport, or planetary, rollers* are responsible for the transportation of film and most often have a diameter of 1 inch. They usually are mounted in pairs, either staggered or directly opposite each other (Fig. 4-7).
- *Master, or solar, rollers* are larger rollers with a 3-inch diameter. These rollers are found at the bottom of each solution tank, where the film must bend and turn back upward.
- Rollers can be made of acrylic plastic (Plexiglas), stainless steel, polyester plastic, rubberized plastic, and phenolic resin. The phenolic rollers are orange-brown and wooden in appearance. Care must be taken in cleaning phenolic rollers (no abrasive pads). Because these rollers are made of relatively soft material that can be scratched, liquid can be absorbed into the roller and subsequent warping can occur. For these reasons, rollers made of phenolic resin are normally found in the dryer section.

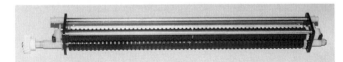

FIGURE 4-6 Entrance rollers for automatic film processor.

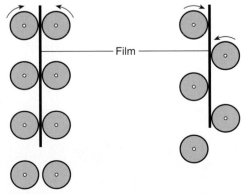

FIGURE 4-7 Transport rollers for automatic film processor.

Transport Rack Subsystem. The transport rack subsystem is the rack or frame containing the rollers, guide shoes, and associated hardware. There are four types of transport racks.

- *Entrance rack.* The entrance rack contains the entrance rollers, guide shoe(s), and a microswitch to activate the replenishment system (in volume replenishment systems) (see Fig. 4-6).
- *Vertical or deep racks.* Vertical or deep racks contain the transport rollers that transport the film into or up out of the tank (Fig. 4-8). Side plates and tie bars hold the rollers in place. The side plates and tie bars can expand and contract over time and cause misalignment.
- *Turnaround rack.* The turnaround rack is found at the bottom of the tank and contains a master roller, transport rollers, and two to three guide shoes (Fig. 4-9).
- *Crossover rack.* Crossover racks move from developer to fixer, fixer to wash tank, and wash tank to dryer transition. The crossover rack for the wash tank to dryer transition is often called a *squeegee rack* because it helps to remove water from the film and faster drying occurs. Usually, these racks contain a master roller, transport rollers, and two guide shoes, but they can vary from manufacturer to manufacturer. These racks are out of solution and

therefore must be cleaned before use because chemical residue can crystallize on the rollers during downtime. If the processor is on standby for longer than 2 hours, then the crossover racks should be cleaned before use.

Drive Subsystem. The drive subsystem is the portion of the transport system that supplies the mechanical energy to move the film (Fig. 4-10). This subsystem includes the following:

- *Drive motor.* The drive motor is a 1/20- to 1/8-hp electric motor that runs at 1725 to 1750 rpm.
- *Main drive chain.* The main drive chain is a no. 25 chain that attaches the drive motor to the gear system (similar to a bicycle chain). It is located on the side of the deep racks.
- *Gear reduction mechanism.* The gear reduction mechanism is a series of gears of different sizes that reduce the speed to between 10 and 20 rpm.
- *Gears.* Gears transfer the mechanical energy from the motor to the rollers. The two types of gears are "drive" gears, which normally are attached to the ends of the rollers, and "worm" gears, which are located on the main drive shaft and used to power the drive gears (Fig. 4-11). The gears can be made of plastic or metal.
- *Main drive shaft.* The main drive shaft connects the gear reduction mechanism to the drive gears with a system of worm gears.

Gears out of solution can be coated lightly with grease. Sprockets and chains out of solution require a light coating of oil, but care must be taken to avoid getting petroleum-based products in chemical solutions or on rollers. In the dryer section, lubricants must be avoided; therefore, the gears must be kept clean to minimize friction.

The average transport system speed for a 90-second processor is about 60 inches of film per minute.

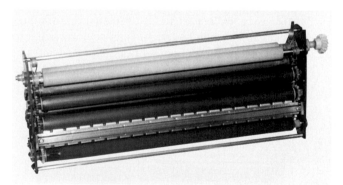

FIGURE 4-8 Vertical rack assembly.

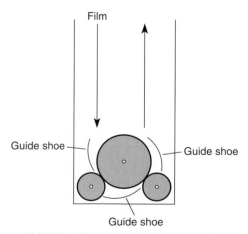

FIGURE 4-9 Turnaround rack assembly.

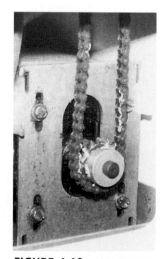

FIGURE 4-10 Drive system.

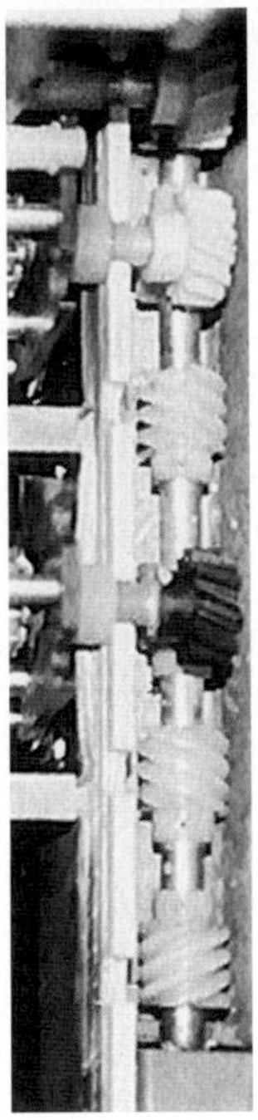

FIGURE 4-11 Worm and drive gears.

Temperature Control System

The temperature control system is also called the *tempering system* and regulates the temperature of each solution. The two basic types of this system currently in use are water- controlled systems and thermostatically controlled systems.

Water-Controlled System. This is often called a *warm-water processor* and uses the wash water temperature to regulate the solution temperature by circulating the water around the outside of the stainless steel processing tanks. This method requires a large supply of hot water and a mixing valve to regulate water temperature (Fig. 4-12).

Thermostatically Controlled System. Processors with this type of system are often called *cold-water processors* because they require only cold wash water to enter the unit. These systems use either an electronic heater for each tank or a heat exchanger, with a thermostat to regulate the system. The heat exchanger is a thin-walled, stainless steel tube located at the bottom of each tank (Fig. 4-13). When a heat exchanger is used, the dryer air is used to heat the solutions in each tank. Because the dryer air temperature can exceed 120° F, the cooler wash water is pumped through the heat exchanger tube to keep the solution temperature in the proper range (typically 85° to 95° F). This system is much more practical than the others because it does not require the large hot water heater and associated utility cost to maintain the supply necessary for the water-controlled system. For this reason, most of the newer processors are of this type. Regardless of the type of temperature control system used, the system must maintain the developer temperature to within ± 0.5° F (0.3° C) of the manufacturer's specifications.

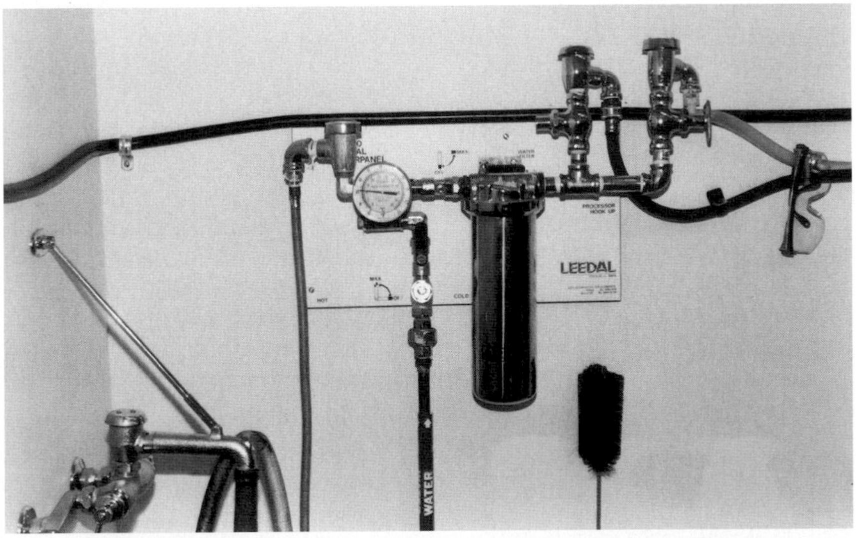

FIGURE 4-12 Mixing valve for warm-water automatic processors.

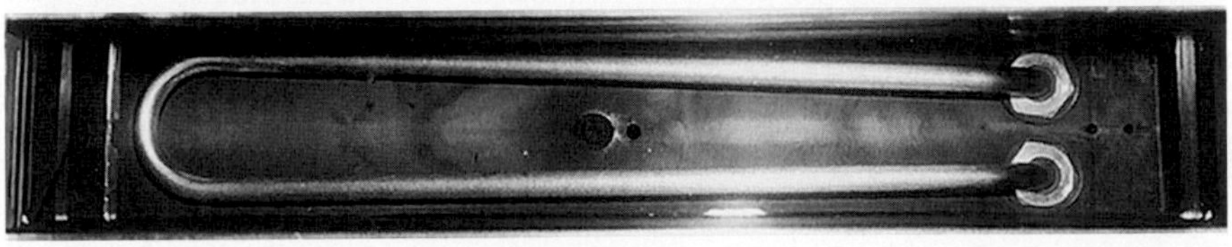

FIGURE 4-13 Heat exchanger located in bottom of water tank in thermostatically controlled temperature system.

Circulation System

The circulation system also can be referred to as the *recirculation and filtration* system. It uses a series of pumps to constantly circulate the solution in each tank and serves the following functions:

- *Ensures complete chemistry mixing.* During processor downtime, chemicals inside the tanks may begin to separate, with the water rising to the top and the chemicals dissipating to the bottom (a condition known as *stratification*). Swirling of the solutions by the circulation system ensures uniform concentration.
- *Provides uniform temperature.* Because the heating or heat exchanging elements are typically on the bottom of the tank, uneven regions of temperature can develop unless the solutions are continuously being circulated.
- *Provides the equivalent of agitation performed in manual processing.*

In manual film processing the halide ions that have been separated from the silver leave the emulsion in the form of bromine gas. This gas can cause a layer of bubbles to form on the outside surface of the film. This can block developing agents from reaching the inner portion of the emulsion, and areas of uneven development called *streaking* occur. **Agitation** in manual processing involves "jiggling" the film every 30 seconds to shake this layer of bubbles on the film. With the developer swirling over the surface of the film in an automatic processor, the layer of bubbles is removed in much the same way as agitation in manual processing.

A 25-μm filter is often located in the developer loop of this system to remove gelatin and other impurities that become dissolved in the developer during processing (Fig. 4-14). This filter must be replaced periodically as part of a processor maintenance program. Most manufacturers recommend replacement of this filter on a monthly basis or after the processing of 5000 films. A filter is not required for the fixer portion of this system. The circulation rate of this system is roughly 3 to 5 gal/min for the developer tank and 1 to 3 gal/min for the fixer. Failure of this system generally results in uneven development of the resulting image.

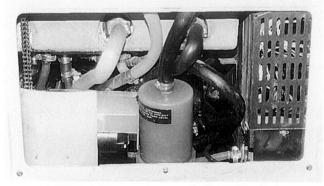

FIGURE 4-14 Developer circulation system filter.

Replenishment System

The replenishment system is also called the *regeneration system* and is responsible for replenishing processor solutions. It consists of a series of pumps, plastic tubing, and plastic storage tanks. The plastic tubing linking the replenishment solution storage tanks to the processor should be inspected periodically because it may be pinched or twisted, which may block the flow of fresh solution (resulting in under-replenishment). The two different types of replenishment systems available in film processors are volume replenishment and flood replenishment.

Volume Replenishment. With the **volume replenishment** system, a volume of chemicals is replaced for each film that is fed into the processor. This is the most common type of replenishment system. A microswitch usually is placed at either end of the entrance rack that senses the film and then activates this system so that the size of the film controls the amount of replenishment that takes place.

The average replenishment rates for this system are as follows:

- *Developer:* 4 to 5 mL/in of film, or roughly 60 to 70 mL per sheet of 14 × 17 inch film (35 × 43 cm)
- *Fixer:* 6 to 8 mL/in, or roughly 100 to 110 mL per sheet of 14 × 17 inch film

The volume replenishment system is used for relatively busy processors that process at least 25 to 50 sheets of 14 × 17 inch film or equivalent per 8-hour workday.

Flood Replenishment. **Flood replenishment** is also called *timed or standby replenishment* and is used for processors that are not in constant use or that process less than 25 to 50 sheets of 14 × 17 inch film or equivalent per day. With the low volume of patient films processed per day, there may be a considerable gap in time between films entering the processor. This allows the developer solution inside the automatic processor to become oxidized, and subsequent films are underdeveloped. This can cause the radiographer to either increase technical factors (the result is a higher patient dose) or increase the replenishment rate of a volume replenishment system (the results are higher department costs). With a flood replenishment system, the replenishment is controlled by a timer, which periodically replenishes the solutions, regardless of the number of films processed. This system was developed by Donald E. Titus of the Eastman Kodak Company. The replenishment pump should operate for approximately 20 seconds out of every 5 minutes and deliver about 65 mL of each solution. This maintains a total replenishment rate of 780 mL/hr. All developer in the processing tank should be replaced every 16 working hours.

Most processors have a replenishment rate indicator on them, so monitoring is easy. In the case of other types of processors, special test paper is available for testing certain concentrations in the developer and fixer.

For developer, the special test paper estimates the levels of bromide ions that are dissolved in the solution. Stable developer should have a bromide level of about 6 g/L. Levels above 8 g/L indicate underreplenishment, which can cause underdevelopment and lead to a lack of optical density and contrast of the resulting image. This is most often caused by a pinched or blocked replenishment line, pump failure, microswitch failure, or failure of the timer circuit during flood replenishment. Levels below 4 g/L indicate overreplenishment, which can result in overdevelopment that causes increased optical density and fogging. This is most often caused by a microswitch that fails to shut off or a pump that does not shut off.

Fixer replenishment can be estimated with silver estimating paper, which estimates the dissolved silver content in the solution. Normal fixer contains about 4 to 6 g/L (0.4 to 0.6 troy oz/gal). Levels above 8 g/L indicate underreplenishment (which causes a lack of clearing and a possible lack of hardening in the resulting film), whereas levels below 4 g/L indicate overreplenishment, which does not adversely affect film quality but wastes fixer (and therefore money).

Dryer System

The dryer system consists of two or three heating units between 1500 and 2500 watts that are used to dry the film. This can draw at least 10 amperes (A) of electric current; the result is that this system consumes 60% to 80% of the electrical power going into the processor. A hot-air blower moves the air at a rate between 100 and 300 ft^3/min over the film. A series of air fins and air tubes are used to direct the air onto the film (Fig. 4-15). These fins and tubes must be kept clean for maximum efficiency. Most automatic processors also require an exhaust tube (which is similar to one found on a clothes dryer) to empty the hot air out of the

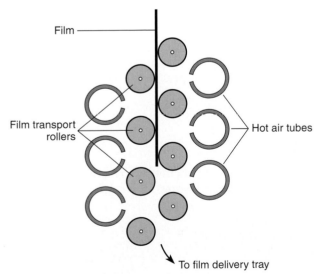

FIGURE 4-15 Dryer air tubes.

processing area. This air can have a temperature exceeding 100° F (37.8° C) and relative humidity values between 25% and 100%, which are not conducive to proper film storage.

Electrical System

The electrical system consists of a solid-state circuit board or microprocessor that distributes electrical power to the other systems. In some newer processors, the microprocessor can be accessed to disclose quality control information such as solution temperature and replenishment rate. It usually handles 4 to 5 kilowatts (kW)/hr and between 15 and 25 A of current. This system requires periodic replacement because of the heat, humidity, and corrosive environment inside of the processor.

TYPES OF AUTOMATIC PROCESSORS

Automatic processors are of several types, and they usually are named according to the time it takes to fully process the film, often called the *dry-to-drop time.*

- *7-minute:* the original Kodak automatic processor from the 1950s; processes about 100 films per hour.
- *3-minute:* also called a *double-capacity processor* because it processes 200 films per hour.
- *90-second:* also called a *fast-access processor* because the film is available in 90 seconds and the processor has a capacity of 300 films per hour. This was developed by Kodak in the mid-1960s and is still the most commonly used film processor.
- *60-second:* a newer type of processor that can process up to 350 films per hour.
- *45-second:* the newest type of processor; it requires special film and chemistry to function properly.

Many newer processors come with a variable speed option so that processing time can be varied according to the type of film used. In other words, the radiographer may select a 90-second processing time, a 180-second processing time, and so on. An example of this is the "extended processing" used in mammography, which increases normal processing time to increase the film contrast. This is covered more completely in Chapter 11. Some processors also have a stand-by option that is useful for low-volume facilities. The drive system and dryer blower are shut off and the water flow rate is reduced, but the chemical and the dryer temperatures are maintained. This occurs when 2 minutes pass without a film entering the unit.

Processor Size

Automatic film processors come in three basic sizes according to the number of films processed in a given period.

Floor-Size Processor. The floor-size processor is the largest processor and, as its name implies, sits on the floor of the darkroom or lightroom. It has heavy-duty rollers, gears, and a drive motor so that it can handle a high volume of operation. This size of processor is normally found in the main radiology department of hospitals.

Intermediate-Size Processor. The intermediate-size processor is a smaller version of the floor-size processor and usually sits on four support legs. It is about the size of a single laundry sink. This processor is lower in cost than the floor-size model and is often found in physicians' offices and clinics and in specialized areas of hospitals such as surgery.

Tabletop-Size Processor. The tabletop-size processor is the smallest and least expensive processor. It is designed for low-volume operation such as in a mobile facility and is small enough to fit on the countertop of a darkroom.

Processor Location

A processor can be installed in the darkroom in one of four methods: totally inside, bulk inside, bulk outside, or daylight processing.

Totally Inside. With totally inside installation, the processor is completely inside the darkroom, and noise, heat, and humidity are generated; therefore, this is the least desirable method of installation. An advantage of this method, however, is easy retrieval of film that has jammed in the processor because it can be removed in safelighting.

Bulk Inside. With bulk inside installation, most of the processor is inside the darkroom and only the drop tray is on the outside. This method minimizes the heat and noise in the darkroom but still allows easy retrieval of jammed film.

Bulk Outside. Bulk outside installation places the feed tray inside the darkroom but all other components outside. This method eliminates the heat, noise, and humidity inside the darkroom but makes retrieval of films more difficult because they must be removed in white light.

The minimum space on all sides of the processor must be 24 inches, to allow for servicing.

Daylight Processing Systems and Processors. Daylight processing systems and processors are designed to eliminate the need for a darkroom. They are discussed in detail in Chapter 5.

SUMMARY

Even though most hospitals have switched to digital radiographic image acquisition, many (along with most smaller sized clinics and physician offices) have not

and, therefore, require film/screen systems. For radiographers working in nondigital imaging departments, a basic understanding of film processing and automatic processing systems is essential for the performance of the quality control activities that are discussed in Chapter 5.

Refer to the Evolve website at https://evolve.elsevier. com for Student Experiments 4.1: Hyporetention Test and 4.2: Automatic Processor Inspection.

REVIEW QUESTIONS

1. When mixing developer solution from concentrate, which part should be placed into the tank first?
   a. Part A
   b. Part B
   c. Part C
   d. Water
2. What would cause an ammonia-like odor in a darkroom?
   a. Contamination of the fixer by the developer
   b. Oxidation of the developer
   c. Improper mixing of the developer
   d. Overreplenishment of the developer
3. In an automatic processor, which of the following is not considered part of the three principal subsystems of the film transport system?
   a. Microswitch
   b. Rollers
   c. Transport racks
   d. Drive motor
4. According to ANSI standards, the maximum amount of hyporetention allowed is _____ _____ $\mu g/cm^3$.
   a. 2
   b. 5
   c. 8
   d. 10
5. If the developer temperature is set at 96° F, then the wash water temperature should be set at _____ ° F.
   a. 86
   b. 91
   c. 96
   d. 101
6. Which processing chemical is responsible for creating the optical densities above 1.2 on a diagnostic image?
   a. Phenidone
   b. Hydroquinone
   c. Elon
   d. Metol

7. Which system of the automatic processor consumes the greatest amount of electrical power?
   a. Transport
   b. Replenishment
   c. Circulation
   d. Dryer
8. Which of the following is located at the bottom of each processing tank?
   a. Entrance rack
   b. Vertical rack
   c. Turnaround rack
   d. Crossover rack
9. Which of the following materials are used in the construction of an entrance roller?
   a. Acrylic plastic (Plexiglas)
   b. Stainless steel
   c. Polyester
   d. Rubberized plastic
10. Hydrogen ions (H^+) that constitute 1/10,000 of a molar of a liquid would have which of the following pH values?
    a. 2
    b. 4
    c. 6
    d. 8

Processor Quality Control

OBJECTIVES

At the completion of this chapter the reader should be able to do the following:

- Understand the importance of a processor quality control program in diagnostic imaging
- List the main components of a processor quality control program in diagnostic imaging
- Describe the factors that affect chemical activity
- Indicate the proper processor cleaning procedures

- Describe the basic types of processor maintenance and appropriate maintenance procedures
- Perform sensitometric tests to monitor processor function and chemical activity performance
- Describe the importance of quality control in daylight systems

The most important part of a quality management program in departments utilizing film/screen image receptors is the quality control of the film processor. This is due to the large degree of variability that can occur with processing systems. Daily monitoring of processor operation and function is required to keep these variables from degrading the image quality. There are four components to a processor quality control program: chemical activity, cleaning procedures, maintenance, and monitoring.

CHEMICAL ACTIVITY

As mentioned in Chapter 4, **chemical activity** refers to how well the processing chemicals are functioning. Many variables affect chemical activity including the solution temperature, processing time, replenishment rate, solution pH, and specific gravity and proper mixing.

Solution Temperature

Variations in developer temperature can significantly affect image contrast, optical density, and the visibility of recorded detail; therefore, developer temperature should not vary by more than $\pm$ 0.5° F (0.3° C) from the manufacturer's recommendations. It should be monitored at the beginning of the workday and then periodically throughout the day. Many film processors have either an analog thermometer or a light-emitting diode (LED) indicator of solution temperature built into the front panel. If this is unavailable, a digital thermometer with a remote probe (Fig. 5-1) is the best instrument to monitor solution temperature because it is the most accurate and works quickly. A glass, alcohol-filled thermometer is an adequate alternative. A mercury thermometer should never be used because mercury is a toxic substance and poses a difficult and potentially hazardous cleanup problem in the event of breakage. Mercury also can sensitize film, even in small quantities. The accuracy of any built-in thermometer should be checked monthly with a digital thermometer and should be within $\pm$ 0.5° F (0.3° C).

Fixer activity is not as temperature sensitive as developer activity, but the temperature should be maintained within $\pm$ 5° F (3° C) of the developer temperature to avoid reticulation marks (discussed in Chapter 10) and to clear the film properly. Wash water temperature should be the same as that of the fixer in order to complete washing.

To check the solution temperatures, place the probe in each tank, starting with the developer. Be sure the probe is clean to avoid contamination. Next, check the wash water and then the fixer. Afterward, rinse the probe with water so that it is ready for the next inspection.

Processing Time

Variations in developer time can have the same effect on image quality as solution temperature; therefore, developer time should be maintained to within $\pm$ 2% to 3% of the manufacturer's specifications. As mentioned in Chapter 4, the transport system is responsible for maintaining processing time. Most of this system is made up of moving parts (and experiences the most wear and tear of any system), so it is subject to the most variability and breakdown. Processing time should be checked daily at the beginning of each workday (or more often if a malfunction is suspected). This can be checked with a stopwatch or digital timer. For the developer time, the film should be fed into the processor with the top open. When the leading edge of the film enters the solution, the timer should be started, and when the leading edge first emerges from the solution, the timer should be stopped. For a 90-second processor, the time should be between 18 and 22 seconds, with a margin of error of roughly 0.5 seconds. Total processing time can be evaluated by using the stopwatch to measure the time when the leading edge of the film enters the processor to when it begins to appear in the drop section and comparing it with the manufacturer's specification. For help with this procedure, a time-in-solution test (TIS) tool is available (Fig. 5-2). It consists of a strip of clear film base with two white tape strips that form the letter T. A black line is drawn about halfway on the first strip as a "get ready" line, to alert the person performing this test to get ready to start the stop watch. Timing begins when the cross of the T enters the solution.

Replenishment Rate

As film is processed during the course of the workday, the processing solutions are being depleted. If they are not adequately replenished, a decrease in image contrast and optical density occurs. Excessive replenishment has the opposite effect. Most film processors have replenishment rate **flow meters** that indicate the replenishment rate for each solution. The values indicated should be within $\pm$ 5% of the manufacturer's specification for the type of replenishment system in use (volume vs. flood replenishment). These values for most processors are described in Chapter 4. The amount of replenishment also should be within 5% of these values. A stopwatch and a graduated cylinder can be used to verify replenishment rate and flow meter accuracy. With the top of the processor open, an 8 × 10 inch (20 × 25 cm) film should be fed lengthwise. The graduated cylinder should be placed under the opening of the replenisher line so that

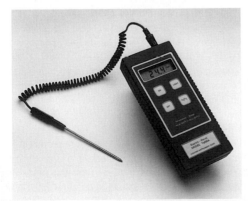

FIGURE 5-1 Digital thermometer for monitoring solution temperatures. *(Courtesy Gammex/RMI, Middleton, Wis.)*

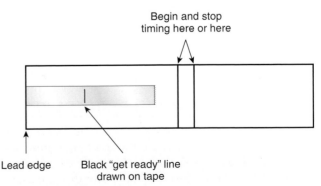

Begin and stop timing here or here

Lead edge   Black "get ready" line drawn on tape

FIGURE 5-2 Time-in-solution (TIS) test tool.

the fresh solution pumps directly into the cylinder. When the film has passed through the entrance rack, the replenisher pump shuts off, stopping the flow of solution. When this happens, the volume of solution should be divided in milliliters by 10 to get the milliliters per inches value (or divide by 25 to obtain milliliters per centimeters) and compared with the manufacturer's values.

Solution pH

Most developer solutions must function in a pH range between 10 and 11.5 to convert the latent image into a visible image. A developer pH that is too low (caused by underreplenishment or contamination) decreases image contrast and optical density, whereas excessive pH has the opposite effect. Fixer solutions should maintain a pH between 4 and 4.5 for proper clearing. Although not as critical as the other factors affecting chemical activity, pH should be checked daily to avoid potential problems. A digital pH meter is recommended for evaluating pH because of its accuracy. If one is not available, litmus paper or similar commercially available test strips are an inexpensive alternative. These are dipped into the solution and change color to indicate the pH value. Care should be taken (by wearing rubber gloves) not to get processing chemicals on one's skin with this method.

Specific Gravity and Proper Mixing

Processing chemicals must be mixed to the manufacturer's specifications of concentration to function within operating parameters. The easiest method of evaluation of solution concentration is the measurement of specific gravity.

$$\text{Specific gravity} = \frac{\text{Density of X liquid}}{\text{Density of water in equal amount}}$$

A **hydrometer** is the instrument used to measure specific gravity. It resembles a large glass thermometer (Fig. 5-3). When placed into a liquid, it sinks to a certain depth in the solution, and the level of the liquid indicates the specific gravity on the stem of the hydrometer. The developer should be measured first, the hydrometer rinsed with water, and then the fixer measured. Developer specific gravity should be in the range of 1.07 and 1.1 and should not vary by more than ± 0.004 from the manufacturer's specifications. Fixer solutions should be in the range of 1.077 to 1.11 and should not vary by more than ± 0.004 from the manufacturer's specifications.

PROCESSOR CLEANING PROCEDURES

Processors that are dirty cannot function according to established parameters and are the most common cause of processor breakdown; therefore, proper cleaning procedures should be performed daily, monthly, quarterly, and yearly.

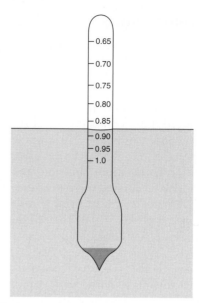

FIGURE 5-3 Floating hydrometer for measurement of specific gravity (indicating value of 0.87 g/cm^3).

Daily

These procedures should be performed daily at start-up.

PROCEDURE

1. Open the top of the processor to see if the crossover racks were removed on the previous night (which should be the case, as shown later in this section). However, the use of the processor may have been necessary during the night on an emergency basis. If the racks are present, remove the splash guards and crossover racks and rinse with water. Be sure the rollers and guide shoes are free of dirt, debris, gelatin, or crystallized processing chemicals. A soft sponge or plastic cleaning pad may be used for cleaning, but steel wool pads or other metallic scrubbers should be avoided. The rollers should be turned by hand so that all surfaces can be reached.

2. Remove the deep transport racks from each solution and rinse with water. Care must be taken not to drip one solution into the next (especially fixer into developer) when lifting the racks out of the solution tanks. Stubborn dirt or residue can be removed with a soft sponge or plastic scrubber. Inspect the rollers and gears for any obvious defects. Carefully replace the racks back into the solutions to avoid contamination.

3. Activate the transport system and observe the rollers and gears for asymmetry, rotation, and hesitation during operation. Replace the crossover racks and again observe the rollers and gears during operation. Replace any defective parts (especially gears and roller tension springs) and be sure that all mounting screws are tightened.

4. Observe the level of processing solutions to be sure that they are within 1 mm of specified level. Activate the replenisher pump or pour fresh solution from the storage tank if low.

5. At shutdown, remove the crossover racks and store adjacent to the processor (if practical) to minimize the formation of chemical residue. The top of the processor should be raised so that a 2- to 4-inch gap exists to allow chemical fumes to escape and avoid condensation of chemicals onto the various processor components.

The procedure just mentioned normally requires 15 to 20 minutes daily but can add several years to the life expectancy of the processor in addition to eliminating most processor artifacts.

Monthly

> **PROCEDURE**
>
> 1. Drain all processing tanks and wash the inside with water. A soft sponge or plastic scrubber can be used to remove stubborn dirt or residue.
> 2. Rinse all tanks with water and refill with the proper amount of chemical solution. The developer solution must be "seasoned" before any films can be processed because typical replenisher solution is too concentrated. This involves the addition of a starter solution, which is stabilized potassium bromide. This raises the bromide level to between 4 and 8 g/L, which is the normal level of a developer solution as it is processing films. Fresh developer replenisher that is used to refill the tank has levels far below this, which can increase the fog level of the film. The amount of starter solution required is about 100 ml/gal of solution.

Quarterly

> **PROCEDURE**
>
> 1. Drain, wash, and rinse all replenishment tanks with water. Be especially careful to remove the oxidized developer from the sides of the developer replenisher tank.
> 2. Refill tanks with fresh solution and check the specific gravity with a hydrometer.

Yearly

Replenisher and circulation system pumps and tubing can experience a build-up of dirt and chemical residue, which can reduce the efficiency of these systems; therefore, some manufacturers suggest the use of a system cleaner to reduce these deposits. The developer system cleaner has an acid pH level to counteract the alkaline developer, whereas the fixer system cleaner has an alkaline pH to counteract the acid fixer. The transport racks should be removed before a system cleaner is used because phenolic and soft rubber rollers can absorb the cleaner and slowly contaminate future processing solutions. Most system cleaners are either chlorine based (which can break down hydroquinone) or sulfamic based (which also breaks down hydroquinone and dissolves metallic silver). Great care also should be taken to flush systems with water to remove residual cleaner. Some manufacturers do not recommend the use of a system cleaner in their processors because of the risk of contamination, so it is best to check with a technical representative.

PROCESSOR MAINTENANCE

Poorly maintained processors (in addition to dirty ones) cannot function according to established parameters and can degrade image quality. They also can lead to premature replacement of the processor, which is a large capital expense ($5000 to $50,000). A film processor should last for at least 10,000 hours of operation or a minimum of 5 years; therefore; a proper maintenance schedule must be maintained by the diagnostic imaging department to ensure continued satisfactory operation of the film processor. A log of any maintenance procedures should be kept for documentation. There are three types of processor maintenance: scheduled, preventative, and nonscheduled.

Scheduled Maintenance

Scheduled maintenance includes procedures that are performed daily, weekly, and monthly. It includes proper lubrication of moving parts; observation of all moving parts; replacement of filters in the water and developer circulation system; adjustment or replacement of tension springs, pulleys, and gears; and correction of any mechanical problems.

Preventative Maintenance

Preventative maintenance is a planned program whereby certain specific parts of the processor are replaced regularly. It includes such items as gear and roller replacement after a certain number of hours of operation.

Nonscheduled Maintenance

Nonscheduled maintenance is required when a system failure occurs. Necessity for this type of maintenance can be minimized by proper cleaning of the processor, along with performing the scheduled and preventative maintenance procedures covered in this chapter.

A processor maintenance schedule should include maintenance procedures daily at start-up; daily during operation; daily at shutdown; and weekly, monthly, quarterly, and yearly.

Daily at Start-Up

> **PROCEDURE**
>
> 1. Follow daily cleaning procedures covered earlier in this chapter.
> 2. Make sure the processor feed tray and darkroom countertops are clean.
> 3. Feed four 14 × 17 inch (35 × 43 cm) green, unprocessed films into the processor. This cleans the rollers of any residual matter and also allows assessment of transport system operation. Do not use preprocessed radiographs because they may contain residual fixer and have a hardened emulsion, which causes extra stress on the transport system. This residual fixer also may contaminate the developer solution.

Daily During Operation

> **PROCEDURE**
>
> 1. Assess any changes in the normal operation of the processor including noise level, vibration, odors, indicator buzzer, and film-feeding characteristics.
> 2. Shut down the unit after 2 hours if no films have been processed (unless it is equipped with a stand-by option). If the unit has been shut down for 30 minutes or longer, run another 14 × 17 inch piece of green film to clean the rollers.

Daily at Shutdown

> **PROCEDURE**
>
> 1. Follow cleaning procedure for shutdown mentioned previously in this chapter.
> 2. Note any obvious problems or changes observed in the unit (abnormal odors or residues).

Weekly

> **PROCEDURE**
>
> 1. Using a thermometer, evaluate the solution temperature and dryer thermostats for accuracy. Compare the stated value on the thermostat with the indicated value on the thermometer. Solution temperatures must be maintained at the previously mentioned parameters. The dryer thermostat should be accurate to within ± 5° F (3° C).
> 2. Evaluate replenishment rates for accuracy, using the previously mentioned procedure.
> 3. Lubricate main driveshaft bearings, motor, and drive chain with motor oil.
> 4. Inspect replenishment system microswitches on the entrance rack for proper operation on units equipped with volume replenishment.
> 5. For units equipped with flood replenishment, drain the developer tank, rinse with water, and fill with fresh solution.
> 6. Inspect and service silver reclamation unit (discussed in Chapter 6).

Monthly

> **PROCEDURE**
>
> 1. Follow monthly cleaning procedures mentioned previously in this chapter.
> 2. Using a large bottlebrush, remove, clean, and inspect all dryer air tubes.
> 3. Replace the filter in the developer circulation. This filter removes dissolved gelatin and other impurities from the developer, down to 75 μm. Before installation, it is best to soak the filter in fresh developer solution to remove any air from the system.
> 4. Replace water filters if the flow rate decreases by more than 10% of the accepted amount.
> 5. Flush the floor drain with a commercial drain cleaner.
> 6. Perform a safelight test (see Chapter 3).

Quarterly

> **PROCEDURE**
>
> 1. Follow the quarterly cleaning procedure mentioned previously.
> 2. Inspect all transport racks, rollers, gears, and guide shoes for wear or malfunction.
> 3. Check the integrity of all electrical connections and remove any dirt or corrosion.
> 4. Perform a hyporetention test on processed films using an American National Standards Institute (ANSI) test kit (see Chapter 4) to evaluate the archival quality of images.

Yearly

> **PROCEDURE**
>
> 1. Disassemble each transport rack and replace worn rollers, gears, or mounting springs.
> 2. Disassemble the drive motor and gearbox, lubricate internal components, and replace worn parts.
> 3. Disassemble all replenishment and circulation system pump heads and replace worn parts including rubber diaphragms and seals.
> 4. Replace the tubing in the circulation and replenishment system with $1/8$-inch-wall, clear polyvinyl chloride tubing. New clamps also should be installed because of the corrosive environment inside of the processor.

PROCESSOR MONITORING

Processor monitoring is accomplished with the performance of daily sensitometric tests. These evaluate the performance of both the processor systems and processing chemicals. **Sensitometry** measures the relationship between the intensity of radiation absorbed by the film and the optical density that is produced. Two British amateur photographers, F. Hurter and U. Driffield, developed the current system of comparing these quantities (hence the Hurter and Driffield curve, which demonstrates film contrast). The following equipment is required to perform sensitometric tests: sensitometer, **densitometer**, either a control chart or graph paper, and quality control film.

Sensitometer

The **sensitometer** is an instrument designed to expose a reproducible, uniform, optical step-wedge pattern onto a film (Fig. 5-4). It contains a controlled-intensity light source with a standardized optical step-wedge image (also called a *step tablet*). These patterns are available in 11- and 21-step versions (Fig. 5-5). The 11-step pattern increases the optical density by a factor of 2 times (100%) between each step. The 21-step pattern increases optical density by a factor of 1.41 (41%) between each step and is more useful in sensitometric

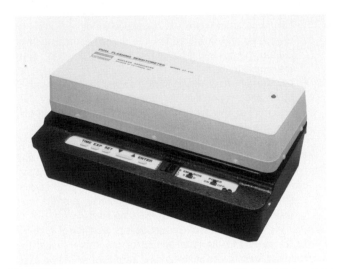

FIGURE 5-4 Sensitometer. *(Courtesy Gammex/RMI, Middleton, Wis.)*

X-Rite®

FIGURE 5-5 Twenty-one–step sensitometry film image. *(Courtesy Nuclear Associates, Carle Place, N.Y.)*

tests. A radiograph taken with an aluminum step wedge or penetrometer should not be used in processor sensitometric tests because x-ray generators are subject to too much variation from day to day and the origin of any differences in radiographic images cannot be determined (i.e., the problem could be with the processor or with the x-ray generator). The controlled light source of the sensitometer eliminates these variations.

Most sensitometers have settings that allow the selection of blue-violet light emission or green light emission to match the spectral response of the film being tested. They also should have an option for exposing single emulsion film or double emulsion (duplitized) film.

These settings must be properly selected to match the type of film that is to be used. Sensitometers remain fairly consistent in their operation until the light bulb burns out. The main concern for quality control technologists is to make sure that the exposure window of the sensitometer (where the light exposes the film) is kept clean and free of dirt and dust. These windows should not be touched by human hands or wiped clean with any type of cloth or gauze pad because they are fragile. Instead, a can of compressed air (which is free of moisture and therefore prevents condensation) should be obtained from a photographic supply store and used to remove any dirt or debris.

Densitometer

The densitometer, also known as *a transmission densitometer*, measures the optical density of a portion of an image with a 0 to 4 scale (Fig. 5-6). It is a photographic light meter that measures the amount of light transmitted (**transmitted light**) through a portion of film and compares it with the original amount of light incident on the film (Fig. 5-7). The 0 to 4 value is then calculated with the following equation:

$$\text{Optical density} = \log_{10} \frac{\text{Incident light}}{\text{Transmitted light}} \text{ or } \log_{10} \frac{I_i}{I_t}$$

If the transmitted light were 10% of the incident light, the optical density would be 1 because the equation would be the following:

$$\text{Optical density} = \log_{10} \frac{100}{10}$$

Because the **incident light** is the full amount of light striking the film, it has a relative value of 100%. The $\log_{10}$ symbol (meaning log to the base 10) in the equation asks the question, "10 to what power equals the number in the equation?" Because 100 divided by 10 equals 10, the $\log_{10}$ of the number 10 is 1 ($10^1 = 10$);

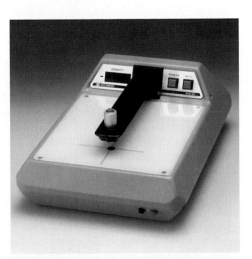

FIGURE 5-6 Densitometer for measurement of optical density. *(Courtesy Gammex/RMI, Middleton, Wis.)*

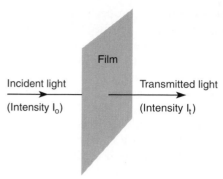

FIGURE 5-7 Diagram of incident and transmitted light. I_o, Original intensity; I_t, transmitted intensity.

therefore, if only 1% of the incident light is transmitted through the film, that portion of the image has an optical density of 2, because $100/1 = 100$ and $10^2 = 100$. A difference in the optical density scale of 0.3 is equivalent to a difference of 2 times in the amount of light transmission through the film because $10^{0.3} = 2$. This means that an optical density of 1.3 is twice as dark as an optical density of 1, and so on. The anatomic structures displayed on a diagnostic image normally have optical density values ranging from approximately 0.25 to 2.5 when measured with a densitometer; this is known as the *diagnostic range*. Optical densities outside of this range do not contain diagnostic information when viewed on a standard viewbox illuminator.

Control Chart

A control chart is a graph that has predetermined upper and lower thresholds indicated (see Chapter 2) and is used to plot the data obtained in the sensitometric test (Fig. 5-8). Most control charts are designed to have these data recorded each day, for an entire month.

PROCEDURE

1. Place an 8 × 10 inch (20 × 25 cm) sheet of unexposed film in the sensitometer and expose according to the manufacturer's instructions.
2. Feed the exposed film into the processor as soon as possible. Avoid variability by keeping the time between the exposure of the sensitometer film and the processing consistent. Be sure to feed the film into the processor correctly (see "Locational effect" later). This helps avoid the following variables:
   - **Bromide drag,** also called *bromide flow* or *directional effect,* is caused by the release of halide ions by the emulsion during development and then their coating the trailing areas of the film, which decreases the optical density of these areas. To minimize this effect, feed the least dense end of the sensitometric strip first, with the long axis of the wedge pattern parallel to the entrance rollers. The steplike image created by the sensitometer is usually created at the edge of one side of the film, along the 10-inch (25-cm)

dimension, as in Figure 5-5. The opposite side of the film is unexposed and should be fed into the processor first. This reduces the number of halide ions that are "dragged" over the remainder of the film.
   - **Locational effect** results from a difference in the location of the test film insertion into the processor. To minimize this effect, try to always insert the film on the same side of the feed tray each time a sensitometric test is performed.
   - **Time of day variability** is important because chemical activity and processing system parameters can vary considerably during the course of the workday; therefore, sensitometric test films should always be processed at the same time each day, preferably early in the morning after the processor has reached optimum operating levels.
3. After the film is processed, optical density readings of each of the 21 steps and the clear portion of the image should be measured with a densitometer and recorded. After the first day, when the operating parameters of the processor are established, it should not be necessary to measure all 21 steps in succeeding days' test films.
4. From these optical density readings, the following indicators of processor performance are to be established:
   - *Base + fog.* Often abbreviated B + F, **base + fog** is the optical density of the clear portion of the image and is the result of the blue tint added to the base of the film and any black metallic silver grains that were created by aging of the film or background radiation exposure. The B + F value for most film ranges from 0.1 to 0.2 and should never exceed 0.25. Once the accepted operating level is established, it should never vary by more than an optical density value of ± 0.05 for dual emulsion films and 0.03 for single emulsion films during subsequent days' sensitometric test films. An above-normal developer temperature, an above-normal developing time, overreplenishment, contaminated solution, improper film or solution storage conditions, improper safelights, an incorrect starter solution in the developer, and fogged film can increase the B + F value above accepted limits.
   - **Speed indicator** or *mid-density point* (MD). This is a measure of the amount of exposure energy necessary to produce an optical density of 1 above the B + F. Once the B + F is determined, find the step with an optical density closest to 1 above this value. The value of this step is always measured and recorded as the speed indicator, regardless of the value obtained. For example, if the B + F is 0.2 on the first day and step 8 of the sensitometry image yields an optical density of 1.2 on the same day, then the optical density of step 8 is always used to determine the speed indicator for all future days' tests. This value should not vary by an optical density of ± 0.15 from the accepted operating level. An increased developer temperature, an increased developer time, overreplenishment, excessive concentration of developer or replenisher (usually due to incorrectly mixed developer where not enough water is added to the concentrate), no starter solution in fresh developer, or a contaminated solution can increase this value above the established limits. A reversal decreases the speed indicator below accepted limits.
   - *Minimum density* (D_{min}) or *low density* (LD). D_{min}, or LD, is the optical density of the step closest to 0.25 above the B + F, which approximates the low end of the diagnostic

(Continued)

range of optical densities. Again, once this indicator is established, the same step is used in future days' testing, regardless of the optical density reading. The optical density of this step should not vary by more than ± 0.05 for dual emulsion films and 0.03 for single emulsion films from the accepted operating level during any future test. The optical density value of this indicator is primarily created by the action of phenidone, which is less sensitive to variability than hydroquinone. Essentially, the same factors affecting the B + F indicator also affect the D_{min}.

- *Maximum* density (D_{max}) or *high density* (HD). D_{max}, or HD, is the optical density of the step closest to 2 above the B + F, which is close to the upper value of the diagnostic density range. This value should stay within ± 0.15 from the accepted operating level. This optical density value is created primarily by hydroquinone, which is more sensitive to variability than phenidone. A rise in developer time, temperature, pH, overreplenishment, or overconcentration of developer solution can increase this value above the upper limit and vice versa.

- *Contrast indicator* or *relative density difference* (DD). Because *contrast* is defined as the difference among optical densities on the processed image, a **contrast indicator** can be obtained by calculating the difference between the D_{max} and D_{min} values during each day's sensitometry test. Once the accepted operating level is initially determined, it should not vary by more than ± 0.15 during any subsequent tests. An increased developer temperature, developer time, overreplenishment, or overconcentration of developer solution can increase the contrast indicator above the upper limit. A decrease below the lower limit occurs if the given factors are decreased.

Before sensitometric tests are performed, ensure that the processor is clean and functioning properly; that fresh, properly mixed chemicals are available; and that a safelight test has been performed with satisfactory results. The processor also should be in operation for at least 20 minutes so that the temperatures are at optimum levels.

Once all of the previously mentioned values are determined, they should be plotted on a control chart (see Fig. 5-8). This helps monitor chemical activity and processor performance and document the quality control activities for accreditation or government agencies. Because control charts have data plotted for an entire month, any trends in processor performance may appear and need to be addressed. The minimum number of data points in one direction that constitutes a trend that should be investigated is 5 for general radiography and 3 for mammographic processors. A processor quality control documentation form and daily sensitometric test form are included on the accompanying Evolve website. If a processor quality control program has not been previously implemented, the accepted operating level or base control number for each indicator has to be established. This established operating level is the value plotted at the centerline of the control chart for each indicator. To establish the accepted operating level for each indicator, establish the control box of film (see later discussion on quality control film) and expose a sheet of film with a sensitometer for 5 consecutive days. Determine the B + F, MD, and DD for each day. At the end of the fifth day, average the B + F, MD, and DD values for all 5 days. These averages are the accepted operating levels or base control numbers that are used on the control chart.

Quality Control Film

When a processor quality control program is implemented, a fresh box of film should be selected and dedicated to sensitometric testing only. This box of film is known as the *control box* and should be clearly labeled and stored under ideal conditions (e.g., no light, ionizing radiation, or chemical fumes). Once all but a few sheets of film in the control box have been used, a crossover procedure to a new box of control film should be performed to minimize any variation that may occur from one batch of film to another (Fig. 5-9).

CHARACTERISTIC CURVE

In addition to the control chart, many diagnostic imaging departments also may benefit from the daily creation of a characteristic curve (also known as the *sensitometric curve, Hurter & Driffield curve, H & D curve,* or *D log E curve*) to monitor processor performance. Because the characteristic curve demonstrates film contrast, changes in the curve from day to day can indicate problems in the processing solutions or processor system performance. The characteristic curve also can demonstrate B + F and film speed or sensitivity (Fig. 5-10).

PROCESSOR TROUBLESHOOTING

As mentioned earlier in this chapter, an automatic film processor is subject to considerable variability during the course of operation, resulting in visible changes in image quality. The troubleshooting guide in Table 5-1 is designed to identify specific processor problems or conditions, or both, and details the necessary corrective action.

DAYLIGHT SYSTEMS

Many diagnostic imaging departments have eliminated traditional darkrooms in favor of **daylight systems,** which automatically load cassettes with fresh sheets of film and unload exposed cassettes directly into a processor (Fig. 5-11). Because the film is loaded and unloaded

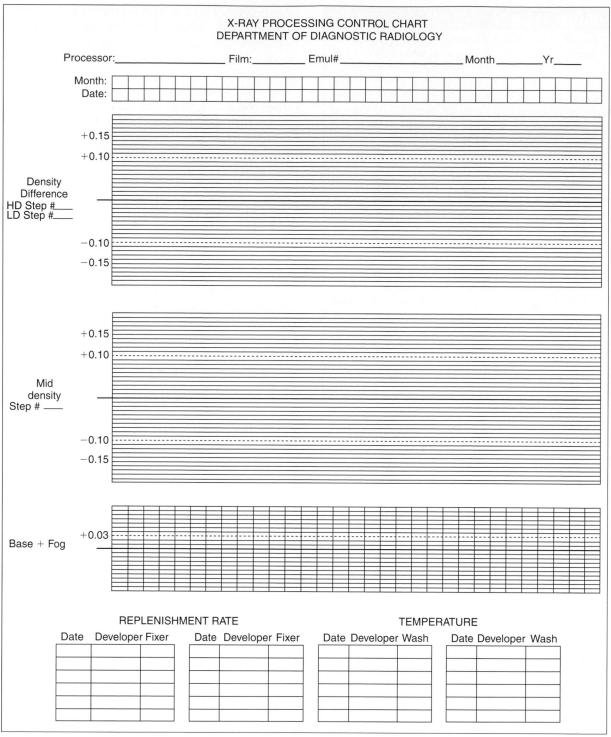

FIGURE 5-8 Processor control chart.

from the cassette mechanically, a regular maintenance program is essential for continued proper operation. This includes cleaning and lubrication of moving parts and replacement of parts as needed. Excessive dirt or dust in the loading section of these systems may enter the cassettes, causing artifacts to appear on subsequent images. It also may result in excessive friction between the sheets of film and the inside of the cassette.

Improper loading may occur, and films may possibly become stuck inside. The cassette-unloading section of these systems also must be kept clean and free of dirt so that films unload cleanly and do not become stuck in the unit where white light exposure ruins any image that may be present. Separate areas for loaded and unloaded cassettes should exist and be clearly marked. The processing section should be cleaned, maintained,

CROSSOVER WORKSHEET

Site _____   Date _____
Film type _____   Technologist _____

New Emulsion # _____   Old Emulsion # _____

Film #	Low Density (LD) Step #____	Mid Density (MD) Step #____	High Density (HD) Step #____	B+F	Film #	Low Density (LD) Step #____	Mid Density (MD) Step #____	High Density (HD) Step #____	B+F
1					1				
2					2				
3					3				
4					4				
5					5				
Average					Average				

Average Density Difference: DD = HD − LD = _____   Average Density Difference: DD = HD − LD = _____

MD difference between new and old film (New MD − Old MD)	
DD difference between new and old film (New DD − Old DD)	
B+F difference between new and old film (New − Old)	

	MD	DD	B+F
Old operating levels			
Difference between new and old film			
New operating levels			

CROSSOVER WORKSHEET
EXAMPLE

New Emulsion #   24578   Old Emulsion #   23456

Film #	Low Density (LD) Step #10	Mid Density (MD) Step #11	High Density (HD) Step #13	B+F	Film #	Low Density (LD) Step #10	Mid Density (MD) Step #11	High Density (HD) Step #13	B+F
1	0.49	1.25	2.39	0.18	1	0.46	1.27	2.33	0.17
2	0.50	1.23	2.43	0.18	2	0.48	1.30	2.30	0.17
3	0.49	1.26	2.40	0.17	3	0.46	1.27	2.28	0.18
4	0.53	1.28	2.41	0.18	4	0.48	1.28	2.32	0.17
5	0.49	1.28	2.43	0.18	5	0.47	1.31	2.35	0.18
Average	0.50	1.26	2.41	0.18	Average	0.47	1.29	2.31	0.17

Average Density Difference: DD = HD − LD = 1.91   Average Density Difference: DD = HD − LD = 1.84

MD difference between new and old film (New MD − Old MD)	−0.03
DD difference between new and old film (New DD − Old DD)	+0.07
B+F difference between new and old film (New − Old)	+0.01

	MD	DD	B+F
Old operating levels	1.34	1.90	0.17
Difference between new and old film	−0.03	+0.07	+0.01
New operating levels	1.31	1.97	0.18

FIGURE 5-9 Crossover worksheet for determining new operating levels.

PROCEDURE

1. Expose and process five films from the old and new boxes of film with a sensitometer. This should be done at the same time, and the films should be processed one after the other. Be sure that you identify which five films are from the old box and which five are from the new box.

2. From each film, determine the B + F, MD value, and DD indicators as described previously. Determine an average of these values for the old box of film and the new box of film (see Fig. 5-9).

3. Determine the difference between the boxes of film by subtracting the average of the old box of film from the average of the new box of film.

4. Determine the new operating level for each indicator (e.g., B + F, MD, or DD) that is to be used as the accepted value. This is done by taking the original operating level (the accepted value of each indicator that was used for the original box of film) and adding to it the difference between the boxes that was determined in step 3. In other words, the new indicator operating level = original operating level + difference.

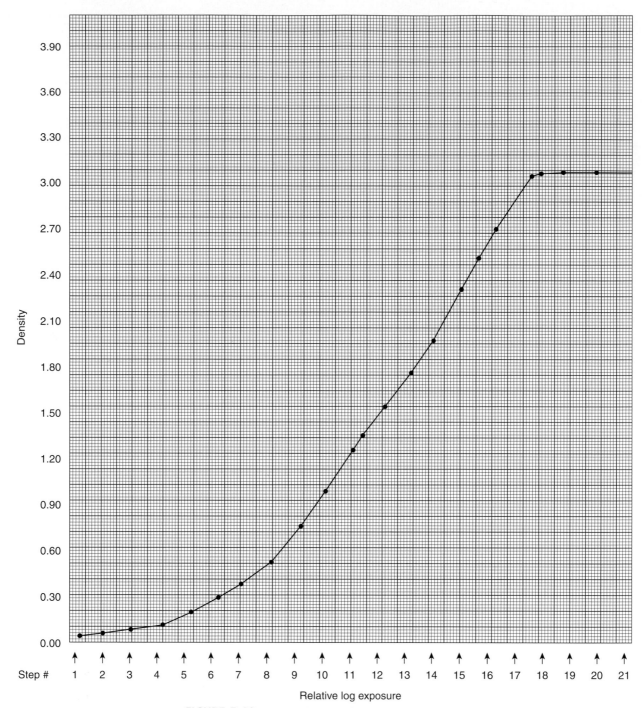

FIGURE 5-10 Sample plotting of a characteristic curve.

PROCEDURE

1. Remove a sheet of 8 × 10 inch (20 × 25 cm) film from the film bin and expose it with a sensitometer. Process the film.
2. Using a densitometer, take optical density readings of each step of the 11- or 21-step pattern.
3. On a sheet of graph paper, plot the optical density of each step on the y-axis and the step number (beginning with the least dense step) on the x-axis. Connect the points on the graph. The resulting curve should have the characteristic S or sigmoid shape (see Fig. 5-10).

4. Calculate the average gradient (slope) of the straight-line portion of the curve, using the optical density points of 0.25 and 2 above the B + F. This yields the contrast indicator of DD. The speed indicator or MD step also should be plotted as the step closest to 1 above the B + F. These values should not vary by more than ± 0.15 from the established value. More information on characteristic curves is available in Appendix A.

TABLE 5-1	Processor Control Chart Troubleshooting Guide		
Processor Problem	**Trend in Graph**	**Image Appearance**	**Corrective Action**
Unsafe darkroom	Sharp rise in B + F with a sudden decrease in the contrast indicator but no change in developer temperature	Increased fog level	Check safelight filter; check for light leaks; check film type and safelight type; check film storage conditions
Developer temperature too high	Sharp rise in speed and contrast indicators, with a smaller increase in B + F	Excessive optical density	Check incoming water temperature or developer thermostat setting
Developer temperature too low	Slight decrease in B + F, with sharp drops in speed and contrast indicators	Optical density too low	Check incoming water temperature or developer thermostat setting
Developer concentration or pH too high	Same as developer temperature too high	Excessive optical density	Check replenishment rates or mix fresh solutions, or both
Developer concentration or pH too low	Same as developer temperature too low	Optical density too low	Check replenishment rates or mix fresh solutions, or both
Underreplenishment	Gradual decline in contrast and speed indicators, with normal values for B + F and developer temperature	Decreased fog level and overall decrease in optical density	Check replenishment rates
Overreplenishment	Increase in B + F level and speed indicator, with a decrease in contrast indicator	Increased fog level and decrease in image contrast	Check replenishment rates
Oxidized developer	Slight increase in B + F with a decrease in speed and contrast indicators	Loss of image contrast	Drain developer tank and mix fresh solution; add correct amount of starter solution

B + F, Base + fog.

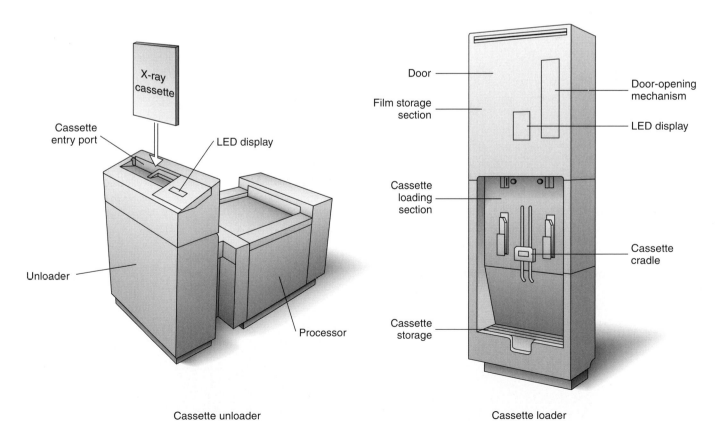

Cassette unloader   Cassette loader

FIGURE 5-11 Daylight systems. *LED*, Light-emitting diode.

and monitored the same way as conventional film processors. For sensitometric tests to be performed, a sensitometry image should be created in a darkroom area as previously discussed. This film then must be manually placed into a cassette (obviously in a darkroom) and then unloaded into the system so that it can be processed by the daylight system's automatic film processor. The indicators of processor performance (e.g., B + F or D_{min}) can then be determined. Temperature and humidity in the area where the daylight system is in use must be maintained to the manufacturer's specifications because high humidity results in films sticking together and jamming inside of the unit. Humidity that is too low could result in static artifacts on the resulting images.

SUMMARY

A properly instituted processor quality control program should reduce variability to a minimum, which should reduce the number of repeat images and maintain the acceptable level of image quality established by the facility.

Refer to the Evolve website at https://evolve.elsevier. com for Student Experiments 5.1: Quality Control of Mechanized Processors and 5.2: Daily Processor Quality Control.

REVIEW QUESTIONS

1. What is the margin of error for the specific gravity of processing solutions?
   a. 0.002
   b. 0.004
   c. 0.006
   d. 0.1
2. Which of the following cannot be determined by an H and D curve or a processor control chart?
   a. Film sensitivity
   b. Film contrast
   c. Recorded detail
   d. B + F
3. What type of films does the presence of bromide drag produce?
   a. Overdeveloped
   b. Underdeveloped
   c. Underfixed
   d. Overfixed

4. When is the best time to process sensitometric films?
   a. Morning, after the processor is warmed up
   b. Late morning or midday, after peak-demand period
   c. Late afternoon, during low-demand period
   d. Evening, during the lowest-demand period
5. Which of the following terms best describes a device designed to give precise, reproducible, and graded light exposures to a film?
   a. Densitometer
   b. Photometer
   c. Sensitometer
   d. Penetrometer
6. Which of the following values is the maximum variation allowed for the contrast indicator in daily sensitometric films?
   a. ± 0.01
   b. ± 0.05
   c. ± 0.15
   d. ± 0.2
7. Which of the following characteristics explains why daily quality control activities are normally required for film processing systems?
   a. High degree of complexity
   b. High degree of variability
   c. High degree of consistency
   d. None of the above
8. What is the principal purpose of the washing process?
   a. Stoppage of the fixation process
   b. Stoppage of the development process
   c. Maintenance of the solution activity
   d. Removal of fixer solution
9. Temperature variations in older models of automatic processors are often related to changes in which of the following variables?
   a. Temperature of the dryer section
   b. Incoming water supply
   c. Replenisher rate
   d. Film transportation rate
10. Which of the following terms defines the relationship between the intensity of radiation absorbed by the film and the optical density produced?
    a. Densitometry
    b. Dosimetry
    c. Sensitometry
    d. Sensitivity

Silver Recovery

OBJECTIVES

At the completion of this chapter the reader should be able to do the following:

- List the reasons for silver recovery in diagnostic imaging
- Describe the methods of recovering silver from processing solutions
- List the factors that affect the efficiency of silver reclamation devices
- Describe the methods of recovering silver from film

Before the digital revolution in diagnostic imaging, the recovery of silver from film and film processing has been a standard practice in most hospitals and medical centers for at least 30 years. In 1967 the federal government lifted previous regulations governing the sale of silver, which escalated the price and therefore increased the demand on worldwide markets. Despite the common use of digital imaging, the photographic industry is still the largest single user of silver worldwide, consuming approximately 30% of the total used; all film used in diagnostic imaging, which is estimated to be roughly one half of all photographic film, is included. Manufacturers of medical radiographic film are the largest consumers of silver in the medical field. Approximately 85 million troy oz of silver are used in the photographic film consumed in the United

States each year. A **troy oz** is a unit for measuring precious metals such as silver. There are 14.58 troy oz in 16 **avoirdupois oz,** or standard ounces.

The next largest industrial consumer of silver is the electronics industry, which uses approximately 20% of all silver. Silver conducts electricity better than most substances and also resists oxidation and rusting. For this reason, most electronic devices, from the smallest electronic watch to the space shuttle, contain some quantity of silver.

The sterlingware industry consumes approximately 15% of all silver. Pure silver is relatively soft (much like lead) and is mixed with copper to create sterling silver. Generally, 925 parts of pure silver are mixed with 75 parts of copper to make sterling silver.

Some medical uses of silver (other than film) include the construction of metal prostheses used in repairing broken bones or joint replacement and the 1% solution of silver nitrate sometimes put into the eyes of newborns by physicians to prevent infection.

Other uses of silver include water treatment filters, in which silver is used as a bactericide, and the catalytic converters of some automobiles. The federal government stopped minting silver coins for general circulation in 1964 but still issues special edition or commemorative coins on a limited basis.

JUSTIFICATION FOR SILVER RECOVERY

The three basic reasons for a diagnostic imaging department to institute a silver recovery program are the dwindling worldwide supply of silver, monetary return back to the diagnostic imaging department, and compliance with federal and state laws.

Worldwide Supply of Silver

The current worldwide shortage of silver is the result of little silver being mined because of low prices and high refining costs. Political instability in countries where silver is abundant also contributes to this shortage. Currently, 120 million more troy oz of silver is consumed than are produced annually in the United States. At this rate, current silver supplies may not last through this century. Even with the advent of digital cameras (used by the general public) and digital imaging for diagnostic purposes, the demand for silver in film still exceeds the supply. The economic downturn of 2008 has lead to a dramatic increase in the price of silver. The photographic industry can recover approximately one half of what is required annually, but eventually a serious shortfall will exist. Because diagnostic imaging constitutes a large portion of the photographic use of silver, efforts to recover as much silver as possible are the responsibility of all diagnostic imaging department managers. It is estimated that 10% to 20% of all hospitals and 30% to 40% of doctors' offices and clinics do not have silver recovery protocols in place.

Monetary Return to Department

Money obtained from silver recovery procedures can be returned to the diagnostic imaging department to help offset the cost of processing supplies, materials, and equipment. Many studies have demonstrated that about 10% of the purchase price of film can be recovered through proper silver reclamation procedures; therefore, if a department spends $50,000 annually for film, then about $5000 can be returned to the department's budget to help offset costs.

When silver reclaimed from processing chemistry or films is sold, bids should be solicited from several dealers so that the best price can be negotiated. Familiarity with the current market prices according to the *Wall Street Journal* or similar business publications and websites is also helpful. It is also better to sell only once a year so that a higher volume price can be obtained, and shipping and handling costs can be reduced.

Federal and State Pollution Laws

The chemical solutions' undergoing of continual replenishment through film processors means that used solutions must be disposed of in some manner. The used fixer and wash water contain silver in some form, which is a toxic heavy metal and therefore subject to strict pollution guidelines by the Environmental Protection Agency (EPA) and many state regulations. California has particularly strict pollution guidelines. Some of the important federal pollution laws are described in Box 6-1.

BOX 6-1   Important Federal Pollution Laws

Water Pollution Control Act of 1972
The Water Pollution Control Act of 1972 bans the placement of toxic substances in public waterways and sewer systems.

Resources Conservation/Hazardous Waste Act of 1976
The Resources Conservation/Hazardous Waste Act of 1976 requires available devices be used to remove toxic substances from waste water.

Clean Water Act of 1984
The Clean Water Act of 1984 amends the previous law (Clean Water Act of 1977), in that it requires the best available methods be used to remove toxic substances from waste water. Silver is classified as a "priority pollutant" under this law, and the Act prohibits the discharge of these pollutants into surface waters.

Resource Conservation and Recovery Act of 1987
The Resource Conservation and Recovery Act (RCRA) of 1987 contains many guidelines affecting film processing and silver recovery methods including the following:

1. The Act limits liquid waste to a level of no more than 5 mg/L or 5 parts per million (ppm) of silver. Used fixer and wash water may exceed this amount. Silver is considered a "characteristic hazardous material" under this law (Environmental Protection Agency [EPA] Hazardous Waste Number D011). Solid wastes containing 5 ppm or more of silver also are given the same classification. This may include processed and unprocessed radiographic film.

2. Special permits are required to dump more than 27 gallons of waste per month into public sewers. For private septic systems, a permit from the National Pollutant Discharge Elimination System (NPDES) and/or the EPA is required.

3. Shipping manifests are required to ship material such as silver recovery cartridges, scrap film, silver flake, or silver-laden fixer. The manifest forms required are EPA Forms 8700-12 and 8700-22.

A silver recovery system is required for most hospitals to remove silver from used processing solutions to meet the requirements of these laws. Some states and municipalities require that used wash water also be collected and disposed of through approved disposal companies because about 5% of the silver may be carried into the wash water.

Silver recovery in a diagnostic imaging department can occur through recovery from processing solutions and recovery from film.

SILVER RECOVERY FROM PROCESSING CHEMICALS

One function of the fixer solution is to remove the unexposed and undeveloped silver halide crystals from the film. These crystals are suspended in the solution and eliminated with the used fixer by the replenishment system. Silver may accumulate at a rate of 100 mg/m^2 of film that is processed. This dissolved silver averages about 50% of the silver that was originally on the film and can be recovered by a variety of methods.

Metallic Replacement

This method is sometimes called the *displacement method* and is the simplest and least expensive method for a diagnostic imaging department. It is the most widely used method of silver recovery from processing chemicals. The metallic replacement system incorporates a plastic bucket that also may be referred to as a canister or cartridge (Fig. 6-1). These canisters are available in a variety of sizes including 3.5 gallons, 5 gallons (most popular in diagnostic imaging), 7.5 gallons, and 10 gallons, depending on the amount of film processed per month. Inside the canister is iron in some form, which reacts chemically with the acid and silver ions in the fixer through ion exchange (an oxidation-reduction reaction). When the acid in the fixer oxidizes the iron, electrons are released and used by the silver ions to form metallic silver. The more active iron ions replace the less

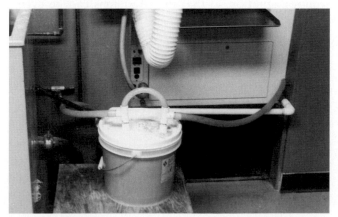

FIGURE 6-1 Metallic replacement silver recovery unit.

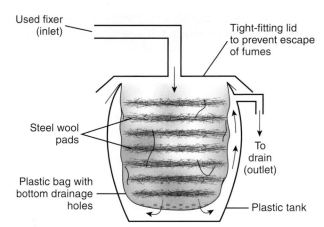

FIGURE 6-2 Diagram of metallic replacement cartridge.

active silver ions, which remain in the canister as the ions are picked up and washed out in the used fixer, hence the name **metallic replacement** (Fig. 6-2). The metallic replacement process is summarized in the following equation:

$$2Ag(S_2O_3)_2^{-3} + Fe^0 \rightarrow 2Ag^0 + Fe^{+2} + 4S_2O_3^{-2}$$

The two types of iron cartridges that can be used inside the canister are the steel wool cartridge and the iron-impregnated foam cartridge.

Steel Wool Cartridge. Because the primary component of steel is iron, the packing of the inside of the cartridge with steel wool can yield a large surface area in which metallic replacement can occur. One pound of steel wool can collect 3 to 4 lb of silver. This is the more common type of cartridge insert because of its lower cost, but it is subject to three potential problems: channeling, rusting, and drain stoppage.

Channeling. **Channeling** occurs when an intermittent or low volume of fixer is used or when a fixer that is too acidic is used. In these situations, the fixer concentrates in almost a straight path, or channel, into and out of the cartridge, rather than moving uniformly throughout the steel wool. Because the solution comes in contact with very little steel wool, not much silver is reclaimed. This can be avoided by filling the cartridge with fixer or water at the time of installation and allowing the fixer to dissipate throughout the cartridge as it enters.

Rusting. Iron that is exposed to moisture and air undergoes a chemical reaction that forms iron oxide, or rust. This rust forms a barrier between the silver ions and the iron ions that prevents the metallic process from occurring or, at the very least, reduces the efficiency of the unit. This occurs with units that are used infrequently.

Drain Stoppage. As the steel wool is dissolved by the acid that is present in the fixer, the iron ions may become deposited on the inside of the drainage pipes, which can cause obstruction. A commercial drain cleaner composed of sodium bisulfate should be used monthly, as mentioned in Chapter 5, to prevent this buildup.

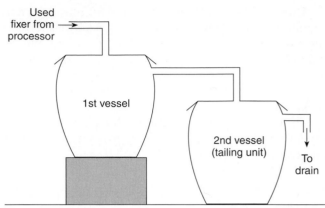

FIGURE 6-3 "Piggybacking" or "tailing" of metallic replacement units.

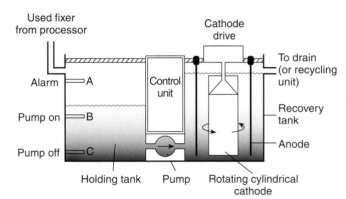

FIGURE 6-4 Diagram of electrolytic silver recovery unit.

Iron-Impregnated Foam Cartridge. An iron-impregnated foam cartridge uses a fine iron powder that is impregnated in a tightly wound piece of plastic foam, similar to a plastic sponge. This design helps minimize channeling and rusting because the foam helps distribute the fixer more evenly. The suspended iron powder also provides 50% more surface area, and the efficiency of the unit is increased. The advantages and disadvantages of the metallic replacement method are discussed in Boxes 6-2 and 6-3.

Electrolytic Silver Recovery

The electrolytic silver recovery method is based on **electrolysis,** or electroplating, and uses an electric current to reclaim the silver (Fig. 6-4). Because unexposed, undeveloped silver halide is removed from the film by the fixer, the suspended silver is in the form of a positive ion (Ag^+). This means that it is attracted to a metal electrode that has a negative charge imparted on it (cathode). As these Ag^+ ions come in contact with the metal cathode, the silver collects in a layer that can be removed at a later time. The chemical reaction occurring at the cathode is summarized in the following equation:

$$Ag(S_2O_3)_2^{-3} + e^- \rightarrow Ag^0 + 2(S_2O_3)^{-2}$$

The cathodes in the electrolytic recovery units are usually made of stainless steel and are either drum shaped (Fig. 6-5) or disk shaped. For best results the solution requires agitation so that the silver ions can be evenly distributed over the cathode surface. This can be accomplished by rotating the cathode with a stationary anode or a stationary cathode with rotating anodes. Another design that is available keeps the cathode and anode stationary and uses a self-contained pump to swirl the solution. Systems are available that recover 3 troy oz of silver or more per hour at 98% efficiency. The purity level of the silver ranges from 92% to 98%. The cathodes are removed periodically, and the silver is stripped off. The silver-laden cathodes can be replaced immediately with cathodes that are clean so that only a minimal interruption in film processing should occur. Once the silver-laden cathodes are cleaned (usually by scraping them with a screwdriver or paint scraper), they can then

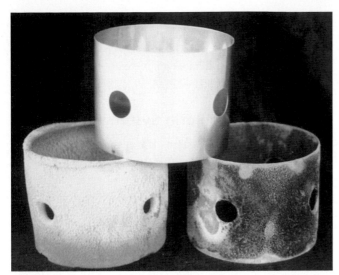

FIGURE 6-5 Cathodes from electrolytic silver recovery unit. Top cathode is clean and unused. Left cathode contains more than 20 lb of silver flake after correct amperage has been used. Right cathode contains silver that has been "burned" by too high of an amperage setting.

be reused at a later date. The anodes also should be cleaned at this time because they may develop a layer of sulfate that may reduce efficiency. The chemical reaction that takes place at the anode of an electrolytic silver recovery unit is summarized in the following equation:

$$SO_3^{-2} + H_2O \rightarrow SO_4^{-2} + 2H^+ + 2e^-$$

The silver that is removed from the cathode is in the form of silver flake (Fig. 6-6), and the color can range from cream or light colored to black. This silver flake should be cream or light colored for maximum purity.

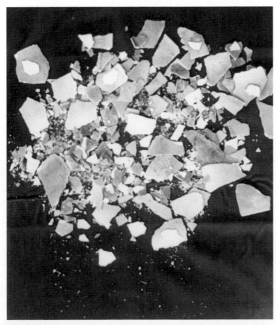

FIGURE 6-6 Silver flake that has been removed from a cathode after correct amperage has been used.

The darker the flake, the less pure the silver that has been recovered. An amperage control switch that is located on the unit regulates the amount of charge on the cathode so that the flake's color and purity are controlled. The amount of this current is usually around 8 amperes (A) for most systems. If the flake is too dark, too much amperage is being used and is "burning" the silver. Too much amperage also causes the fixing agent to be converted into sulfide, which results in a foul-smelling (like rotten eggs), yellow-brown deposit of sulfur on the cathode. This is known as *sulfating* or **sulfurization.** If the silver flake coating is very light or silver, the amperage is too low. A computerized timer and current selector that are available on some models of electrolytic silver reclaimers adjust the current according to the time of day or use.

The two types of electrolytic silver recovery units are the terminal electrolytic system and the recirculating electrolytic system.

Terminal Electrolytic System. The **terminal electrolytic unit** is connected to the fixer overflow line from the processor replenishment system. Once this unit recovers the silver, the used fixer is flushed down the drain. Most processor manufacturers recommend this type of electrolytic unit.

Recirculating Electrolytic System. The **recirculating electrolytic unit** (sometimes referred to as an *inline electrolytic unit*) is designed to recover silver from used fixer and then recirculate the fixer back into the processor. This normally does not conserve much fixer because electrolysis destroys the preservative in the fixer. Fixer replenishment is decreased by no more than 20%. The main advantage of this method is that the overall concentration of silver in the fixer tank is decreased; therefore, the amount of silver transported into the wash water through the fixer is decreased, and the wash water may have a low enough silver content to avoid the thresholds of certain pollution standards. Most film manufacturers do not recommend this method because of decreased archival quality of the processed films. The advantages and disadvantages of the electrolytic silver recovery method are discussed in Boxes 6-4 and 6-5.

BOX 6-4	Advantages of Electrolytic Silver Recovery

- Electrolytic silver recovery is more efficient than metallic replacement, without the problems of channeling, rusting, or drain stoppage.
- The silver recovered is in the form of silver flake, which is 92% to 98% pure, as opposed to sludge (30% to 50% pure).
- Payment for the silver can be received on delivery of the flake to the refiner because the content is immediately apparent.
- Shipping costs of materials to the refiner are minimal.
- The system produces no new pollutants (as opposed to the sludge produced by metallic replacement).
- The system is reusable because the cathodes can be cleaned and reused.

Direct Sale of Used Fixer

Roughly 0.5 to 0.8 troy oz of silver is in each gallon of used fixer. In small-volume facilities (<10 gal/wk), metallic replacement or electrolytic units may not be practical. In this case, used fixer can be collected in storage drums and sold to a refiner who reclaims the silver from the solution. The advantages of this method are that no capital outlay for equipment is required by the facility and no pollutants other than the used developer and wash water are discharged into a sewer system. The disadvantages are that considerable handling or storage and a fee for the pickup and hauling of the solution (as much as $2 to $6 per gallon of used solution) may be required, and the profit margin from the sale of the silver may be reduced.

Chemical Precipitation

Chemical precipitation is the oldest form of silver recovery. In this method the mixing of such compounds as sodium sulfite and zinc chloride with used fixer can cause a chemical reaction. This results in the silver precipitating, or sinking, to the bottom of the tank or drum, where it can be removed. This is a fairly efficient method but has many disadvantages including the following:

- The chemicals used are hazardous and require special precautions.
- Toxic fumes such as chlorine gas and hydrogen are created by the chemical reaction.
- A large drum or vat with adequate space is required.
- The process is labor intensive, which reduces the profit margin.

Because of these disadvantages, this method should not be attempted by diagnostic facilities and should be carried out only by licensed silver refiners or commercial photographic laboratories. The silver in fixer sold directly to a silver refiner is usually reclaimed in this fashion.

Ion Exchange or Resin Systems

Ion exchange or resin systems use resin particles treated with an acid to give them a negative ionic charge. This is similar to the resin system of a water softener that is found in many homes. The silver (Ag^+) is attracted to the negative charge in the resin, where it remains. A regeneration cycle is used to release the silver from the resin. This method requires a large amount of space (because of the resin columns) and is labor intensive (for the regeneration cycle). The resin can only be regenerated for so many cycles and then must be replaced. The old resin column can be sent to a silver refiner for further recovery of silver. This method is best used for recovering silver from the used wash water (the acid in the fixer may mimic the regeneration cycle) and can reduce the amount of silver in the wash water to as little as 0.1 to 0.5 parts per million (ppm).

Box 6-6 lists factors affecting silver recovery from processing solutions.

SILVER RECOVERY FROM FILM

As previously mentioned, 50% of the silver is dissolved in the fixer. This means that the other 50% remains on the film. For images that are not of diagnostic quality (and therefore not kept for the patient's files), the sheets of film can be stored in a bin and then sold to a silver refiner. Film of this nature is sometimes referred to as *pete*. A price per pound is negotiated for the film and the money paid to the facility. The three basic categories of film that hospitals and medical centers can release for sale are green film, scrap exposed film, and archival film.

Green Film

Green film is film that has not been processed such as film that has expired or film that was accidentally exposed to white light (such as an open film bin). This is the most valuable film because all of the silver is in place (usually about 0.4 troy oz per sheet of 14 × 17 inch [35 × 43 cm] film). Because of this higher value, it is recommended that this film be separated from other categories of film to be sold and that a higher price per pound be negotiated.

Scrap Exposed Film

Scrap exposed film is film that has been exposed and processed such as rejects, old sensitometry films and even dry laser print films obtained from digital systems. This film contains about 0.11 troy oz of silver per 14 × 17 inch (35 × 43 cm) sheet and is therefore of least value.

Archival Film

Archival film is film that has been exposed and processed and has outlived its use as a patient record. Most hospitals and associated medical facilities retain images for a minimum of 5 years (except for mammograms, which must be kept by a facility for either 10 years if the patient never returns for another exam or 5 years if the patient returns regularly). Generally, the film is released for sale, except for film containing certain pathologic conditions or those required for litigation or pending litigation. Any film dated before 1974 contains 20% more silver (0.13 to 0.18 troy oz per 14 × 17 inch sheet) than film manufactured since then. The reason is that the price of silver escalated in 1974, and manufacturers responded by developing emulsions that could maintain image quality with less silver. Any film in this category should be separated from newer archival film and scrap exposed film so that a higher price per pound can be negotiated.

Once a refiner obtains films from a diagnostic imaging department, the silver is reclaimed through either incineration (which burns the film and removes the silver from the ash) or chemical treatments (which use chemicals to remove, or leach, the silver from the film).

SUMMARY

In many diagnostic radiology departments, the quality control technologist is given the responsibility of determining the type of silver reclamation to be used, as well as maintaining and servicing the unit during operation. A basic understanding of these systems is essential to fulfilling this responsibility.

Refer to the Evolve website at https://evolve.elsevier. com for Student Experiment 6.1: Silver Recovery.

REVIEW QUESTIONS

1. Which of the following units is used for measurement of precious metals such as silver?
   a. Standard ounce
   b. Avoirdupois ounce
   c. Troy ounce
   d. None of the above
2. Which of the following is the largest worldwide consumer of silver?
   a. Photographic industry
   b. Electronics industry
   c. Sterlingware industry
   d. Space program
3. The Resource Conservation and Recovery Act (RCRA) of 1987 limits liquid waste to a toxic level of no more than _____ ppm.
   a. 2
   b. 5
   c. 10
   d. 100
4. From which of the following components do most silver recovery systems reclaim the silver?
   a. Developer solution
   b. Fixer solution
   c. Wash water
   d. Dryer section
5. Which of the following is the simplest and least expensive method of silver reclamation?
   a. Metallic replacement method
   b. Electrolytic method
   c. Chemical precipitation
   d. Resin method
6. Problems with steel wool metallic replacement cartridges include (1) channeling, (2) rusting, and (3) drain stoppage:
   a. 1 and 2 only
   b. 2 and 3 only
   c. 1 and 3 only
   d. 1, 2, and 3

7. When electrolytic silver recovery units are used, the silver is deposited on which of the following?
   a. Anode
   b. Cathode
   c. Both cathode and anode
   d. Neither cathode nor anode
8. The oldest form of silver recovery is the _____ method.
   a. metallic replacement
   b. electrolytic
   c. chemical precipitation
   d. resin

9. Which of the following are factors that affect the efficiency of silver reclamation systems: (1) dwell time, (2) agitation, or (3) surface area?
   a. 1 and 2 only
   b. 2 and 3 only
   c. 1 and 3 only
   d. 1, 2, and 3
10. What percentage of the silver is normally dissolved in the fixer solution during film processing?
   a. 10%
   b. 25%
   c. 50%
   d. 90%

Quality Control of X-Ray Generators and Ancillary Radiographic Equipment

KEY TERMS

actual focal spot
automatic exposure control
comparator
coulomb/kilogram
detector
effective focal spot
focal spot blooming
grid latitude
grid uniformity
half-value layer
high-frequency

homogenous phantom
ion chamber
kilowatt rating
Law of Reciprocity
linear tomography
line focus principle
linearity
mobile x-ray generator
objective plane
photodetector
pluridirectional tomography

portable x-ray generator
reciprocity
reproducibility
roentgen
sensor
single-phase
solid state detector
three-phase
voltage ripple

OBJECTIVES

At the completion of this chapter the reader should be able to do the following:

- Explain the difference between single-phase, three-phase, and high-frequency x-ray generators
- Recognize the voltage waveform characteristics of the three types of x-ray generators
- List the voltage ripple values for the three types of x-ray generators
- Calculate the power output rating for the three types of x-ray generators
- List the three main parts of a quality control program for radiographic equipment
- List and describe the performance tests for radiographic equipment

- List the main components of an **automatic exposure control** (AEC) system
- Perform quality control testing of various AEC parameters
- Describe the quality control parameters for conventional tomographic systems
- Discuss the importance of grid uniformity and alignment on image quality
- Explain the quality control tests performed on mobile equipment

OUTLINE

Several of the previous chapters have dealt with film/screen image receptors (digital image receptors are discussed in a later chapter) and the importance of quality control testing to avoid poor quality images. However, many other components of diagnostic imaging departments are subject to variability and must have separate quality control protocols established to ensure safe operation and function. One such component is the equipment used as the x-ray source in conventional radiography. This includes the x-ray generator, control or operating console, x-ray tube, and accessory devices such as the x-ray table and support mechanism.

X-RAY GENERATORS

The x-ray generator is the largest component of the radiographic unit. It contains the high-voltage transformers, rectifiers, timing circuitry, and milliampere (mA) and kilovolt (peak) (kVp) selectors. Single-phase, three-phase, and **high-frequency** x-ray generators are available.

Single-Phase Generator

A single source of alternating current is used to power the generator in a **single-phase** unit. A graphic representation of single-phase alternating current is shown in Figure 7-1.

The graph in Figure 7-1 plots the voltage on the y-axis versus time on the x-axis. The peaks in the graph represent the flow of electricity changing direction throughout the circuit. Voltage values range from zero volts to a peak value (hence the term *kilovolts [peak]*) and back to zero volts. The two types of single-phase

generators used in diagnostic radiography are half-wave rectified and full-wave rectified.

Half-Wave Rectified. In a half-wave rectified generator, one half of the normal alternating current wave is used to power the x-ray tube, and the other half is shut off by the addition of one or two rectifiers. This causes the normal single-phase alternating current waveform graph to appear as shown in Figure 7-2.

Because the standard frequency of alternating current in the United States is 60 Hz, or 60 cycles per second (c/s) (a cycle represents the current flowing in each direction one time), only 60 pulses of electricity per second can be used to create radiographs. This means that the radiographs are emitted in pulses, or spurts, and therefore a longer amount of time is required to obtain a specific quantity of radiographs. For this reason, half-wave rectified units are generally used in dental x-ray units and some small portable x-ray units.

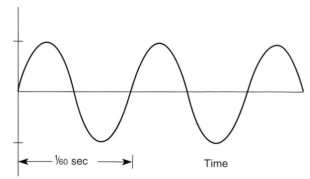

FIGURE 7-1 Voltage waveform graph of single-phase alternating current.

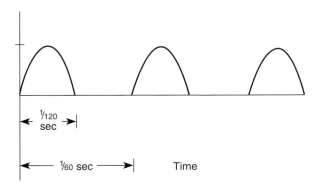

FIGURE 7-2 Voltage waveform graph of half-wave rectified, single-phase current.

Full-Wave Rectified. Full-wave rectified generators use a combination of four rectifiers to channel all of the pulses through the x-ray tube during x-ray production. The resultant waveform graph for this type of unit appears in Figure 7-3.

Because 120 pulses of electricity per second can be used to create x-rays, twice as many x-rays can be created in a given period as compared with the half-wave unit. This allows full-wave rectified units to be used for many conventional radiographic procedures. However, the x-rays are still emitted in pulses (as demonstrated by the number of times the pulses reach zero on the waveform graph) and therefore still require some time to achieve a specific quantity of x-rays. The shortest exposure time available for single-phase x-ray generators is $^1/_{120}$ second. For this reason, full-wave rectified units are seldom found in larger hospitals but are frequently found in doctors' offices and small clinics because of their relatively low purchase price and installation cost (in comparison to 3-phase generators discussed below).

Three-Phase Generator

Three-phase x-ray generators are powered by three separate sources of alternating current that have been staggered so that they are "out of phase" with each other by 120 degrees or one third of a cycle. The voltage waveform graph for three-phase alternating current appears in Figure 7-4.

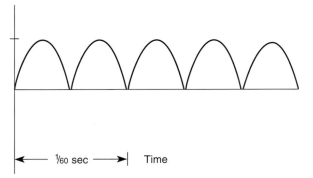

FIGURE 7-3 Voltage waveform graph of full-wave rectified, single-phase current.

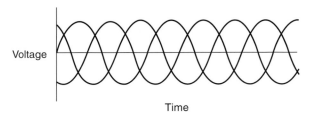

FIGURE 7-4 Voltage waveform graph of 3-phase alternating current.

By the time one pulse of current begins to drop toward zero voltage, another pulse is heading back up to the maximum value, so the voltage never reaches zero and x-rays are continuously produced (eliminating the pulsed effect of single-phase units). This allows exposure time values as low as $^1/_{1000}$ second (1 ms). The x-rays created with three-phase units also have a higher average energy than those of single-phase units because the voltage is near the peak value for a higher percentage of the time during x-ray production (which can lower patient dose compared with single-phase units). The main disadvantages of three-phase equipment are higher capital cost (at least twice as expensive as single-phase) and the size of the unit (because of the additional electronic components required). The advantages have generally outweighed the disadvantages because the three-phase x-ray generator has been the most common type of unit in major hospitals and medical centers since the 1970s. The two types of three-phase generators are 6-pulse and 12-pulse generators.

Three-Phase, Six-Pulse. The six-pulse type of three-phase unit uses six rectifiers and one half of the three-phase alternating current pulses. The resulting voltage waveform appears in Figure 7-5.

As mentioned previously, one cycle of single-phase alternating current referred to one pulse of electricity traveling each direction one time so that two pulses are found in one cycle. Because 60 cycles occur each second, one cycle requires a time of $^1/_{60}$ second. In a three-phase, six-pulse x-ray generator, six pulses of electricity exist during the same cycle or $^1/_{60}$-second time interval (instead of two pulses per $^1/_{60}$ second in single-phase), hence the name *three-phase, six-pulse*. This means that 360 voltage pulses are now available per second.

Three-Phase, 12-Pulse. The 3-phase, 12-pulse type of x-ray generator uses 12 rectifiers (four rectifiers per phase) that direct all of the three-phase alternating current pulses through the x-ray tube during x-ray production. This yields 12 pulses of electricity per one-cycle

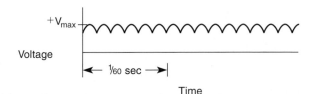

FIGURE 7-5 Voltage waveform graph of 3-phase, 6-pulse current.

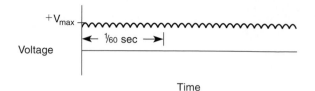

FIGURE 7-6 Voltage waveform graph of 3-phase, 12-pulse current.

($^{1}/_{60}$-second) time interval, for a total of 720 voltage pulses available per second. This unit is more efficient than the three-phase, six-pulse unit but is more expensive in capital cost. The voltage waveform for a 3-phase, 12-pulse x-ray generator appears in Figure 7-6.

High-Frequency Generator

Developed in the late 1970s, high-frequency x-ray generators are the newest generator equipment available. They are sometimes referred to as *medium-frequency generators,* depending on the design and manufacturer. Most of these units use a single source of alternating current that is first fed into a microprocessor circuit before entering the high-voltage section. This microprocessor changes the frequency of the alternating current from the standard 60 Hz to as much as 100,000 Hz in some of the more recent models. It is then rectified and smoothed with capacitors before application across the x-ray tube. This causes the pulses to merge together and results in a voltage waveform that appears in Figure 7-7.

High-frequency generators and three-phase generators produce similar voltage waveforms. However, the capital cost and power requirements for high-frequency units are far less than those for three-phase units. The transformers in high-frequency units can be smaller because they are much more efficient at higher frequencies (according to Faraday's law of electromagnetism), which accounts for the lower capital cost. The transformers also lower the space requirement for installation. Because these units yield most of the advantages of a three-phase unit but at a fraction of the cost, they are becoming more common in hospitals, medical centers, clinics, and doctors' offices.

Voltage Ripple

Voltage ripple is a term often used to distinguish the voltage waveforms of each type of x-ray generator. This

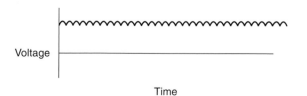

FIGURE 7-7 Voltage waveform graph showing resultant current through the x-ray tube in a high frequency x-ray generator.

is the amount of variation from the peak voltage that occurs during x-ray production. For single-phase units, the voltage ripple is considered to be 100% because the voltage drops from its peak all the way to zero before rising again, so 100% of all possible voltages are obtained. For three-phase equipment, the voltage does not fall all the way to zero. One pulse is rising as soon as the previous one is falling, which yields a voltage ripple of 13% for a 3-phase, 6-pulse generator and 3.5% for a 3-phase, 12-pulse unit. High-frequency generators can create voltage ripple values between 1% and 15%, which are comparable to those of 3-phase units.

Power Ratings

The power output of an x-ray generator is used to measure the capacity of x-ray production from the individual unit. This value is measured in kilowatts (kW) and is called the **kilowatt rating.** It is usually calculated by determining the maximum combinations of kVp and mA that can be achieved by a particular generator, at an exposure time of 100 ms. These kVp and mA values are then placed into the following equations:

$$\text{Three-phase and high frequency} \quad kW = \frac{kVp \times mA}{1000}$$

$$\text{Single-phase} \quad kW = \frac{kVp \times mA \times 0.707}{1000}$$

The rippling effect of the single-phase alternating current requires that the 0.707 multiplier be added to the equation.

CONTROL OR OPERATING CONSOLE

The control or operating console contains all of the various controls to operate the x-ray machine (e.g., kVp selector, mA selector) and various meters to monitor the production of x-rays. Guidelines of the Food and Drug Administration (FDA) mandate that diagnostic x-ray machine-operating consoles must indicate what the conditions of exposure (kVp, milliampere-second [mAs]) are and when the x-ray tube is energized. The conditions of exposure usually are indicated by the mA and kVp selection mechanism (i.e., the mA or kVp buttons or computer touch pad keys that are pushed). There is also either an analog or a digital milliampere-second meter to indicate the quantity of x-rays produced by the x-ray unit. These meters also are used to indicate energized x-ray tubes and to detect lights or audible signals. Characteristics for the control booth area, which house the operating console of a radiographic x-ray unit, include the following:

1. The floor of the control booth must not have an area less than 7.5 sq ft.
2. The exposure switch should be fixed within the booth at a position at least 30 inches from any open

edge of the booth wall and should be closest to the examining table.

3. X-ray photons must scatter at least twice before they can enter any opening in the control booth. Each time an x-ray photon scatters, its intensity from the scattering object is $^1/_{1000}$ of the original intensity, at a distance of 1 m.

4. The control booth window must have the same shielding requirements as the walls (usually 1.5 mm lead equivalent), be at least 1 sq ft in size, and be mounted at least 5 feet above the floor. There should be no obstructions blocking the view of the patient table.

5. The wall of the control booth, facing the radiographic examination table, must be at least 7 feet high and fixed to the floor.

6. Any door on the control booth that is an entrance to the examination room must be interlocked with the control panel so that an exposure cannot be made unless the door is closed.

HIGH-VOLTAGE GENERATOR

This section of the radiographic unit is responsible for converting the relatively low voltage values that are supplied by the power companies (usually 220 to 440 volts) to the kilovolt levels necessary for the production of diagnostic radiographs. Included in this section is a high-tension transformer, which is a shell-type step-up transformer that will increase the voltage level that was selected with an autotransformer to the kilovoltage selected on the control console. Also included in the high-voltage generator is a filament (step-down) transformer that feeds a stepped-down voltage level to the filament of the x-ray tube. This section also may contain rectifiers that will convert the alternating current of the incoming power supply to a pulsating direct current that will be fed to the x-ray tube for x-ray production. These can range in number from 4 to 12 depending on the type of x-ray generator and are usually solid state in nature. The high-voltage generator is normally housed in a metal box that may be found in the x-ray room or in a nearby area such as the control booth. High-voltage cables (one going to the cathode of the x-ray tube and another to the anode) will connect the high-voltage generator to the x-ray tube.

X-RAY TUBE, TUBE ACCESSORIES, AND X-RAY TABLE

The third main part of any radiographic x-ray unit is a combination of the x-ray tube, x-ray tube support mechanism, x-ray examination table, and x-ray tube accessories such as the collimator and added filtration. Most radiographic x-ray tubes are rotating anode x-ray tubes that can withstand higher kVp and mAs combinations than the stationary anode x-ray tubes used in dental and small portable x-ray machines. The x-ray

tube must be equipped with metal housing to prevent leakage of radiation. This housing must confine the leakage amount to less than 100 milliroentgen (mR)/hr when measured at a distance of 1 m away from the housing. The x-ray tube also must be equipped with a variable-aperture collimator to control the size of the x-ray field (discussed in detail later in this chapter). The x-ray tube support mechanism that holds the x-ray tube in position over the Bucky device must have the following characteristics:

1. The support mechanism must be strong because the x-ray tube, insulating coil, collimator, and metal housing are heavy.

2. The support mechanism should be counterbalanced to help offset the weight of the x-ray tube and accessory devices.

3. Immobilization locks must be incorporated into the support mechanism to hold the x-ray tube in position.

4. The x-ray tube position, in relation to the image receptor, must be clearly indicated (source-to-image distance [SID] indicator). This must be accurate to within 2% of the SID.

In addition, if a radiographic examination table is present (as opposed to an upright Bucky or chest unit), the maximum tabletop thickness over the Bucky assembly is 1 mm of aluminum equivalent. This is to prevent the tabletop material from absorbing excessive amounts of radiation before reaching the image receptor (which would therefore increase patient dose).

QUALITY CONTROL PROGRAM FOR RADIOGRAPHIC UNITS

The three parts of a quality control program for radiographic equipment are visual inspection, environmental inspection, and performance testing.

Visual Inspection

Visual inspection includes checking the main components of the equipment for proper function, mechanical condition, and safety. This inspection should be performed at least annually (monthly for American College of Radiology [ACR] accreditation) with a checklist for documentation. An example of this checklist is provided on the Evolve website. The inspection should include the control panel, overhead tube crane, radiographic table, protective lead apparel, and miscellaneous equipment.

Control Panel. The control panel contains all of the selectors for controlling x-ray production (mA, kVp, and exposure time) and the various meters that monitor the operation of the generator. The control panel inspection should include verification of the proper function of x-ray tube heat sensors and the overload protection indicator (procedure discussed later in this chapter). There also should be verification that all panel lights, meters, and switches are functioning as designed. The inspection should ensure a proper view of the exposure room through the window (unobstructed), correct exposure switch placement, and the presence of an up-to-date technique chart.

Overhead Tube Crane. The overhead tube crane is the mounting bracket that holds the x-ray tube over the x-ray table. Items to evaluate in this section include the condition of the high-voltage cables and other wires (are they discolored or frayed?); the condition of the cable brackets, clamps, or tie-downs (are they intact and functioning normally?); the stability of the system; proper movement; SID and angulation indicator function (procedure discussed later in this chapter); detent operation; lock function; the Bucky center light; collimator light brightness (procedure discussed later in this chapter); and interlock function.

Radiographic Table. A patient is usually in contact with the x-ray table throughout the diagnostic procedure, so the table must be kept clean and safe. Items to inspect include surface condition and cleanliness of tabletop, power top and angulation switches, Bucky tray and cassette locks, stability, table angulation indicator (use a protractor to verify that the indicator is accurate to within ± 2 degrees), and the condition of any footboard or shoulder braces.

Protective Lead Apparel. Lead aprons and gloves should be present in the radiographic room and have a minimum 0.5 mm of lead–equivalent thickness. Standards set forth by The Joint Commission (TJC) dictate that healthcare organizations must perform routine inspections on protective lead apparel. They should be radiographed or viewed fluoroscopically (with remote fluoroscopy if possible) on acceptance and then every 6 months thereafter to determine if any cracks or holes are present (Fig. 7-8). A log should be kept of when these inspections are performed as well as the results and any corrective action. Software programs are available for maintaining inspection reports. When not in use, they should be properly hung to prevent cracks. Lead vinyl sheets and gonadal shields also should be evaluated in the same manner. If a piece of lead protective apparel is no longer usable, it must be disposed of in an appropriate manner. According to the Health Physics Society, lead and other heavy metals meet the criteria for a hazardous material under the Resource Conservation and Recovery Act. The best option for disposal is to recycle the protective apparel so that the lead can be re-used.

Miscellaneous Equipment. A measuring caliper should be present in radiographic rooms where the manual technique is used. The caliper and a technique chart aid in establishing the correct exposure factors. Positioning sponges and other patient position aids should be clean and free of contrast media. A check of the manual integrity of any step stools or intravenous fluid stands also should be included.

Environmental Inspection

Environmental inspection should be performed annually and involves checking for mechanical and electrical safety. Often, it can be performed along with the visual inspection. One item included in the environmental inspection is evaluation of the condition of the x-ray tube high-tension cables. This is accomplished by checking the covering on the outside of the cables (or any other wires that are visible on the outside of the unit). Any discoloration of the outside insulation, especially where the wire or cable bends, could be an indicator of internal heat and a potential short circuit. A service engineer should be consulted if this is present.

The mechanical condition of the x-ray tube counterweights and tracks (especially in overhead tube stands) also should be included in the environmental inspection. Proper lubrication of moving parts also should be provided at this time.

Electrical safety is critical for the safety of both the patient and the equipment operator. All radiographic equipment should be grounded, and all obvious electrical connections should be intact.

Should the possibility of a short circuit exist, never touch an electrical device with one hand while the other hand is touching any type of conductor. This helps prevent the direct flow of electricity through the heart. If someone is experiencing an electric shock, do not grasp the person directly. Instead, either open the main switch (turn the power off) or use some type of insulator (dry wooden board) to separate the person from the source of the electricity. A good rule of thumb to remember when dealing with electric current is that the combination of high voltage and low amperage tends to throw a person, whereas a combination of low voltage and high amperage tends to hold a person and is potentially

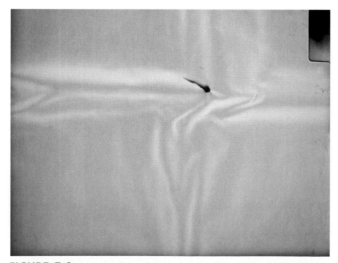

FIGURE 7-8 Image of lead apron demonstrating a large hole in the center.

more dangerous. For older equipment or equipment that has a history of problems with electrical safety, a service engineer should be consulted for environmental inspections. Many states require that an electrical inspection record be posted on the equipment.

Performance Testing

Performance testing evaluates the performance of the x-ray generator and x-ray tube with specialized test instrumentation, which can range from simple phantoms and test tools to sophisticated computerized systems such as the Noninvasive Evaluation of Radiation Output (NERO) system (Fig. 7-9) or similar devices available from various manufacturers. These computerized systems make the data gathering for performance evaluations quick and easy, but they can cost thousands of dollars. It is more common for facilities to use several smaller devices to gather the necessary data. The results of these tests should be documented for governmental and accreditation agencies. Many states and the ACR require that these performance tests be performed by a medical physicist. However, radiographers should know how the tests are performed and how to interpret the results. Sample forms for many of these tests are provided on the accompanying Evolve website.

Radiation Measurement. Much of the data obtained during performance testing includes radiation measurement; therefore, some type of radiation detector is a standard piece of equipment for many of these tests. The more common type of detector used in performance testing is the gas-filled chamber. As radiation enters this chamber, it ionizes the gas along its path (Fig. 7-10).

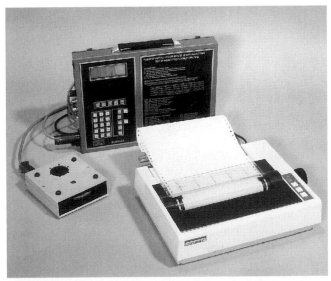

FIGURE 7-9 The Noninvasive Evaluation of Radiation Output (NERO) is a microprocessor that can be programmed to acquire and analyze exposure data, providing quality control test results for numerous parameters. *(From Ballinger PW: Merrill's atlas of radiographic positions and radiologic procedures, ed 9, St Louis, 1999, Mosby.)*

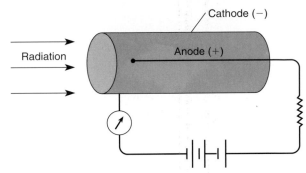

FIGURE 7-10 Schematic diagram of an ion chamber.

This produces a trail of ions that allows the flow of current through the chamber for a split second. This current is converted to a voltage pulse that is amplified and counted. The size of the voltage pulse is proportional to the energy expended in the chamber by the incident radiation. A quenching material may be added to the chamber to speed the return of ions to a stable state. There are three types of gas-filled chamber detectors, which vary according to the chamber voltage (Fig. 7-11).

Ion Chamber. With 100 to 300 V placed on it, the ion chamber is the least sensitive of the three chambers. The ion chamber is useful for measuring x-rays because a high sensitivity is not required for their detection and ion chambers often are used in performance testing. They usually are available as pocket ionization chambers (also called *pocket dosimeters*) and analog or digital dosimeters (Fig. 7-12). They also can be used as the sensor in automatic exposure control systems and as the detectors in computed tomography (CT) scanners.

Proportional Counter. A voltage of 300 to 900 V placed on the chamber increases the sensitivity. Proportional counters are often used in stationary laboratory counters to measure small quantities of radioactive material.

Geiger-Müller Counter. A voltage of 900 to 1200 V placed on the chamber yields the greatest sensitivity. Geiger-Müller counters often are used for contamination control in nuclear medicine departments.

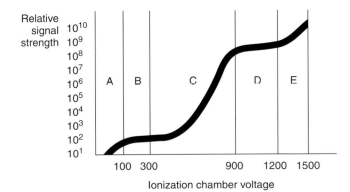

FIGURE 7-11 Graph showing how the intensity of the signal from a gas-filled detector increases as the voltage across the chamber increases. **A,** Region of recombination. **B,** Ionization region. **C,** Proportional region. **D,** Geiger-Müller region. **E,** Region of continuous discharge.

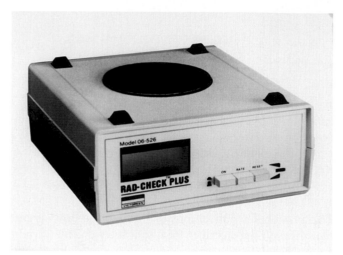

FIGURE 7-12 Digital dosimeter. *(Courtesy Gammex/RMI, Middleton, Wis.)*

Some newer types of radiation-monitoring devices use a solid-state or semiconducting detector instead of an ionization chamber. This incorporates a crystal of either silicon or germanium with selected impurities (such as lithium) added to detect the incident radiation. When the crystal is attached to an electric current, little or no current can flow through the crystal because no free electrons are available.

If the crystal is exposed to radiation, electrons are dislodged within its matrix and electric current can flow through it. This increase in current is proportional to the amount of radiation incident on the crystal and is registered with an analog or digital meter. This type of detector is relatively small and accurate but can be higher in cost than ionization chambers. It is also more sensitive than a gas-filled chamber. In most gases, an average energy of 30 to 40 electron volts (eV) is expended per ion pair produced. In a silicon semiconductor, an ion pair is produced for each 3.5 eV deposited by the incident radiation. For germanium detectors, only 2.9 eV are required to produce an ion pair. This means that many more ion pairs are produced in semiconductor detectors (as compared with ion chambers) for a given amount of energy absorbed.

The value obtained from the radiation detector is most often the radiation intensity, which can be measured in a special unit called the **roentgen** (R) or in an SI unit called the **coulomb/kilogram** (C kg^{-1}).

$$1\ R = 2.58 \times 10^{14}\ C\ kg^{-1}$$
$$1\ C\ kg^{-1} = 3.88 \times 10^{3}\ R$$

Because both units measure a relatively large amount of radiation, smaller increments of mR or microcoulomb/kilogram (μC/kg^{-1}) most often are obtained during performance testing. Some detectors are designed so that the exposure rate (intensity of radiation/unit of time) can be displayed in addition to the radiation intensity; these are known as *rate meters*. Detectors also can

be calibrated to measure absorbed dosage in rad or gray (Gy). One rad is equivalent to 0.01 Gy or 1 centigray (cGy). Rad or gray also is used to measure a value known as *air kerma*, which is discussed in Chapter 9.

Reproducibility of Exposure. An x-ray generator should always produce the same intensity of radiation each time that the same set of technical factors is used to make an exposure. For example, if a technique of 80 kVp, 500 mA, and 0.02 second yields 100 mR of radiation when measured with a dosimeter, then at any future time that the same technical factors are entered into the same x-ray generator, the yield, when tested, should be 100 mR. This concept is known as **reproducibility**. ❻ *The maximum variability allowed in reproducibility is ± 5% according to (1020.31(b)), 21 CFR Subchapter J.* Evaluation of the reproducibility variance requires a dosimeter (unless a computerized noninvasive system is used). Reproducibility testing should be performed upon acceptance, after a major system repair, and then annually.

PROCEDURE

1. Place a lead apron on top of a radiographic tabletop, with the center of the lead apron in the approximate center of the tabletop. Place a dosimeter on top of the lead apron, in the center of the tabletop. The lead apron absorbs backscatter from the tabletop material, which can reduce the accuracy of any readings obtained. If a lead apron is unavailable, a sheet of lead vinyl may be substituted. Center the central ray of the x-ray beam to the dosimeter; use a SID distance of 40 inches. Collimate the beam so that the x-ray field is just slightly larger than the dosimeter or remote probe.

2. Make a series of three to five separate exposures of the dosimeter at 80 kVp, 100 mA, and 100 ms. The dosimeter must be cleared (reset to zero) after each exposure. Record each reading on some type of documentation form such as the Radiographic Survey Form found on the Evolve website.

3. Use the readings obtained to determine the reproducibility variance with the following equation:

$$\text{Reproducibility variance} = \frac{(mR_{max} + mR_{min})}{(mR_{max} + mR_{min})}$$

The calculated variance should be less than 0.05 (5%) for a properly functioning x-ray generator. This test should be performed on acceptance of new equipment and then annually or when service is performed on the x-ray generator or x-ray tube. Variations in x-ray generator performance (e.g., kilovolt [peak] selector, milliampere selector, rectifier failure) or x-ray tube operation (e.g., filament evaporation, arcing) can cause the reproducibility variance to exceed accepted limits. This can cause radiographs of inconsistent quality and necessitate repeat exposures.

Radiation Output. X-ray generators should emit a specific amount of radiation (mR or μC/kg) per unit of x-ray tube current and time (mAs). In addition, similar types of x-ray generators and tubes within a department should emit the same values of mR per mAs (μC/kg/mAs) so that technique charts can be valid in all rooms and the number of repeat examinations can be reduced. The original value of mR per mAs (μC/kg/mAs) value is determined on acceptance of the unit or at the start of the quality control program. The radiation output is then measured annually and compared with this original value.

Many states and TJC require the posting of this value to guarantee that the x-ray generator does not emit excessive amounts of radiation exposure for a given combination of kVp per mAs.

The ACR specifies a maximum entrance exposure for chest and abdominal views obtained with an ACR phantom. Chest views should not exceed a maximum exposure of 50 mR (measured with a dosimeter), and abdominal views should not exceed 1100 mR.

PROCEDURE

1. Place a dosimeter on the radiographic tabletop on a lead apron or sheet of lead vinyl, using a source-to-detector distance of 40 inches (just as in step 1 of the procedure for determining reproducibility).
2. Make an exposure at 80 kVp, 100 mA (large focal spot), and 100 ms (10 mAs). Some physicists recommend that the dosimeter be placed under a homogenous phantom of aluminum or acrylic plates or in the Bucky for this measurement. Either method is satisfactory, but the test must always be performed the same way so that the values can be compared for variation.
3. Divide the radiation measurement recorded from the dosimeter by 10 mAs to obtain the value of mR/mAs, or μC/kg/mAs. This value should be recorded and the test repeated at least annually (with the same procedure and exposure factors). The current and previous readings should be compared, and the percent deviation should be determined with the following equation:

$$\text{Percent mR/mAs variation} = \frac{(mRm/As_{min} - mR/mAs_{min})}{(mRmAs_{max})} \times 100$$

ⓖ *The original acceptance value and future values should be within ± 10% of each other in a properly functioning x-ray generator.* In addition, values obtained in different radiographic rooms with similar x-ray generators and tubes also should be compared and should fall within ± 10% of each other to establish room-to-room consistency. If these rooms exceed the 10% variation limit, they should have separate technique charts provided for each room. Variation in mR/mAs (μC/kg/mAs) for a single room can occur over time from problems in the x-ray generator calibration, timer circuit inaccuracy, and filament evaporation from the cathode of the x-ray tube (some of the tungsten from the filament deposits on the inside of the window of the x-ray tube and causes additional filtration of the beam).

Filtration Check. Proper filtration is necessary to remove low-energy photons from the x-ray beam (1020.30(m)), 21 CFR Subchapter J. A patient's skin dose can increase by as much as 90% if the photons are not removed. This test should be performed on acceptance and then annually or whenever service is performed on the x-ray tube or collimator. The best method to determine if adequate filtration exists is to measure the **half-value layer** (HVL) (the amount of filtration that reduces the exposure rate to one half of its initial value) because normally it is not possible to measure inherent filtration. This is due to filament evaporation that is continually taking place, which adds a layer of tungsten onto the inside of the x-ray tube window. By measuring the HVL (which measures beam quality) instead of the total amount of filtration, it doesn't matter how much material is in the path of the beam, as long as sufficient beam quality is measured and obtained. Using HVL for determining sufficient filtration is also relatively easy to obtain and noninvasive. The HVL should not vary from its original value (which is established at acceptance) or its value at the beginning of the quality control program. It is dependent on the kVp used, the total beam filtration, and the type of x-ray generator (Fig. 7-13, Table 7-1).

PROCEDURE

1. Place a dosimeter on the radiographic tabletop on top of a lead apron or lead vinyl (to prevent backscatter).
2. Adjust the tube-to-dosimeter distance between 60 and 80 cm and collimate the x-ray beam to an area slightly larger than the dosimeter.
3. Make an exposure at 80 kVp and 50 mAs and record the amount of radiation from the dosimeter on a documentation form such as the HVL Evaluation Form found on the Evolve website.
4. Clear the dosimeter and add a 1-mm-thick aluminum plate between the bottom of the collimator and the dosimeter and expose. Record the reading and clear the dosimeter. Repeat this procedure, adding aluminum plates in 1-mm increments until a total of 6 to 8 mm are in place.
5. Use semilog graph paper and plot a graph of x-ray intensity (dosimeter readings) on the y-axis versus absorber thickness on the x-axis (see Fig. 7-13). Draw in a curve by connecting the dots in the graph. The HVL is determined by taking one half of the maximum dosimeter reading and then drawing a line from this point on the y-axis to the curve and then another line from this point on the curve, down to the x-axis. This value on the x-axis represents the HVL. This should be greater than or equal to 2.3 mm because this is the minimum HVL at 80 kVp, according to the FDA. The HVL amounts at various kilovolt (peak) values are given in Table 7-1.

A quick test to determine if adequate filtration is present can be performed in cases in which HVL value measurement cannot be made. However, this indicates only the presence of adequate filtration and not the actual amount of filtration; therefore, it should not take the place of HVL measurement during formal quality control testing. In this method a dosimeter and a 2.3-mm-thick aluminum plate are used.

Kilovolt (Peak) Accuracy. The x-ray tube voltage (kVp) has a significant effect on the image contrast, the optical density, and the patient dose. Therefore the kVp stated on the control panel should produce an x-ray beam with a

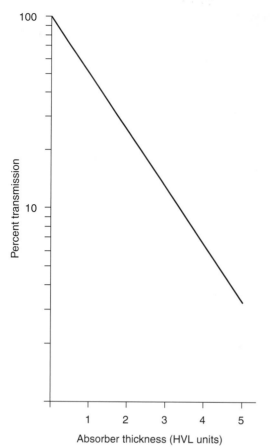

FIGURE 7-13 Semilog plot of radiation intensity versus attenuator thickness for determination of half-value layer (HVL).

PROCEDURE

1. Place the dosimeter on the radiographic table on top of a lead apron.
2. Make an exposure at a source-to-detector distance of 40 inches at 80 kVp and 50 mAs and record the reading.
3. Clear the dosimeter and make a second exposure using the same technical factors but with the aluminum plate between the detector and the x-ray source.
4. Place the readings obtained into the following equation:

$$\frac{\text{Exposure with aluminum plate}}{\text{Exposure without aluminum plate}}$$

If adequate filtration is present, the number obtained from the equation should range from 0.5 to 0.75. If less than 0.5, the beam filtration is inadequate. If the number is greater than 0.75, excessive filtration exists, which is legally acceptable but can be an indicator of pending x-ray tube failure because of excessive tungsten deposits on the x-ray tube window resulting from filament evaporation.

comparable and consistent amount of energy. **ⓖ** *Variations between the stated kVp and the x-ray beam quality must be within ± 5%.* For example, if 80 kVp is selected on the control panel, the maximum x-ray beam energy should fall within ± 4 kVp of this value. The kVp accuracy can be determined with either a specialized test cassette such as the Wisconsin Test Cassette (Fig. 7-14), Ardan and Crook's cassette, or a digital kVp meter (Fig. 7-15), according to the respective manufacturer's instructions. The digital meters are usually more accurate and easier to use (because when they are exposed, the measured kVp appears automatically with a light-emitting diode [LED] readout) but are more expensive than the test cassettes. The test cassettes require that a film be placed inside and exposed to a specific set of technical factors. The resulting image is then analyzed

TABLE 7-1	Minimum HVL Values for Diagnostic X-Ray Units		
X-Ray Tube Voltage (kilovolt peak)		**Minimum HVL (mm of Al)**	
Designed Operating Range	**Measured Operating Potential**	**Specified Dental Systems**	**Other X-Ray Systems**
Below 50	30	1.5	0.3
	40	1.5	0.4
	49	1.5	0.5
50 to 70	50	1.5	1.2
	60	1.5	1.3
	70	1.5	1.5
Above 70	71	2.1	2.1
	80	2.3	2.3
	90	2.5	2.3
	100	2.7	2.7
	110	3.0	3.0
	120	3.2	3.2
	130	3.5	3.5
	140	3.8	3.8
	150	4.1	4.1

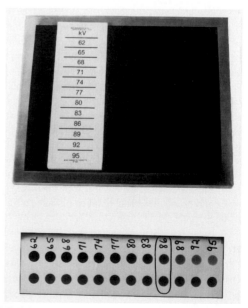

FIGURE 7-14 Wisconsin Test Cassette. (*Courtesy Gammex/RMI, Middleton, Wis.*)

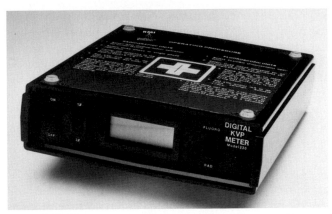

FIGURE 7-15 Digital kilovolt (peak) meter. *(Courtesy Gammex/RMI, Middleton, Wis.)*

visually or with a densitometer to obtain the measured kVp. Whichever device is used for this test, it should estimate the peak voltage at various kVp stations that are available for the particular x-ray generator being evaluated. This can be done in 10- to 20-kVp increments, usually beginning with 50 kVp. This test should be performed on acceptance and then annually or when service is performed on the x-ray generator or tube. Variations in kVp output may be caused by variations in the line voltage supplying the x-ray generator, by faulty high-voltage cables, or by problems with the autotransformer/kVp selection circuitry.

Timer Accuracy. Exposure time directly affects the total quantity of radiation emitted from an x-ray tube; therefore, an accurate exposure timer is critical for properly exposed radiographs and reasonable patient radiation exposure. ❻ *The variability allowed for timer accuracy is ± 5% for exposure times greater than 10 ms and ± 20% for exposures less than 10 ms.* Timer accuracy should be determined on acceptance and then annually or when service is performed on the x-ray generator or if technique problems arise suddenly. The easiest method to validate timer accuracy is the use of a digital x-ray timer available from various manufacturers (Fig. 7-16). These usually incorporate a solid-state detector that measures the total time of x-ray production and then displays the time by means of a digital LED readout. Because these devices cost several hundred dollars, other lower-cost methods can be used. One of the oldest methods is the spinning top test. This test includes a spinning top consisting of a metal disk with a hole or slit cut into the outside edge. If a single-phase x-ray unit is being evaluated, a manual spinning top can be used (Fig. 7-17). Single-phase generators emit x-rays in pulses, and therefore each pulse creates a dot on the radiograph made of the spinning top (Fig. 7-18). The number of dots appearing on this radiograph is then compared with the number that should theoretically appear at the particular time station selected on the control panel for each exposure. The number of dots that should theoretically appear is determined by the following equations:

Half-wave rectified:

Correct number of dots = Exposure time (seconds) × 60

Full-wave rectified:

Correct number of dots = Exposure time (seconds) × 120

Exposures should be made at $^{1}/_{10}$, $^{1}/_{20}$, $^{1}/_{30}$, and $^{1}/_{40}$ of a second for single-phase equipment.

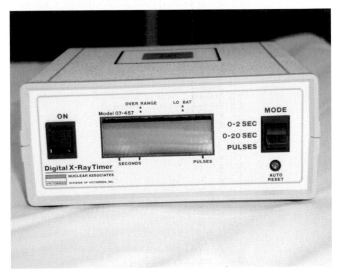

FIGURE 7-16 Digital timer for radiographic units. *(Courtesy Nuclear Associates, Carle Place, N.Y.)*

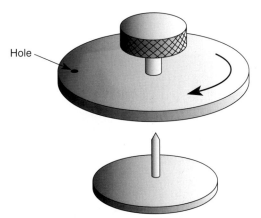

FIGURE 7-17 Manual spinning top.

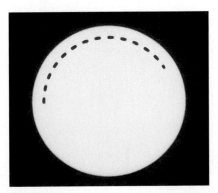

FIGURE 7-18 Image from manual spinning top on a single-phase x-ray generator.

For three-phase and high-frequency generators, x-ray production is constant, so a solid line or arc appears instead of a series of dots. For this reason, a manual spinning top cannot be used; a synchronous or motor-driven spinning top is used instead (Fig. 7-19). The synchronous spinning top also may be used to evaluate single-phase equipment. The electric motor in the synchronous spinning top rotates at a constant speed of 1 rps (revolution per second) so that at the end of 1 second,

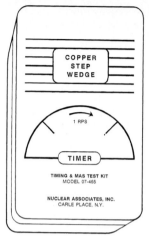

FIGURE 7-19 Synchronous spinning top. *(Courtesy Nuclear Associates, Inc., Carle Place, N.Y.)*

a 360-degree circle is made. When placed on an image receptor and exposed with a three-phase or high-frequency x-ray generator, this device creates an arc on the processed image that is some fraction of 360 degrees at exposure times less than 1 second. The arc size on the image is measured with a protractor (Fig. 7-20) and then inserted into the following equation to determine the actual exposure time (as a fraction) that occurred:

$$\text{Actual exposure time} = \text{Arc size}/360$$

For example, if the image yields an arc size of 72 degrees, $^{72}/_{360}$ equals a $^{1}/_{5}$-second exposure time (0.2 sec or 200 ms). At least four different time stations should be tested for three-phase equipment.

Many of the newer high-frequency units come equipped with mAs timers instead of separate mA and time stations. Because the exposure time is regulated by the internal microprocessor circuitry, the actual time is unknown. A digital mAs meter must be used instead of the digital timer or spinning top test. These devices have electrical probes that must be attached to the circuitry of the unit to obtain a reading. Only a person with adequate training on the use of these devices should attempt to access the circuitry.

Another option to determine timer accuracy is the use of an oscilloscope to display the voltage waveform, which is discussed in the next section.

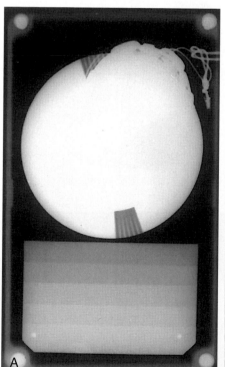
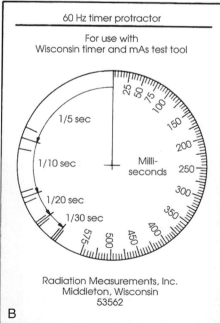
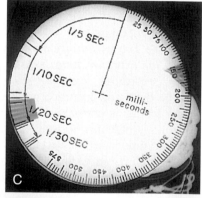
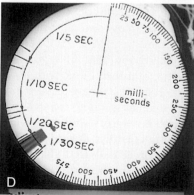

FIGURE 7-20 A, Radiograph produced at 200 mA and 1/20-second exposure. **B,** RMI protractor template. **C,** Radiograph A with template showing acceptable results for a 1/20-second exposure. **D,** Radiograph produced at 200 mA and 1/30 second showing unacceptable results. *mAs,* Milliampere-second. *(From Ballinger PW: Merrill's atlas of radiographic positions and radiologic procedures, ed 9, St Louis, 1999, Mosby.)*

Voltage Waveform. As discussed previously, each type of x-ray generator creates a distinctive voltage waveform. If the waveform could be displayed on an oscilloscope screen during x-ray production, considerable information could be obtained concerning timer accuracy, rectifier malfunctions, loading characteristics, contactor or switching problems, and high-voltage cable or connector arcing (Fig. 7-21) because these variables affect the size or shape of the waveform. The oscilloscope can be hooked up electronically (only by personnel with extensive electronics backgrounds such as physicists, biomedical engineers, or service engineers) to specific areas of the x-ray generator, or it can be attached to a commercially available x-ray output detector (Fig. 7-22). This detector is placed in the x-ray beam, and the output cable is connected to the oscilloscope input. The display is then analyzed for potential problems. This test should be performed on acceptance and then annually or after x-ray generator service and documented with a form such as the Radiographic Survey Form on Evolve website.

Milliampere and Exposure Time Linearity and Reciprocity. The mA selector in an x-ray generator is used to regulate the x-ray tube filament temperature, which, along with the exposure time, ultimately determines the quantity of x-rays in the x-ray beam. Therefore, the accuracy of the mA selected is equally important to the accuracy of the exposure timer. One method of testing mA accuracy is to make a 1-second exposure while watching the mAs meter on the control panel. A better method is to determine the mA **reciprocity** and linearity.

Reciprocity refers to the same mAs being selected but with different combinations of mA and exposure time. The radiation output should be the same as long as the kVp is kept constant. For example, an exposure of 70 kVp, 50 mA at 1 second should produce the same amount of radiation as an exposure of 70 kVp, 100 mA at $^1/_2$ second because both yield 50 mAs. ❻ *Any variation in reciprocity must be ± 10%.*

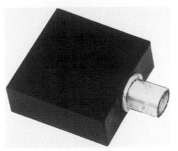

FIGURE 7-22 Output detector for obtaining voltage waveforms. *(Courtesy Nuclear Associates, Inc, Carle Place, N.Y.)*

PROCEDURE

1. Place a dosimeter on the radiographic tabletop on top of a lead apron or lead vinyl, 40 inches from the focal spot.
2. Make three to five exposures at 80 kVp and 20 mAs. Each exposure should be at a different mA and time combination. Be sure to reset the dosimeter after each exposure.
3. Record the dosimeter readings from each exposure and then divide each by 20 mAs to yield the mR per mAs, or µC/kg/mAs, value.
4. The minimum, maximum, and average of these three to five values are then used to determine the reciprocity variance with the following equation:

$$\text{Linearity variance} = \frac{[\text{mR/mAs}_{max} - \text{mR/mAs}_{min}]}{\text{mR/mAs}_{average}} \div 2$$

Adequate reciprocity exists when the variance is less than 0.1 (10%).

If a dosimeter is unavailable, images of an aluminum step wedge or homogenous phantom made of aluminum or acrylic can be created with the use of a similar procedure to the one described earlier. Using a 10 × 12 inch image receptor, make three to five exposures at 80 kVp and 5 mAs (be sure to use lead vinyl strips so that you can fit all three to five images on a single image receptor). Once the image is processed, optical density readings are then taken of the same area from each of the three to five images with a densitometer and then compared. The readings should be within an optical density value of ± 0.1.

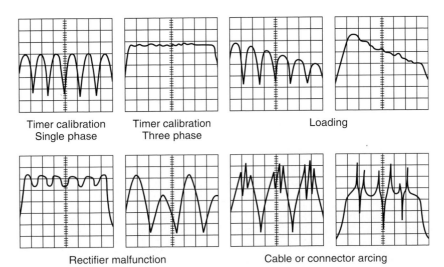

Timer calibration Single phase	Timer calibration Three phase	Loading	
Rectifier malfunction		Cable or connector arcing	

FIGURE 7-21 Voltage waveforms indicating various conditions within the x-ray generator.

Linearity means that sequential increases in mAs should produce the same sequential increase in the exposure measured. In other words, if factors of 70 kVp and 10 mAs were to produce 50 mR of exposure on a dosimeter, then factors of 70 kVp and 20 mAs on the same x-ray generator should produce an exposure of 100 mR if the mA station and timer are accurate. ● *Any variation must be within ± 10% according to (1020.31(c)), 21 CFR Subchapter J.* This can be evaluated in a manner similar to reciprocity.

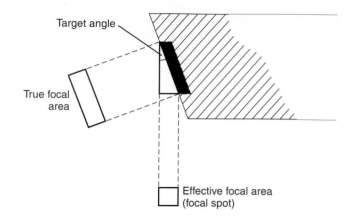

Relationship between true and effective focal areas

$$\text{Sine of target angle} = \frac{\text{Opposite}}{\text{Hypotenuse}}$$

FIGURE 7-23 Line focus principle.

PROCEDURE

1. Place the dosimeter on the radiographic table on a lead apron or strip of lead vinyl, just like in the reciprocity procedure.
2. Make four exposures using 70 kVp, 0.1 second (100 ms), and mA stations of 50, 100, 200, and 400. These yield mAs values of 5, 10, 20, and 40 (each exposure twice the previous one). These factors can be modified if the x-ray generator does not have these mA stations.
3. Record each reading and determine the mR/mAs for each exposure, along with the maximum, minimum, and average mR/mAs values, which are then placed into the following equation:

$$\text{Linearity variance} = \frac{[\text{mR/mAs}_{max} - \text{mR/mAs}_{min}]}{\text{mR/mAs}_{average}} \div 2$$

Adequate linearity exists when the variance is less than 0.1 (10%). (This variance also can be determined without a dosimeter, with a step wedge or homogenous phantom and image receptor. Make an exposure of the phantom or step wedge onto an image receptor using the mentioned technical factors. After the image is processed, compare the optical density readings of the same area to see if they are within ± 0.1 of each other.) Problems in the x-ray generator such as the mA selector, timer circuitry, or rectifier failure can cause the linearity variance to exceed accepted limits.

Focal Spot Size. The area of the anode that is bombarded by projectile electrons is called the *focal spot.* Because these projectile electrons lose their kinetic energy at this point, this is also the source of x-ray photons. This area can be viewed from two perspectives: the actual rectangular surface on the target where electrons strike, called the **actual focal spot,** and the actual focal spot viewed from the perspective of the image receptor, called the **effective** (apparent or projected) **focal spot.** The effective focal spot always appears smaller than the actual focal spot because of the angle of the **line focus principle** (Fig. 7-23). This effect is the result of the angle of the anode surface (the smaller the anode angle, the smaller the effective focal spot size). The effective focal spot size has a significant impact on the amount of recorded detail in a radiographic image because an increase in the effective focal spot size decreases the amount of recorded detail. Therefore focal spot size should remain relatively constant over the life

of the x-ray tube. However, focal spot size can increase with age and use and with increases in the mA station selected. This phenomenon is known as **focal spot blooming.** To evaluate the degree of focal spot blooming, one can use several performance tests.

Pinhole Camera. As shown in Figure 7-24, a pinhole camera is made up of a plate of gold platinum alloy with a tiny hole of a specified shape and size cut into its center. A 0.03-mm hole is used for measuring focal spots smaller than 1 mm. A 0.075-mm hole is used for measuring focal spot sizes from 1 to 2.5 mm, and a 0.1-mm hole is used for measuring focal spot sizes greater than 2.5 mm. When placed on a stand over an image receptor (preferably a fine-grain film placed in a non-screen holder or an extremity cassette) and then exposed, an image of the focal spot is projected on the film and can be measured with a ruler or micrometer after processing. This then can be compared with the stated, or nominal, focal spot size that is supplied by the x-ray tube manufacturer.

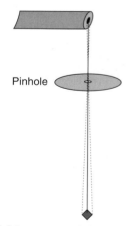

FIGURE 7-24 Concept of the pinhole camera.

PROCEDURE

1. Place the pinhole camera stand on the radiographic tabletop and align with the central ray and image receptor. If computed radiology (CR) is used, set the preprocessing image data recognition to fixed mode (the CR image receptor acts like a film/screen cassette).
2. Adjust the pinhole-to-image receptor distance and SID to obtain the proper enlargement factor. For focal spots less than 2.5 mm, an enlargement factor of 2 should be selected. This means that the pinhole-to-image receptor distance should be 60 cm, and the x-ray source-to-pinhole distance should be 30 cm. For focal spots larger than 2.5 mm, the enlargement factor should be 1. This is obtained with a source-to-pinhole distance of 40 cm and a pinhole-to-image receptor distance of 40 cm.
3. Expose the image receptor to 75 kVp and 50 mAs (100 mAs if a nonscreen image receptor is used). This should yield an optical density between 0.8 and 1.2 on the resulting image.
4. Measure the pinhole area on the processed image with a ruler or calipers in both the x-axis and y-axis (with the long axis of the x-ray table and transverse to the long axis of the x-ray table). If CR is used, you either may use the measuring software or print a hard copy of the image using a dry laser printer.
5. Divide the measurements by the enlargement factor obtained in step 2 to obtain the dimensions of the focal spot.

Focal Spot Test Tool. As shown in Figure 7-25, an image of this test tool is obtained, and the resulting image is compared with a chart supplied by the manufacturer (Table 7-2).

Resolution Chart. Resolution charts are tools that project a chart pattern of various shapes or lines onto a film when radiographed. These charts can be used to estimate focal spot size. The two basic types are star (Fig. 7-26) and slit charts. Slit charts normally yield the amount of spatial resolution in line pair per millimeter,

TABLE 7-2	Guide to Accompany Focal Spot Test Tool*	
Smallest Group Resolved	**lp/mm of Group**	**Dimension of Effective Focal Spot (mm)**
1	0.84	4.3
2	1	3.7
3	1.19	3.1
4	1.41	2.6
5	1.68	2.2
6	2	1.8
7	2.38	1.5
8	2.83	1.3
9	3.36	1.1
10	4	0.9
11	4.76	0.8
12	5.66	0.7

lp/mm, Line pairs per millimeter.
*The accuracy of this test is limited to 16% because the group sizes change by steps of 16%.

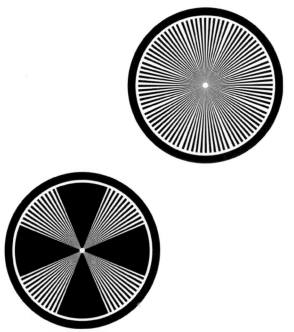

FIGURE 7-26 Star resolution patterns.

which then corresponds to a certain focal spot size being used to create the image (this was discussed in detail in Chapter 3 because this also determines the spatial resolution of imaging systems). When a star pattern resolution chart is used, the pattern is imaged on a fine-grain film (preferably in a nonscreen holder) and the image diameter (D_i) is measured from the resulting film. When this is compared with the actual diameter of the star pattern (D_o), the magnification factor (M) can be calculated with the following equation: $M = D_i / D_o$.

The diameter of the blur zone, or zero contrast band in millimeters, is measured from the image with a ruler (the diameter measured in both the X and Y dimensions

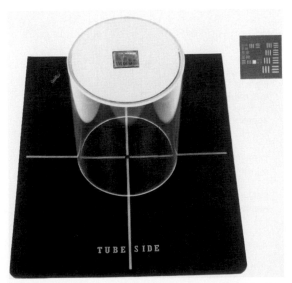

FIGURE 7-25 Image from the focal spot test tool. *(Courtesy Nuclear Associates, Inc, Carle Place, N.Y.)*

can be used to obtain the exact dimensions of the focal spot). This is the diameter of the center of the pattern where the lines appear blurred. A smaller focal spot size should be able to image lines that are closer together (such as in the center of the star pattern), so the blur zone is smaller in diameter. Once the diameter of the blur zone is obtained, the following equation can be used to calculate the focal size:

$$\text{Focal spot size in mm} = \theta\, D/(M-1)$$

where θ is the spoke angle of the star pattern in radians (radians = degrees $\times\ \pi \div 180$) obtained from the star pattern. D is the diameter of the blur zone measured in millimeters, and M is the magnification factor. Both the X and Y dimensions of the focal spot size should be calculated.

The focal spot size should be determined on acceptance and then evaluated annually. The maximum degree of focal spot blooming that is allowable is determined by the National Electronics Manufacturers Association (NEMA). The values for nominal focal spot size variation are listed in Table 7-3.

For example, if a focal spot size is stated to be 0.5 mm by the manufacturer but measures 0.75 mm during an evaluation test, is it within the NEMA guidelines? The answer is yes. Because its stated size is 0.5 mm, it is allowed up to a 50% variation, and 50% of 0.5 mm is 0.25 mm. Therefore the maximum focal spot size would be 0.75 mm, which would be just within the variation allowed.

Beam Restriction System. The beam restriction system is responsible for regulating the size of the x-ray field area. It therefore plays a significant role in patient dosage (because it controls the amount of patient anatomy that is exposed to radiation) and image contrast (because an increase in the area of the field increases the production of scattered radiation). Performance of this system should be evaluated on acceptance and then every 6 months or whenever work is performed on the system. The factors to evaluate within the beam restriction system include light field–radiation field congruence, image receptor–radiation field alignment, accuracy of the X-Y scales, and illuminator bulb brightness, and are covered in (1020.31(e), (f), (g), 1020.32 (b)), 21 CFR Subchapter J.

Light Field–Radiation Field Congruence. The light field–radiation field congruence value measures how well the collimator regulates the field size and if the area illuminated by the positioning light and the area exposed by x-rays are the same. The collimator is made up of two sets of lead shutters that can be opened and closed, along with a small light bulb mounted on the outer edge and a mirror mounted in the center to reflect the light from the bulb through the shutter opening (Fig. 7-27). Over time, this mirror may shift or the mechanism that moves the shutters can malfunction, causing improper performance. This can lead to higher patient dosage and repeat images. ❻ *The light field and radiation field must be congruent to within ± 2% of the SID. Evaluation can be performed by the use of either a collimator test tool with the manufacturer's instructions or the eight-penny (or nine-penny) test* (Figs. 7-28 and 7-29).

TABLE 7-3	NEMA Values for Nominal Focal Spot Size Variation	
Stated Focal Spot Size (mm)	**Focal Spot Blooming Variation Allowed (%)**	
≤0.8	50	
0.8–1.5	40	
≥1.6	30	

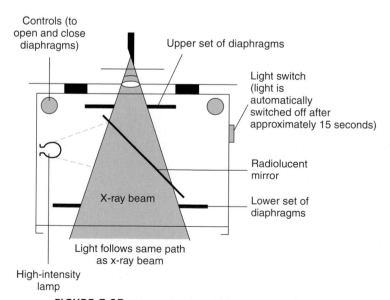

FIGURE 7-27 Schematic of variable aperture collimator.

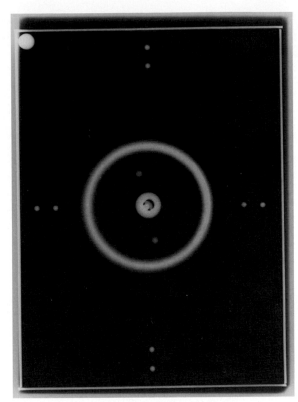

FIGURE 7-28 Image obtained with a collimator test tool showing collimator is within accepted limits.

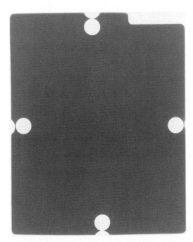

FIGURE 7-29 Image obtained with the eight-penny test.

Image Receptor–Radiation Field Alignment. The image receptor–radiation field alignment value must be determined for x-ray units equipped with positive beam limitation (PBL) or automatic collimation. These systems have sensors in the Bucky tray that detect the size of the image receptor and then automatically adjust the collimator shutters to match. Malfunctions in this system can occur with age and use and can be evaluated with a collimator test tool placed on top of the tabletop with an image receptor in the Bucky. An image is created with the previously described procedure for collimator test tool, light field/radiation field congruence. Testing should

---

PROCEDURE

Collimator Test Tool

The collimator test tool requires an image to be created with the use of an image receptor.

1. Place an image receptor on top of a radiographic table with the x-ray beam centered to the center of the image receptor. Next, place the test tool on top of the image receptor according to the manufacturer's instructions. If CR is used, set the preprocessing image data recognition to fixed mode (the CR image receptor acts like a film/screen cassette).
2. Adjust the collimators to the area outlined on the test tool. Make an exposure with the technical factors supplied by the test tool manufacturer.
3. Process the image and visually determine if the x-ray field and radiation field are congruent (see Fig. 7-28).

PROCEDURE

Eight-Penny (Nine-Penny) Test

1. The eight- or nine-penny test involves laying eight pennies on a 10 × 12 inch (25 × 35 cm) cassette placed on a tabletop but collimated to an 8 × 10 inch field size at a 40-inch SID.
2. Four of the pennies are placed on the inside edge of the light field at the center of each dimension, and the other four are placed on the outside edge in contact with the inner pennies, meeting at the edge of the light field. A ninth penny may be included (hence, the alternate name, *nine-penny test*). This may be placed in the light field toward the cathode end of the x-ray field to demonstrate on the resulting image the direction of any error in x-ray field/radiation field congruence (see Fig. 7-29). If CR is used, set the preprocessing image data recognition to fixed mode (the CR image receptor acts like a film/screen cassette).
3. When a radiograph is made and the image is processed, the collimation line of the x-ray field also should fall in between the pairs of pennies or at least within the shadow of the pennies because the diameter of a penny is 0.8 inches (which is exactly 2% of 40 inches).

---

be done in both the vertical and horizontal position if the x-ray tube is used in both positions. Ⓖ *Variation between the x-ray field and either the length or width of the image receptor must not differ by more than 3% of the SID.* An override switch should be in place to disconnect the PBL in case of malfunction. Ⓖ *The sum of the length and width differences should be no more than ± 4% of the SID used in taking the measurement.*

Accuracy of the X-Y Scales. Modern collimators have two knobs or dials on the front that allow the radiographer to control the x-ray field size during manual collimation. These knobs also have some type of indicator that shows the size of the X and Y dimensions of the x-ray field. Ⓖ *The indicated size on the collimator of the X and Y dimensions and the actual field size measured at the film must correspond to within ± 2% of the SID.* This can be tested with a collimator test tool or a 14 × 17 inch (36 × 45 cm) cassette placed on a 40-inch SID tabletop.

PROCEDURE

1. Set the *X-Y* control knobs on the collimator to a 10 × 12 inch field size (25 × 33 cm) and expose a 14 inch × 17 inch image receptor. If CR is used, set the preprocessing image data recognition to fixed mode (the CR image receptor acts like a film/screen cassette).
2. Process the image and use a ruler to measure the black rectangle in the center of the image. The dimensions should be within 0.8 inch of 10 × 12 inches.

Illuminator Bulb Brightness. The beam restriction system must be equipped with a positioning light and mirror, according to the Center for Devices and Radiological Health (CDRH) (1020.31(d)(2)(ii)) 21 CFR Subchapter J. The distance from the light bulb to the center of the mirror should equal the distance from the x-ray tube focal spot to the center of the mirror. ⦿ *The illumination of the light source must be at least 15 footcandles (ft-cd) or 160 lux when measured at a 100-cm (40-inch) distance.* A photometer such as the one used in Chapter 3 for evaluation of viewbox brightness or a photographic light meter should be used.

PROCEDURE

1. Bring a photometer or photographic light meter into a radiographic room. Set the meter to record illuminance in lux or ft-cd. Adjust the ambient light to the level that would routinely be used in the room during diagnostic procedures.
2. Set the x-ray tube-to-tabletop distance for 40 inches (100 cm) and turn on the illuminator light. Collimate to a 10 × 12 inch field size.
3. The cross hairs should appear in the light field; divide the light field into four equal quadrants. Place the photometer or light meter in the exact center of each quadrant of the light field and record the brightness (be sure to avoid dark bands such as those from the cross-hair images). The reading should be at least 15 ft-cd or 160 lux.

An illuminator bulb with an inadequate level of brightness may lead to positioning errors and subsequent repeat images. This problem usually is corrected by replacing the light bulb or cleaning the mirror inside the collimator.

Beam Alignment. The x-ray beam must be mounted properly in its metal housing and aligned to the Bucky tray. This alignment should be evaluated on acceptance and then annually with a beam alignment test tool (Fig. 7-30). Items to evaluate in this category include perpendicularity and x-ray beam-Bucky tray alignment.

Perpendicular. ⦿ *The x-ray tube must be mounted in its housing so that the central ray of the x-ray beam is within 1 degree of perpendicular.* If not, the image is distorted. Rough handling of the housing during x-ray examinations can cause the x-ray tube to shift slightly within its housing.

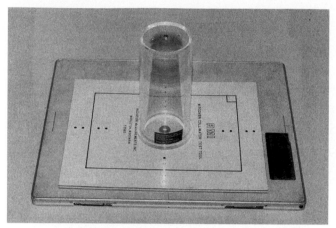

FIGURE 7-30 Beam alignment tool.

PROCEDURE

Beam Alignment Tool
1. Place an image receptor on the radiographic tabletop and center the x-ray beam, using a 40-inch SID.
2. Place the beam alignment tool on top of the image receptor and collimate to the area on the template.
3. Make an exposure using 60 kVp and a mAs appropriate to the speed of the image receptor being used. If CR is used, set the preprocessing image data recognition to fixed mode (the CR image receptor acts like a film/screen cassette).
4. Process the image. Within the test tool, a steel ball is mounted in the center of a disk at each end of the 15-cm-tall plastic container. When the balls are positioned over one another and at a right angle to the image receptor, their images appear as one, if the central ray is perpendicular to the image receptor. If the image of the upper steel ball (which is magnified because it is farther away from the image receptor) intersects the image of the first disk (this appears as a ring), the central ray is approximately 1.5 degrees away from perpendicular.

X-Ray Beam-Bucky Tray Alignment or Central Ray Congruency. The center of the Bucky tray and the center of the x-ray beam must be aligned to avoid clipping important anatomy and to avoid grid cutoff. ⦿ *X-ray beam–Bucky tray alignment must be within 1% of the SID.* The same beam alignment tool that was used to determine perpendicularity also can be used to evaluate this alignment (Fig. 7-31).

Source-to-Image Distance and Tube Angulation Indicators. All medical x-ray units must be equipped with SID and tube angulation indicators, according to the CDRH, because they influence patient dose, optical density, recorded detail, size distortion and shape distortion. ⦿ *The SID indicator must be installed so that it is accurate to within ± 2% of the SID. The tube angulation indicator must be accurate to within ± 5 degrees.* The accuracy of the tube angulation indicator can be

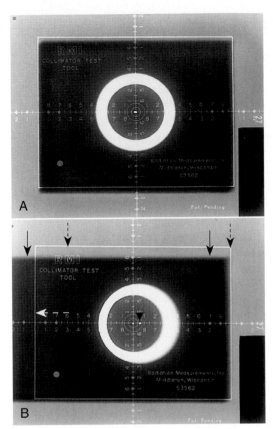

FIGURE 7-31 A, Acceptable beam perpendicularity and beam-light field alignment. **B,** Unacceptable beam perpendicularity and beam-light alignment. Radiation beam *(arrows)* does not agree with collimator light field *(broken arrows)*. Perpendicularity is out of alignment. Note top head is shifted to the right *(arrowhead)*. *(From Ballinger PW: Merrill's atlas of radiographic positions and radiologic procedures, ed 9, St Louis, 1999, Mosby.)*

PROCEDURE

Washer or Coin Method

If a beam alignment tool is unavailable, the following also can be used to determine x-ray beam–Bucky tray alignment.

1. Bring a metal coin, a steel washer, or a lead number zero, along with an 8 × 10 inch image receptor, into a radiographic room. If CR is used, set the preprocessing image data recognition to fixed mode (the CR image receptor acts like a film/screen cassette).
2. Place the image receptor in the Bucky tray (with the long axis of the image receptor in the same direction as the long axis of the radiographic table) and center the x-ray field to the image receptor. Set the SID for 40 inches (100 cm).
3. Turn on the positioning light and place the coin, lead zero, or steel washer in the center of the crosshairs. Place another coin or some other lead number in the light field, near the edge closest to where you are standing. This allows you to determine which direction the alignment may be off when analyzing the resulting image.
4. Make an exposure using 50 kVp and 1 mAs (you may have to increase this amount, depending on the image receptor speed). Process the image.
5. Using a ruler, measure the distance from the middle of the outside of the long axis of the image to the washer, coin, or lead zero (with CR systems you can use the electronic measuring software). If proper beam alignment exists, the distances are exactly the same. If they are not the same, the image of the washer, coin, or lead zero should be within 0.4 inch of the center of the image or a service person should be notified to repair the system.

PROCEDURE

Beam Alignment Test Tool

1. With the x-ray tube centered by means of the centering detent lock, place an image receptor in the Bucky tray and slide it into its proper place. If CR is used, set the preprocessing image data recognition to fixed mode (the CR image receptor acts like a film/screen cassette).
2. Position the test tool so that the metal washer is in the exact center of the x-ray field, using the cross hairs from the positioning light, and expose the image receptor.
3. Process and then visually analyze the resulting image. The image of the washer should be in the center of the film or within 0.4 inch (or ≈ 1 cm) of the center (see Fig. 7-31). A service engineer should be called if the alignment is off by more than this amount.

---

checked with a protractor. The SID indicator accuracy is determined with a simple tape measure or the triangular method and should be checked on acceptance and then annually or when service is performed on the x-ray tube. When evaluating with the triangulation method, use the following procedure.

Overload Protection. Most x-ray generators are equipped with an overload protection mechanism to prevent excessive temperatures inside the x-ray tube during a single exposure. ❻ *The overload protection mechanism should not permit an exposure that exceeds 80% of the tube capacity for a single exposure.* This exposure level can be determined by selecting a kVp and mA combination that exceeds this 80% limit and then engaging the rotor button. This should cause a tube overload indicator light to appear on the control panel; some systems do not allow the rotor to engage in this situation. Should either of these fail to occur, the user should call a service technician to repair the system. No one should engage the expose button because serious x-ray tube damage can result if the overload protection system is malfunctioning. The overload protection mechanism should be evaluated on acceptance and then annually or when service is performed on the x-ray generator.

X-Ray Tube Heat Sensors. As just mentioned, most x-ray generators are equipped with overload protection circuits to prevent excessive tube heat in a single exposure. They generally do not protect against cumulative heat build-up that can occur when several exposures

---

PROCEDURE

1. Place a radiopaque object (e.g., a metal plate about 2 inches long) at a distance from the focal spot mark on the x-ray tube housing. Measure and record the exact distance from the focal spot to the object. This value will be known as d_1 (Fig. 7-32). Also measure and record the exact size of the object.

2. Using a 40-inch SID, make an image of the object using an image receptor. If CR is used, set the preprocessing image data recognition to fixed mode (the CR image receptor acts like a film/screen cassette). Make sure that the object is positioned in the beam such that it is fully covered by the beam, and the image receptor is large enough to contain the image produced.

3. Process the image and measure the size of the radiopaque object recorded in the image. The SID ($d_1 + d_2$) can then be calculated using the similar triangles equation and inserting the measured values of d_1, object size, and image size:

$$\frac{d_1}{\text{object dimension}} = \frac{d_1 + d_2 (\text{SID})}{\text{image dimension}}$$

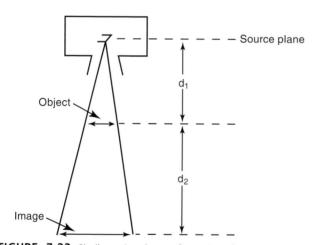

FIGURE 7-32 Similar triangle configuration for determination of SID.

are made within a relatively short period. To guard against this accumulated heat, radiographers can rely on anode cooling charts or housing cooling charts supplied by the tube manufacturer. This is especially critical during fluoroscopy and angiography, in which considerable heat can be produced quickly. Many newer units are equipped with x-ray tube heat sensors that provide an LED readout of the percentage of heat capacity remaining inside the x-ray tube housing. ❻ *Heat sensors should provide a warning when anode heat reaches 75% of the maximum.* These devices should be checked on acceptance and then every 6 months. This involves taking several exposures at a known heat unit value and then comparing the total with the known maximum heat capacity of the x-ray tube provided by the manufacturer.

ANCILLARY EQUIPMENT

The creation of diagnostic radiographs in a modern radiology department requires more than just an x-ray generator, x-ray tube, and x-ray table. Several types of ancillary equipment also are involved in the imaging chain to help create or enhance the radiographic image, regulate x-ray production, and protect the patient and radiographer. These include automatic exposure control systems, tomographic systems, grids, and mobile x-ray systems. Because variation in this equipment can occur during use, quality control protocols must be in place to minimize repeat examinations.

AUTOMATIC EXPOSURE CONTROL SYSTEMS

The AEC system has been used in radiography since the 1960s, and it functions as a regulator for the exposure time. This type of system involves some type of radiation detection device that measures the quantity of x-rays received by the patient or image receptor. When this exposure reaches a level corresponding to a predetermined value, the system causes the x-ray generator to terminate the exposure. This value is set by a service engineer on the basis of the image receptor system that is used in the department. An AEC system has two main parts, the detector and the comparator.

Detectors

The **detector,** also known as the **sensor,** is a radiation detector that monitors the radiation exposure at or near the patient and produces a corresponding electric current that is proportional to the quantity of x-rays detected. Detectors are sometimes referred to as *cells* or *chambers.* Normally, three detectors are available for use by the radiographer, one in the midline and one on either side of the midline (Fig. 7-33). Units also are available with

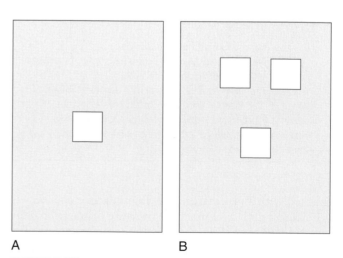

A   B

FIGURE 7-33 Sensor cell location for automatic exposure control (AEC) systems. **A,** Single-cell option. **B,** Three-sensor option.

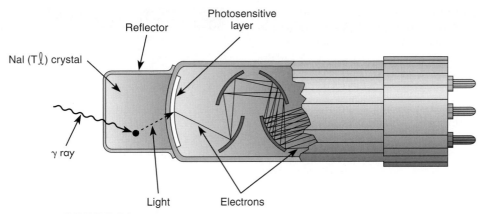

FIGURE 7-34 Schematic for photomultiplier tube and scintillation crystal.

only one or two detectors. Three different types of radiation detectors have been used in AEC systems: photodetectors, ion chambers, and solid-state detectors.

Photodetectors. The **photodetector,** or photocell, uses a scintillation crystal (usually sodium iodide) coupled with a photomultiplier tube (Fig. 7-34). When radiation interacts with the crystal, light is created, and it enters the photomultiplier tube. This light then releases electrons through the process of photoemission. These electrons multiply in number and form an electric current that is proportional to the original amount of radiation that struck the photocell. The photodetector was the original detector used as a sensor and was marketed under the name "phototimer." This name is still commonly used to describe AEC systems, even though the photodetector is seldom used in modern systems. These sensors are placed behind the image receptor to measure the exposure because they are not radiolucent. Care must be taken with these systems so that the lead in the back of the cassettes (normally present to control backscatter) is not excessive.

Ion Chambers. The **ion chamber** (discussed earlier in this chapter) consists of a gas-filled chamber. It is smaller than a photocell and can be made of a radiolucent material. This allows it to be placed between the grid and the front of the image receptor so that any type of cassette design can be used. This is the most common type of sensor found in current AEC systems. It is often marketed under the name "ionomat."

Solid-State Detectors. The **solid-state detector** uses a small silicon or germanium crystal, which is more sensitive but also more expensive than photocells or ion chambers. The crystals are radiolucent and can be placed between the grid and image receptor. The solid-state detector is often marketed under the name "autotimer."

Comparator

The **comparator** is an electronic circuit that receives the current signal sent by the sensor. An internal capacitor stores a voltage as long as this current is flowing. When the voltage in the capacitor becomes the same as a preset reference voltage, a switch is opened, and it terminates the exposure. Changing the density selector switch changes this reference voltage and therefore the quantity of radiographs produced by the generator. Each step on the density selector should change the radiation exposure by 25% to 30%. Typical selector settings are shown in Figure 7-35. The radiographer also must select the proper chamber, kilovolt (peak) (kVp), and milliampere (mA); verify properly positioned patient and x-ray tube; and verify backup time in case of system failure.

Automatic Exposure Control Testing

It is becoming more common for radiographic examinations to be performed with AEC systems. It is estimated that more than 60% of all hospital radiology departments have radiographic equipment that uses an AEC system or anatomically programmed units (which contain a microprocessor circuit with preprogrammed technical factors). The advantage of AEC is that it delivers consistent optical density on radiographs over a wide range of patient thickness and kVp settings. Proper system performance should therefore be monitored through quality control procedures on acceptance and then semiannually or whenever work is performed on the system. Items that should be monitored include backup, or maximum exposure time and minimum exposure time.

	Density setting
Weak, very young Very old, debilitated	−2
Thin Easy to penetrate	−1
Average Normal build	0/Neutral
Muscular	+1/+2

FIGURE 7-35 Automatic exposure control (AEC) density selector settings.

Results should be recorded as pass or fail on a documentation form. A sample form for AEC system evaluation is available on the accompanying Evolve website.

Backup, or Maximum Exposure, Time. Because the exposure is controlled by the sensor and comparator combination instead of a conventional timer, care must be taken to avoid excessive patient exposure and heat in the x-ray tube in the case of system failure or during the examination of an extremely large patient. This is accomplished by setting a backup timer on the control unit. ❻ *The backup timer should terminate the exposure within 6 seconds or 600 mAs, whichever comes first.* This can be checked with the following procedure.

PROCEDURE

1. Place a lead apron over the AEC detector cells and make an exposure at 70 kVp and 100 mA.
2. Watch the mAs meter on the control panel, in addition to using a stopwatch, to see if the backup system terminates the exposure within the 6-second or 600-mAs limit. If not, release the expose button so that the x-ray tube is not damaged.

Minimum Exposure Time. The detector and comparator combination requires a certain period to detect the radiation, compare it with the preset value, and then terminate the exposure (usually around 10 ms). If a particular x-ray examination requires an exposure less than this amount, the AEC system cannot respond in time and the resulting image is overexposed. For this reason, distal extremity radiographs are generally not performed with AEC. Certain lung diseases such as emphysema also can require less than the minimum exposure time, so it is important to lower the mA before making the exposure. The manufacturer's literature should be checked as to the minimum exposure time available, and then the technologists should be instructed as to which radiographic examinations and kVp and mA combinations can and cannot be used with AEC.

Quality Control for Automatic Exposure Control

Consistency of Exposure with Varying Milliampere. The AEC system should be able to adjust the exposure time and maintain optical density with any changes in mA on the control panel. ❻ *Any variation cannot exceed ± 10%.* To evaluate this parameter, use the following procedure (Fig. 7-36).

Consistency of Exposure with Varying Kilovolt (Peak). The AEC system should be able to adjust the exposure time and maintain optical density with any changes in kVp on the control panel. This can be evaluated with the same homogenous phantom mentioned previously.

PROCEDURE

1. Obtain a **homogenous phantom,** which is uniform in thickness, made of acrylic plastic (Plexiglas or Lucite) that is at least 10 cm in thickness (see Fig. 7-36).
2. Make a series of four radiographs of the phantom on a 10 × 12 inch (25 × 30 cm) image receptor using 70 kVp, 40-inch SID Bucky, and normal density setting, with each at a different mA station. If CR is used, set the preprocessing image data recognition to fixed mode (the CR image receptor acts like a film/screen cassette).
3. Process each radiograph and use a densitometer to measure the optical density of the center of each image. For CR images, print a hard copy of the image using a dry laser printer. ❻ *The optical density values should measure the same or be within an optical density of ± 0.2.* If not, inconsistent optical density in the resulting radiographs can occur, leading to repeat exposures. This is usually the result of a malfunctioning comparator.

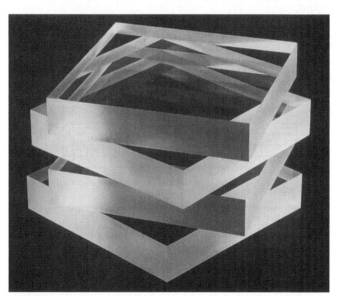

FIGURE 7-36 Automatic exposure control (AEC) test tool consisting of acrylic sheets of varying thickness. *(Courtesy Nuclear Associates, Carle Place, N.Y.)*

PROCEDURE

1. Make four exposures of the phantom on a 10 × 12 inch image receptor, using 100 mA; normal density setting; 40-inch SID Bucky; and values of 60, 70, 80, and 90 kVp. If CR is used, set the preprocessing image data recognition to fixed mode (the CR image receptor acts like a film/screen cassette).
2. Process the four radiographs and take optical density readings of the center of each image, using a densitometer. For CR images, print a hard copy of the image using a dry laser printer. ❻ *The optical density values should measure the same or be within an optical density of ± 0.3.*

Consistency of Exposure with Varying Part Thickness. The AEC system should be able to adjust the exposure time and maintain optical density with any changes in part thickness. System evaluation again uses a homogenous phantom.

PROCEDURE

1. Make three exposures on separate 10 × 12 inch image receptors at 70 kVp, 100 mA, normal density setting, and 40-inch SID Bucky. Make each exposure with a phantom thickness of 10, 20, and 30 cm. If CR is used, set the preprocessing image data recognition to fixed mode (the CR image receptor acts like a film/screen cassette).
2. Process each image and take density readings of the center. For CR images, print a hard copy of the image using a dry laser printer. ❻ *The optical density values should measure the same or be within an optical density of ± 0.2.*

Consistency of Exposure with Varying Field Sizes.

The AEC systems also should be able to compensate for changes in the area of field, provided the detector remains in the field. Radiographs of the homogenous phantom also can be used to evaluate this parameter.

PROCEDURE

1. Make a series of three exposures of the phantom, using factors of 70 kVp, 100 mA, normal density settings, and 40-inch SID. If CR is used, set the preprocessing image data recognition to fixed mode (the CR image receptor acts like a film/screen cassette).
2. Each exposure is made with a different field size of 6 × 6, 10 × 10, and 14 × 14 inches, with an appropriate image receptor size. Be sure that the x-ray beam is centered to the detector chamber.
3. Process the images and record the optical density from the center of each. For CR images, print a hard copy of the image using a dry laser printer. ❻ *The optical density values should measure the same or be within an optical density of ± 0.1.*

Consistency of Automatic Exposure Control Detectors.

Most AEC systems use a configuration of three detectors. Each detector should provide the same exposure or exposure time as the other two. For evaluation, use the following procedure.

PROCEDURE

1. Make a series of three radiographs of the homogenous phantom, using a different detector selection for each. Be sure that the phantom is placed over the appropriate detector. Use exposure factors of 70 kVp, 100 mA, normal density setting, and 40-inch SID Bucky. If CR is used, set the pre-processing image data recognition to fixed mode (the CR image receptor acts like a film/screen cassette).
2. Process the radiographs and compare the optical density readings from the center of each image. For CR images, print a hard copy of the image using a dry laser printer. ❻ *The optical density values should measure the same or be within an optical density of ± 0.2.*

Reproducibility.   Exposures made at the same kVp and mA stations of the same phantom thickness should produce the same optical density on the resulting image. This is referred to as **reproducibility.**

PROCEDURE

1. Make three exposures of the homogenous phantom using 80 kVp, 200 mA, normal density setting, 10 × 12 inch image receptor size, and 40-inch SID Bucky. If CR is used, set the pre-processing image data recognition to fixed mode (the CR image receptor acts like a film/screen cassette).
2. Process each radiograph and compare the optical density readings taken from the center of each image. For CR images, print a hard copy of the image using a dry laser printer. ❻ *The readings should be within an optical density of ± 0.10 of each other*.

An alternative method of evaluating reproducibility is to make the same three exposures but not to use an image receptor to record an image. Instead, a radiation detector and homogenous phantom can be placed over the appropriate sensor chamber and the readings obtained in each exposure can be recorded. For valid results, the radiation detector should be radiolucent. The reproducibility variance can then be calculated with the equation found earlier in this chapter. ❻ *The reproducibility variance must be within = 0.05 (5%).*

Density Control Function.   The density selector switch should allow for changes in radiation exposure of 25% to 30% for each increment. The accuracy can be evaluated by the following procedure.

PROCEDURE

1. Make a series of five radiographs of the homogenous phantom using 70 kVp, 100 mA, and 40-inch SID Bucky and using the density selector settings of normal (0/neutral), +1, +2, −1, and −2 (these settings vary according to manufacturer). Be sure to mark each image with a lead number or some other identifier. If CR is used, set the preprocessing image data recognition to fixed mode (the CR image receptor acts like a film/screen cassette).
2. Take optical density readings from the center of each of the processed images and compare. For CR images, print a hard copy of the image using a dry laser printer. Each should increase in optical density by a value of 0.2 to 0.25, from the lowest to the highest density setting (−2 to +2).

Reciprocity Law Failure

The **Law of Reciprocity** states that the same amount of radiation should be created at any milliampere-second (mAs) value, regardless of the mA/time combination used; therefore, the optical density of any resulting image also should be the same. Film/screen image receptor systems can experience reciprocity failure at very short exposure time values (<10 ms) and very long exposure time values (>1 second).

- Phantom images of either a homogenous phantom or an anthropomorphic (lifelike) phantom should be made at 70 kVp, normal density setting, 40-inch SID Bucky, and the lowest mA station possible on the control panel (so that a long exposure time is made).
- Another image should be made with the highest mA station available (to yield a short exposure time).
- Optical density readings should be obtained from the center of each image and compared. If reciprocity failure exists, the optical density of the images varies by more than a value of ± 0.2.

CONVENTIONAL TOMOGRAPHIC SYSTEMS

Many radiographic units are equipped with a conventional tomographic system that is used to image certain "slices" of the body, whereas all other slices are blurred. This helps remove superimposition and improve the radiographic contrast in the area of interest. There are two basic types of conventional tomography: linear tomography and pluridirectional tomography.

In **linear** (sometimes called *rectilinear*) **tomography** the x-ray tube and image receptor move longitudinally in opposite directions during the exposure (Fig. 7-37). The plane through the fulcrum or pivot point remains in focus, whereas structures that are above and below this plane are blurred by the motion of the tube and film. This plane is called the **objective plane** or tomographic section. The fulcrum level determines the level of the objective plane and is measured from the radiographic tabletop upward. For example, a 5-cm tomographic section means that the objective plane is 5 cm above the tabletop. The thickness of the tomographic section is determined by the tomographic angle. This is the angle between the central ray at the beginning of the exposure and at the end of the exposure. The greater

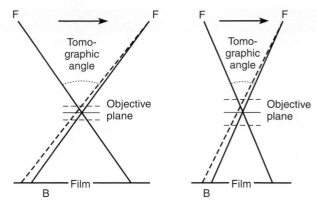

FIGURE 7-38 Effect of tomographic angle on section thickness.

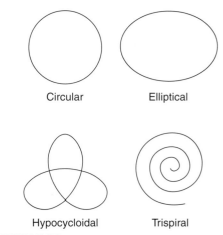

FIGURE 7-39 Pluridirectional tomographic patterns.

the tomographic angle, the thinner the tomographic section because of the greater motion of the tube and film (Fig. 7-38).

In **pluridirectional tomography** the x-ray tube and film move in a variety of patterns such as circular, elliptical, hypocycloidal, and trispiral (Fig. 7-39). These units produce sharper images than rectilinear units because of the increased motion of the tube and film. Because of this complexity of motion, pluridirectional units usually are dedicated to only tomographic imaging. This has limited their use on a widespread basis because most radiology departments cannot afford to have a room dedicated solely to this type of unit, with a relatively small number of patients who might benefit.

Quality Control of Tomographic Systems

Because tomography involves motion of the x-ray tube and image receptor, considerable variation can occur in the performance of these systems with age and use. Mechanical instabilities can manifest in the tube system as a result of the large mass of the x-ray tube and housing. This manifestation can cause inconsistencies in the exposure and asymmetry in tube motion and can lead to poor image quality; therefore, specific quality control

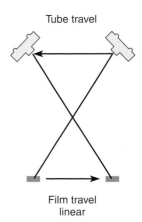

FIGURE 7-37 Principle of linear tomography.

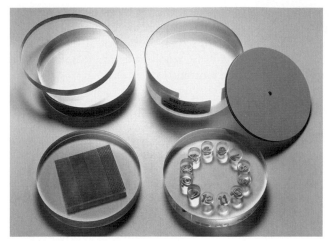

FIGURE 7-40 Tomographic test tool. *(Courtesy Gammex/RMI, Middleton, Wis.)*

tests should be performed on acceptance and then annually. Specialized test tools and phantoms should be used for these evaluations (Fig. 7-40). Factors to evaluate include section level, section thickness, level incrementation, exposure angle, spatial resolution, section uniformity and beam path, and patient exposure.

Section Level

G *The level of the tomographic section (fulcrum level) that is indicated on the equipment and the actual level of the tomographic section that is imaged above the tabletop should be the same or within ± 5 mm (some manufacturers suggest ± 1 mm for pluridirectional units).* Evaluation is made with a test tool that has a series of lead numbers at various depths that are imaged on the image receptor (Fig. 7-41). A tomographic exposure is made of the test tools at various fulcrum levels. The resulting image is then analyzed for the appearance

of the number that appears the sharpest. For example, if the fulcrum for the exposure is set for 5 cm, the number 5 should be the sharpest number visible.

Section Thickness

The thickness of the tomographic section depends on the tomographic angle. Table 7-4 lists the section thickness at various tomographic angles. Evaluation is made with a special test tool according to the manufacturer's instructions (Fig. 7-42).

TABLE 7-4	Section Thickness at Various Tomographic Angles
Tomographic Angle (Degrees)	**Section Thickness (mm)**
50	1.1
40	1.4
30	2
10	6
5	11
0	—

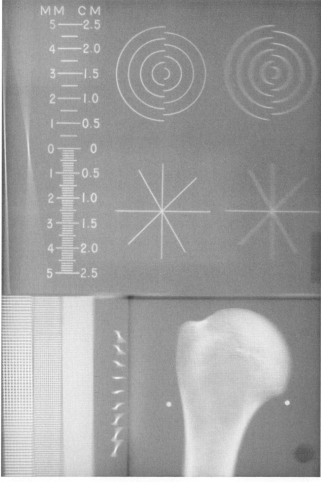

FIGURE 7-42 Multipurpose tomographic test tool with section thickness ruler.

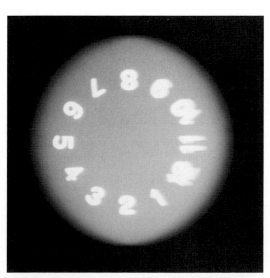

FIGURE 7-41 Image from tomographic test tool indicating the level of tomographic section.

Level Incrementation

All tomographic units have some type of ruler or other device to indicate the level of the tomographic section. ❻ *A ruler should be constructed so that changing from one tomographic section to the next is accurate to within ±2 mm.* Evaluation can be accomplished with the same test phantom and procedure used in section level determination.

Exposure Angle

The exposure angle determines the thickness of the tomographic section. ❻ *It is important that the value indicated on the equipment and the actual angle is the same or within ± 5 degrees for units operating at angles greater than 30 degrees.* For exposure angles less than 30 degrees, the maximum variation allowed is ± 2 degrees. Accurate measurement of this variable is difficult and is best accomplished by evaluating the section thickness with the appropriate phantom. Variations in section thickness are usually the result of improper exposure angles.

Spatial Resolution

Spatial resolution in tomographic imaging is the ability of the tomographic system to resolve objects within the tomographic section. The structures within the tomographic section must be demonstrated with sufficient spatial resolution to make an accurate diagnosis possible. Figure 7-43 shows an image of a tomographic resolution test tool with wire mesh patterns of 20 holes per inch (0.8 holes per millimeter), 30 holes per inch (1.2 holes per millimeter), 40 holes per inch

(1.6 holes per millimeter), and 50 holes per inch (2 holes per millimeter). Most tomographic units should be able to resolve a mesh screen pattern of at least 40 holes per inch. Variations in resolution are usually due to asymmetry in tube motion.

Section Uniformity and Beam Path

The amount of radiation emitted should be consistent throughout the tomographic exposure so that the optical density of the image is uniform. This can be evaluated with a test tool consisting of a lead aperture (Fig. 7-44). When an exposure is made on a linear tomographic unit, a thin line should appear on the resulting image (Fig. 7-45). Optical density readings should be taken throughout the line and compared. ❻ *Any variation should be within an optical density value of ± 0.3.* This

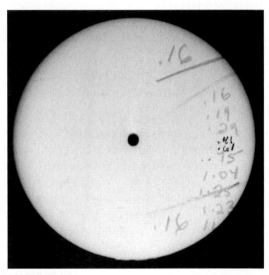

FIGURE 7-44 Lead aperture of tomographic test tool.

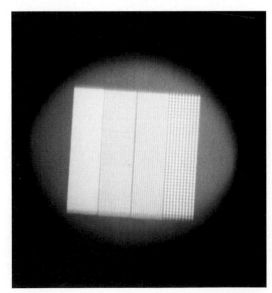

FIGURE 7-43 Image from tomographic test tool indicating the resolution pattern.

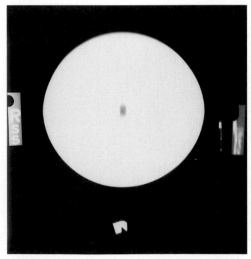

FIGURE 7-45 Image of lead aperture with linear tomography.

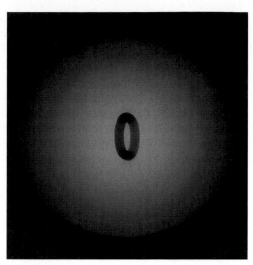

FIGURE 7-46 Image of lead aperture with elliptical motion. *(Courtesy Central DuPage Hospital, Winfield, Ill.)*

same device also can be used for evaluation of beam path. Any asymmetry in motion or inconsistencies in the exposure could alter the normal shape of the beam path. Linear units should demonstrate a straight line, as shown in Figure 7-45. Pluridirectional units should create images that are appropriate to the pattern selected. Figure 7-46 shows an image created with an elliptical pattern. ❻ *Path closure in pluridirectional units should be within ± 10% of the path length.*

PROCEDURE

1. Using either an abdomen or skull phantom, make a nontomographic exposure with an appropriately sized image receptor and the kVp and mAs specified for your particular unit. If CR is used, set the preprocessing image data recognition to fixed mode (the CR image receptor acts like a film/screen cassette).
2. Using the same phantom, make a tomographic image at the same kVp and appropriate mAs specified for your particular unit.
3. Process the images and use a densitometer to obtain density readings of the same anatomic structure from each image (e.g., middle of the L4 vertebra and middle of the sella turcica). For CR images, print a hard copy of the image using a dry laser printer. The readings should be the same or within an optical density value of ± 0.1.
4. If the optical density readings are similar, compare the mAs values used for each exposure. The tomographic exposure should not be more than double the mAs required for the nontomographic exposure.

Patient Exposure

As the x-ray tube and film move in opposite directions during tomography, different patient thicknesses exist at various points within the exposure; therefore, the mAs is greater during conventional tomography than with conventional radiography of the same view.

The tomographic exposure should not exceed two times the nontomographic exposure for the same part. For example, if 50 mAs is required for an anteroposterior (AP) projection of the kidneys, an AP tomographic cut of the same kidneys should be obtained at 100 mAs or less. For departments equipped with more than one tomographic unit, patient exposure should not vary by more than 20% if the units have comparable x-ray tubes and generators. Evaluation can be made by exposing an abdomen or skull phantom to create both tomographic and nontomographic images.

Grids

The grid is the most common device for controlling scattered radiation (assuming collimation to the appropriate field size has been performed). Improper use of a grid can cause grid cutoff (resulting in an underexposed radiograph) or grid artifacts (e.g., grid lines and moiré patterns). These artifacts are discussed in detail in Chapter 10. Grid artifacts also can occur because of imperfections during the manufacturing process or mishandling during clinical use (dropping the grid). Barium or other contrast media also can create artifacts and must be removed. The grid variables that need to be evaluated are grid uniformity and grid alignment, which should occur on acceptance and then annually.

Grid Uniformity

All of the lead strips in the grid must be uniformly spaced or a mottling effect may appear in the image, which can mimic a pathologic condition. Nonuniformity can occur from manufacturing defects or by dropping a grid on its edges. For evaluation of **grid uniformity,** the following procedure may be used.

PROCEDURE

1. Place an image receptor under a grid and make an image of a homogenous phantom (made of either aluminum Lucite or a pan of water), using a kVp comparable for use with the grid ratio and enough mAs to create an optical density of 1.5.
2. After processing, take optical density readings of the center and the four quadrants (and any suspicious areas) of the image and compare. ❻ *All density readings should be within an optical density value of ± 0.10 for proper uniformity.* Stationary grids on grid cassettes may require more frequent evaluation.

Grid Alignment

Grids that are misaligned attenuate more of the primary x-ray beam, and this attenuation results in a loss of image quality and higher patient dosage. Proper alignment refers to the centering of the x-ray field with the focused grid and the maintaining of proper grid focusing

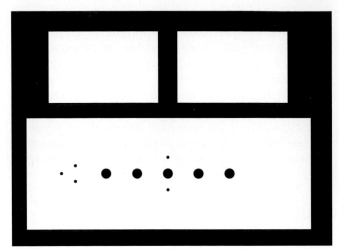

FIGURE 7-47 Grid alignment tool. *(Courtesy Nuclear Associates, Carle Place, N.Y.)*

distance. Grid focusing distance is the proper distance from the x-ray source that a focused grid can be used (because the angle of the lead strips in the grid and the angle of divergence of the x-ray photons being emitted only match at a specific range of distance values). Alignment is more critical with higher grid ratios such as 10:1, 12:1, and 16:1 because grid latitude is less. **Grid latitude** is the margin of error in centering the x-ray beam to the center of the grid before significant grid cut-off appears in the resulting image. The alignment must be within the grid latitude specified by the manufacturer (usually within 1 inch). The grid latitude value can be found either on the grid front or with the literature supplied by the manufacturer. A grid alignment tool is commercially available (Fig. 7-47) and should be used according to the manufacturer's specifications.

PORTABLE AND MOBILE X-RAY GENERATORS

Many radiographic examinations must be performed with mobile x-ray generators in hospitals and medical centers because the patients' conditions may prevent them from being transported to the main x-ray department. Most of the variables mentioned in earlier in this

chapter such as reproducibility, linearity, and focal spot size, can be tested with the same test tools and procedures used for standard radiographic equipment. Testing should occur on acceptance and then annually or when service is performed. Electrical safety and grounding are critical for safe operation of mobile equipment. A policy also must be in place regarding the storage of the keys that are required to operate this equipment. Federal and state regulations prohibit leaving keys in mobile equipment when this equipment is not in use and stored in a public area. This is a safety indicator of TJC. Some type of lockbox with a combination lock, a key storage area within the radiology department, and a key allotment policy for radiographers are just some of the possible ways to address this concern. A distinction should be made between portable and mobile x-ray generators.

Portable X-Ray Generator

A **portable x-ray generator** is small enough to be carried from place to place by one person. It consists of an oil-filled metal tank or casing that contains a stationary anode x-ray tube and transformers. A smaller control unit, containing the exposure switch and timer circuitry, attaches to the casing by means of a 6-foot (1.8-m) cord. A metal stand or tripod holds the casing in place. The maximum output for portable units is 75 kVp and 15 mA, so use is generally confined to chest and extremity examinations in nursing homes, to battlefield use by the military, and to field veterinary use.

Mobile X-Ray Generator

A **mobile x-ray generator** is a smaller version of a radiographic unit that is mounted on wheels and pushed from one location to the next. Mobile units are most often found in hospitals for the examination of patients who are too ill or injured to be taken to the main radiology department. Often, mobile units are mistakenly called "portables." There are several types of mobile x-ray generators (Table 7-5).

Direct-Power Units. Direct-power units are usually equipped with stationary anode x-ray tubes and have a

TABLE 7-5	Comparison of Mobile Radiographic Units		
Direct Power	**Capacitor/Discharge**	**Battery Powered**	**High Frequency**
Single-phase output	Constant potential (x-ray production constant)	Constant potential (x-ray production constant)	Constant potential (x-ray production constant)
Limit of 15 mA	Limited to short exposure time	Unit is relatively large and heavy	Unit is small and lightweight
Subject to power fluctuations	No power fluctuation	No power fluctuation while battery is being charged	High kVp and mAs available
Requires standard outlet in immediate area of operation	Requires standard outlet in immediate area of operation	No need for outlet in immediate area of operation	Requires standard outlet in immediate area of operation

kVp, Kilovolt (peak); *mAs,* milliampere-second.

plug that is placed into a standard 110/120-volt (V) outlet. The maximum output for most of these units is 100 kVp and 15 mA. These units are subject to power fluctuations in line voltage.

Capacitor Discharge Units. Capacitor discharge units are equipped with a high-tension capacitor that must be precharged before each exposure. In order for the unit to operate properly, it must be plugged into the main power supply, and the appropriate kVp and mAs are selected. A charge button is then activated on the control panel, which allows the capacitor to charge up to the selected value. This normally takes about 10 seconds. A green light indicates a full charge. The x-ray exposure should be made immediately after the indicator light appears because the charge on the capacitor begins to leak. If the kVp drops below 2 kVp of the selected value, the green light deactivates and no exposure can be made until the unit is recharged. Because the voltage drops during the exposure (at about 1 kV/mAs), the exposure time should be kept short in order to keep the kVp at the desired level. This effect also makes testing for kVp variation difficult for these units; therefore an average kVp per mAs value should be established on acceptance and then maintained throughout the life of the unit. ❻ *Any variation of the kVp/mAs value must be within ± 5%. X-ray output is constant, much like that of a three-phase or high-frequency x-ray generator.*

Cordless, or Battery-Powered, Mobile Units. Cordless, or battery-powered, mobile units use a series of lead or nickel-cadmium wet-cell batteries (usually three) that must be kept charged when the unit is not in use (with a built-in charger that is plugged into the main power supply). The batteries are used to power a drive motor that propels the unit and a polyphase electric generator that produces the electric current that energizes the x-ray tube. These units can usually attain a maximum output of 100 kVp and 25 mA, with a constant x-ray output. The batteries should be removed from the unit, cleaned, completely discharged, and then recharged every 6 months to maintain a continued optimum charge.

High-Frequency Mobile Units. Like their large counterparts, these mobile units are equipped with a microprocessor circuit that increases the frequency of the alternating current to create a nearly constant potential. They are plugged into a standard outlet and can achieve up to 133 kVp and 200 mAs with a minimum exposure time of 3 ms.

SUMMARY

Through visual inspections, environmental inspections, and performance testing, variation in the functioning of radiographic equipment can be kept to a minimum. This should increase department efficiency, lower the repeat rate, and reduce unnecessary exposure. In addition, ancillary equipment used in conjunction with radiographic units must function within specific parameters to obtain consistent and acceptable quality images. Therefore, quality control testing also is required to monitor this level of performance.

Refer to the Evolve website at https://evolve.elsevier. com for Student Experiments 7.1: Radiographic Unit Visual Check; 7.2: Half-Value Layer Measurement and Filtration; 7.3: Milliampere and Exposure Time Linearity; 7.4: Reproducibility, Milliampere-Second Reciprocity, and Milliroentgen per Milliampere-Second; and 7.5: Collimation, Beam Alignment, and Perpendicularity; 7.6: Automatic Exposure Control Reproducibility; 7.7: Automatic Exposure Control and Patient Positioning; and 7.8: Grid Alignment.

REVIEW QUESTIONS

1. The indicated level of the tomographic section and the actual level of the section must correspond to within ± _____ mm.
   a. 2
   b. 5
   c. 10
   d. 15

2. A three-phase x-ray generator can operate at a maximum of 100 kVp and 500 mA at 100 ms. What is the kilowatt rating of this generator?
   a. 5 kW
   b. 35 kW
   c. 50 kW
   d. 500 kW

3. The backup timer for an AEC system should terminate the exposure at _____ second(s) or _____ mAs, whichever comes first.
   a. 1; 100
   b. 3; 300
   c. 6; 600
   d. 9; 900

4. How large of an arc appears during a spinning top test of a three-phase x-ray generator at 50 ms?
   a. 18 degrees
   b. 20 degrees
   c. 36 degrees
   d. 90 degrees

5. A quality control program for radiographic equipment should include (1) visual inspection, (2) environmental inspection, or (3) performance testing:
   a. 1 and 2 only
   b. 2 and 3 only
   c. 1 and 3 only
   d. 1, 2, and 3

6. The minimum HVL for x-ray units operating at 80 kVp is _____ mm of aluminum.
   a. 1.3
   b. 1.5
   c. 2.3
   d. 2.5

7. The maximum variability allowed for the reproducibility of exposure is ± _____ %.
   a. 2
   b. 5
   c. 10
   d. 20

8. Any variations between the stated kilovolt (peak) on the control panel and the measured kilovolt (peak) must be ± _____ %.
   a. 2
   b. 5
   c. 10
   d. 20

9. The variability allowed for timer accuracy in exposures less than 10 ms is ± _____ %.
   a. 2
   b. 5
   c. 10
   d. 20

10. The variability allowed for mA and time linearity is ± _____ %.
    a. 2
    b. 5
    c. 10
    d. 20

Quality Control of Fluoroscopic Equipment

OBJECTIVES

At the completion of this chapter the reader should be able to do the following:

- List the main components of a modern fluoroscopic system
- Discuss how the brightness of fluoroscopic images is maintained
- Describe the various methods of monitoring fluoroscopic images
- Perform visual and environmental inspections of a fluoroscopic system
- List and describe the performance tests for fluoroscopic equipment

OUTLINE

Fluoroscopic imaging is widely used in radiology to visualize the dynamics of internal structures and fluids. The image produced is a dynamic, or real-time, image compared with conventional radiography, which creates a static image. Because of the real-time image created, fluoroscopy is widely used for gastrointestinal (GI) studies, vascular and cardiac studies, and interventional procedures. Many of these studies and procedures involve a considerable length of x-ray exposure time for the patient. For this reason, fluoroscopy is considered the principle source of medical radiation to the population of the United States. In particular, upper GI tract fluoroscopy is the most commonly conducted fluoroscopic procedure in the United States and contributes the highest effective dose to the U.S. population.

Strict quality control guidelines and protocols should be in place to minimize variation in equipment performance so that the patient's dose is as low as possible. Federal guidelines for fluoroscopic equipment can be found in Title 21 of the Code of Federal Regulations Part 1020 (21 CFR 1020) subchapter J, which uses input from the American College of Radiology (ACR), the American Association of Physicists in Medicine (AAPM), and various other groups. Many states have or will be adopting fluoroscopic protocols developed by the NEXT (Nationwide Evaluation of X-Ray Trends) committee of the Conference of Radiation Control Program Directors (CRCPD). This chapter contains many of the mentioned guidelines and protocols, but regulations in the state of practice also must be checked.

INTRODUCTION TO FLUOROSCOPIC EQUIPMENT

The three main parts of a typical fluoroscopic unit are the x-ray tube and generator, the image intensifier, and the video monitoring system. The x-ray generators in modern fluoroscopic units are either three-phase or high-frequency units, for maximum efficiency. Fluoroscopic units equipped with cinefluorography require fast exposure times, on the order of 5 to 6 ms for a framing rate of 48 frames per second; therefore, the x-ray generators must offer a high output, that is, a 130- to 200-kilowatt (kW) power rating. The x-ray tubes are usually higher-capacity tubes (at least 500,000 heat units) compared with general radiographic tubes (about 300,000 heat units). The x-ray tube and generator generally must perform according to the same standards as radiographic units and are evaluated in a similar way. Factors such as filtration (half-value layer [HVL]), focal spot size, x-ray tube heat sensors, overload protection, kilovolt (peak) (kVp) accuracy, reproducibility, linearity, output waveforms, automatic exposure control (AEC) (for spot film devices), and grid uniformity and alignment all should be tested at least every 6 months with the methods and test tools discussed in previous chapters.

Image Intensifiers

Components. Most fluoroscopic systems use image intensifiers, which electronically brighten the image obtained during fluoroscopy by converting a low-intensity, full-size image into a high-intensity minified image. This type of device was first developed in 1948 by Coltman, who used technology similar to an electron microscope (Fig. 8-1). An alternative to the image intensifier is the flat plate sensor used in some direct-to-digital fluoroscopic systems, which is discussed in Chapter 9. The essential parts of an image intensifier are the glass envelope, input phosphor, photocathode, electrostatic focusing lenses, anode, and output phosphor.

Glass Envelope. A conventional **image intensifier** is a vacuum tube that allows the free flow of electrons from one side of the device (photocathode) to the other (anode). The glass envelope is necessary to contain this powerful vacuum, which can experience as much as a ton of force from the outside air pressure pushing

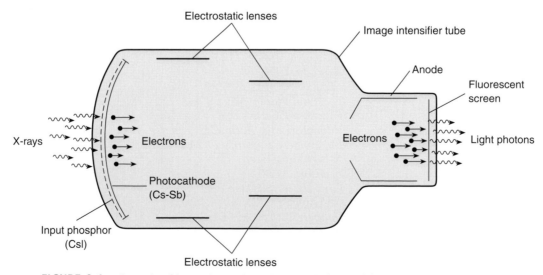

FIGURE 8-1 Schematic of image intensifier tube. *CsI*, Cesium iodide; *Cs-Sb*, cesium antimony.

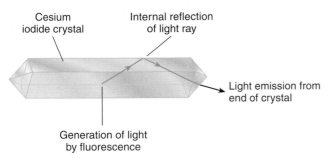

Cesium iodide crystal

Internal reflection of light ray

Light emission from end of crystal

Generation of light by fluorescence

FIGURE 8-2 Cesium iodide light pipe.

against it. Breakdown of the vacuum integrity is the usual cause of limited life of the image intensifier.

Input Phosphor. On entry into the image intensifier, the x-rays strike the input phosphor, which absorbs them and converts their energy into visible light. The image intensifier ranges in diameter from 6 inches to 16 inches (15 to 40 cm) and is curved to maintain an equal distance between all points on the input and output phosphors. An input phosphor consists of either a glass or thin aluminum base (used in most newer input phosphors) with a coating of sodium-activated cesium iodide crystals placed in a layer from 0.1 to 0.2 mm thick. The crystals form long, needle-like shapes that act as light pipes to emit light with minimal divergence (Fig. 8-2). The light emitted has a wavelength of about 4200 angstroms (Å) (420 nanometers [nm]), which places it in the blue portion of the color spectrum.

Photocathode. Light photons from the input phosphor immediately strike the photocathode, which is a thin layer of antimony and cesium compounds. The light photons release electrons from the photocathode through the process of **photoemission**.

Electrostatic Focusing Lenses. Electrostatic focusing lenses are positively charged metal plates that focus and accelerate the electrons as they travel toward the output phosphor.

Anode. The anode is a positively charged electrode that attracts the electrons toward the output phosphor. The potential difference between the anode and photocathode is 25 to 35 kilovolt (kV).

Output Phosphor. Output phosphor is usually a piece of glass or aluminum about 1 inch (2.54 cm) in diameter and coated with a thin layer (4 to 8 μm) of zinc cadmium sulfide (also known as *P20*). When electrons from the photocathode strike these crystals, light is emitted with wavelengths between 5000 and 6500 Å (500 to 650 nm), which places it in the yellow-green portion of the color spectrum. Because the light is placed in the approximate center of the visible light spectrum, video cameras (and the human eye) can easily detect this light.

Image Brightness. The image intensifier increases the brightness of the image by the following two processes:

- The image from the larger input phosphor is condensed onto the smaller output phosphor. Because the image is emitted from a smaller area, it appears to be brighter. This increase in brightness is known as

minification gain and can be calculated with the following equation:

$$\text{Minification Gain} = \frac{\text{Input diameter}^2}{\text{Output diameter}^2}$$

- A high voltage accelerates the electrons from the photocathode, and their kinetic energy is increased, releasing many times more light photons from the output phosphor surface. This increase in brightness is known as the **flux gain**. At 25 kV, one electron incident on the output phosphor releases 50 light photons. The flux gain is then considered 50 times.

The total **brightness gain** is determined by multiplying the minification gain by the flux gain. Brightness gain may be referred to as the amount of brightness of an image-intensified image versus a non-image-intensified fluoroscopic image. The brightness level of a fluoroscopic image is affected by milliampere (mA), kVp, automatic brightness control (ABC), variable tube current, and variable pulse width, as shown in Box 8-1.

BOX 8-1 | **Factors Affecting the Brightness of Fluoroscopic Images**

Milliampere
An increase in the fluoroscopic x-ray tube mA multiplies the number of x-ray photons incident on the image intensifier, and therefore image brightness increases.

Kilovolt (Peak)
An increase in the fluoroscopic x-ray tube potential difference multiplies the number of x-ray photons reaching the image intensifier; also, image brightness increases.

Patient Thickness and Tissue Density
An increase in these factors reduces the number of x-ray photons reaching the image intensifier, thereby decreasing the image brightness.

Automatic Brightness Control or Automatic Brightness Stabilization
Automatic brightness control (ABC), or **automatic brightness stabilization** (ABS), allows the fluoroscopic unit to automatically maintain the brightness level of the image for variations of patient thickness and attenuation. This can be accomplished by one of the following three methods, depending on the manufacturer.

- *Variable kVp.* Variable kVp systems use a motor-driven autotransformer that varies the kVp in response to image brightness-sensing electrodes. These electrodes can monitor the output phosphor directly or use a signal generated by a video camera. This method can cover a wide range of patient thicknesses. However, it is slow, and the images may demonstrate quantum noise and low image contrast at high kVp values.
- *Variable tube current.* This system varies the mA or tube current in response to image brightness-sensing electrodes. This requires a large-capacity x-ray generator.
- *Variable pulse width.* In the variable pulse width method, the x-ray output is pulsed with a grid-controlled x-ray tube at a sequence rapid enough to avoid image flicker. A faster-pulsing sequence is selected by the equipment to increase fluoroscopic image brightness and vice versa.

Multifield Image Intensifiers. The **multifield image intensifier** allows the fluoroscopic image to be magnified electronically. This is accomplished by changing the voltage on the electrostatic focusing lenses, which decreases the amount of the input phosphor image sent to the output phosphor. The resulting image is then magnified (Fig. 8-3). Because the minification gain becomes decreased, the mA must be increased to maintain image brightness. This results in a significantly increased patient dose. Another disadvantage is that the field of view is decreased. This type of image intensifier is used in digital fluoroscopic units and interventional, vascular, and cardiac studies.

The two basic types of multifield image intensifiers are dual focus and trifocus.

Dual Focus. The dual focus multifield image intensifier allows for a choice of two different fields of view to be used. The most common dual focus option is called the 9/6, which means that the input phosphor can vary from a 9-inch diameter for a normal field of view to a 6-inch diameter for a magnified field of view (also called 23/15 for centimeter diameter measurement).

Trifocus. The trifocus option allows the user a choice of three input phosphor diameters, the most common of which is the 10/7/5 (in inches) or the 25/18/12 (in centimeters).

Image Intensifier Artifacts. The use of image intensifiers in fluoroscopic systems may lead to five basic types of artifacts.

Veiling Glare, or Flare. Veiling glare, or flare, is caused by light being reflected from the window of the output phosphor, which reduces image contrast. This most often occurs when moving from one portion of the patient's anatomy to another (such as when imaging the chest and moving down into the abdominal area), causing a sudden increase in image brightness. Most manufacturers incorporate designs to reduce veiling glare to minimize this effect.

Pincushion Distortion. Pincushion distortion is caused by projecting an image from a curved surface (input phosphor) onto a flat surface (output phosphor). This effect is similar to that of a carnival mirror that distorts appearance and is greater toward the lateral portions of the image. With pincushion distortion, magnification increases toward the periphery (Fig. 8-4).

Barrel Distortion. Barrel distortion is similar to pincushion and is caused again by projecting from a curved surface to a flat one (or vice versa), but magnification will be reduced toward the periphery (also seen in Fig. 8-4).

Vignetting. Vignetting is a decrease in image brightness at the lateral portions of the image and is caused by

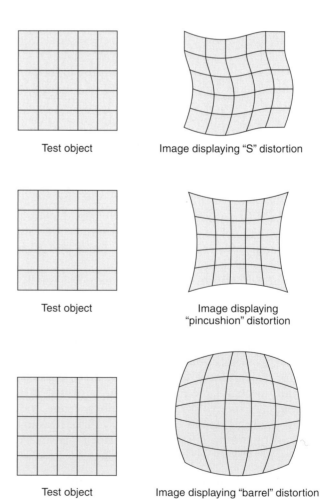

Test object — Image displaying "S" distortion

Test object — Image displaying "pincushion" distortion

Test object — Image displaying "barrel" distortion

FIGURE 8-4 S, pincushion, and barrel distortion.

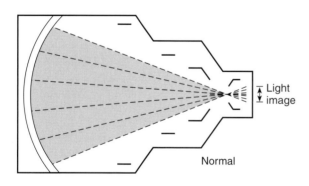
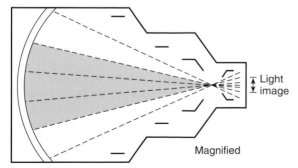

FIGURE 8-3 Multifield image intensifier showing normal and magnification modes.

a combination of pincushion distortion and the coupling of the television camera to the output phosphor.

S Distortion. An **S distortion** artifact is a warping of the image along an S-shaped axis and is the result of strong magnetic fields changing the trajectory of the electrons moving across the image intensifier tube.

Image Monitoring Systems

Because the output phosphor is only 1 inch (2.54 cm) in diameter, the image projected is relatively small and must therefore be magnified and monitored by an additional system. The main methods used include mirror optics, closed-circuit television (CCTV) monitoring, cinefluorography, photofluorospot, and film/screen spot devices.

Mirror Optics. Mirror optics is the oldest method of monitoring the image from an image intensifier. It uses a system of mirrors and lenses. The final image is projected onto a 6-inch-diameter mirror mounted on the side of the image intensifier tower. The field of view is small, so only one person can view the image at a time. Image resolution of this system is 3 to 4 line pairs per millimeter (lp/mm). This method is rarely used today.

Closed-Circuit Television Monitoring. CCTV is the most common method for monitoring the fluoroscopic image. A television camera is focused onto the output phosphor and then displayed on a monitor. The components necessary for television monitoring are a television camera, linkage from the camera to the output phosphor, and a television monitor.

Television Camera. The television camera converts visible light images into electronic signals. Four basic types of television cameras have been in use over the years, namely, the orthicon, plumbicon, vidicon, and charge-coupled device.

Orthicon. The **image-orthicon** is the largest and most sensitive type of television camera and functions as both an image intensifier and a television pick-up tube. Image quality is excellent and is completely free of lag; however, it is expensive, extremely sensitive to temperature changes, and requires a long warm-up time (Fig. 8-5).

Plumbicon. The **plumbicon** camera uses lead oxide as the target phosphor and is often used in digital fluoroscopy because of its short lag time.

Vidicon. The **vidicon** camera is currently the most common type of video camera in fluoroscopic systems. Target material in the camera is antimony trisulfide, which has a relatively long lag time (helpful in GI studies) to help reduce image noise.

Charge-Coupled Device. The **charge-coupled device** (CCD) does not use a photoconductive target inside of a glass tube to convert light images into electronic signals (as in the first three types of cameras). Instead, an array of several hundred thousand tiny (5 to 20 μm) photodiodes on a solid-state computer chip forms pixels to create the signal (Fig. 8-6). When light strikes these photodiodes, electrons are released in direct proportion to the amount of incident light. These electrons build up charges that form electronic pulses. These pulses then form the electronic video signal containing the image information. Most home video cameras use CCD technology, as do digital photographic cameras. More fluoroscopic units are being equipped with CCD cameras, a trend that should increase as the number of pixels increases (which increases resolution). The CCD cameras exhibit virtually no lag and very low electronic noise. They are also more sensitive than video tubes (meaning they can detect lower amounts of light) and have a much longer life than video camera tubes (because they do not have a heated cathode). The CCD cameras also consume less electrical power during operation than tube cameras (operating costs are lowered) and are not as fragile (because there is no glass envelope).

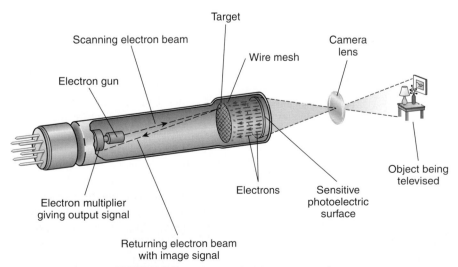

FIGURE 8-5 Orthicon television camera tube.

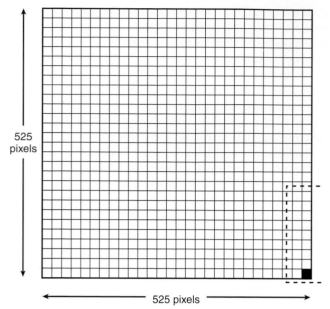

FIGURE 8-6 Representation of photodetector/pixel arrangement in charge-coupled device (CCD).

Linkage from the Television Camera to Output Phosphor. The television camera must be coupled, or linked, to the output phosphor so that image quality is maintained. This can be accomplished by one of two methods, fiber optics and lens coupling.

Fiber Optics. Fiber optics linkage uses flexible glass or plastic fibers, where the total internal reflection occurs (Fig. 8-7). This method is small in size, rugged, and relatively inexpensive but cannot accommodate auxiliary devices such as cine or spot film cameras.

Lens Coupling. The lens coupling method uses a system of lenses and mirrors to split the image so that auxiliary devices can view the image simultaneously with the television camera (Fig. 8-8).

Television Monitor. The television monitor uses a cathode-ray tube (CRT) to display the fluoroscopic image. The type of monitor in most fluoroscopic systems uses the Electronics Industries Association's RS-170 standard for closed-circuit black-and-white television, which uses 525 lines per frame, with 30 separate frames

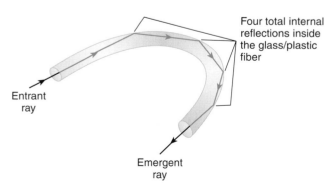

FIGURE 8-7 Principle of fiber optics.

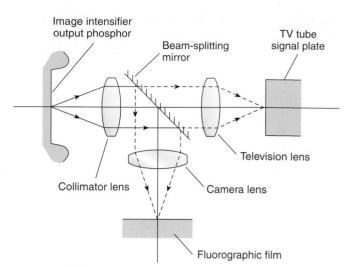

FIGURE 8-8 Split mirror for monitoring fluoroscopic images.

appearing each second, and an aspect ratio of 4:3. Standard monitors use a method called *interlaced horizontal scanning* to avoid flicker. This involves scanning the odd-numbered lines in the first half of the frame and the even-numbered lines during the second half, rather than all 525 at once. This type of monitor can resolve between 2 and 2.5 lp/mm. Noninterlaced, or progressive, scan monitors (which scan all lines in order and have a frame rate of 60 frames/sec) also are available and are used in most personal computer displays. These monitors are preferred in angiographic and interventional procedures because of their reduced flickering. High-resolution CRT monitors with up to 1023 lines per frame are available and demonstrate 2.5 to 5 lp/mm. Digital fluoroscopic systems also are beginning to incorporate high-resolution flat panel monitors in which a liquid crystal display (LCD) is used instead of a CRT. The next chapter contains a more complete discussion of viewing monitors. As high-definition television (HDTV) systems become more cost-effective, they will eventually replace current monitors.

Cinefluorography. With the **cinefluorography** method, a motion picture camera is used to monitor the image from the output phosphor. This high-speed motion picture camera records the image of fast-moving objects, and it is ideal for cardiac catheterization studies (95% of all cine studies involve cardiac studies). The film used is either 16 mm or, most often, 35 mm (98% of all cine studies) black-and-white motion picture film. The larger size yields better image quality but requires a higher patient dose. The camera is capable of recording framing frequencies of 7.5, 15, 30, 60, and 120 frames per second, depending on the motion of the object. The greater the framing frequency, the greater the ability to minimize motion in the resulting image. However, this also results in an increased patient dose. The x-ray beam is pulsed with a grid-controlled x-ray tube to match the framing frequency. Quality control tests on cine equipment are discussed in Chapter 9.

Photofluorospot, or Spot Film, Camera. The photo-fluorospot, or spot film, method uses a spot film camera that takes a static photograph of the fluoroscopic image with a lens-coupling device. The lens has a longer focal length than that of cine cameras to cover a larger film format. These cameras use 70-mm, 90-mm, 100-mm, or 105-mm roll or cut film sizes. The larger the film format, the better the image quality, but with a higher patient dose. The patient dose with this method is lower than that with film/screen spot filming, as is the cost of film and processing. Quality control tests on these cameras are discussed in Chapter 9.

Film/Screen Spot Film Devices. Film/screen spot film devices do not monitor the fluoroscopic image from the image intensifier but rather use the fluoroscopic x-ray tube to create a radiograph on a standard cassette. This cassette is routinely kept in a lead-shielded compartment until the spot film device is activated. It is then placed into the x-ray beam path behind a grid, and a field format is selected (e.g., 1 on 1, 2 on 1) (Fig. 8-9). The fluoroscopic x-ray tube is then changed from approximately 3 mA to as much as 1000 mA, and the exposure is made and then controlled with an AEC system. The images created with this method have a higher contrast and spatial resolution than photofluorospot images. Spot film devices are preferred for most angiographic procedures, air contrast GI examinations, endoscopic retrograde cholangiopancreatography (ERCP), arthrography, and sialography.

Digital Image Recorders. Digital image recorders now are being used in many fluoroscopic systems to view fluoroscopic images at a later time. These systems are discussed in Chapter 9.

QUALITY CONTROL OF FLUOROSCOPIC EQUIPMENT

The procedure for evaluation of fluoroscopic systems involves much of the same process as the evaluation of radiographic systems, with the components of visual inspection, environmental inspection, and performance testing.

Visual Inspection

A fluoroscopic system visual inspection should be performed at least every 6 months with the use of a checklist, by either a quality management technologist or a medical physicist. A sample checklist is found on the Evolve website. The following should be included in the checklist:

- *Fluoroscopic tower and table locks.* Manually operate all locks to verify function.
- *Power assist.* The tower should move smoothly over the tabletop when the power assist is activated.
- *Protective curtain.* A protective curtain or drape must be in place and move freely so that it can be

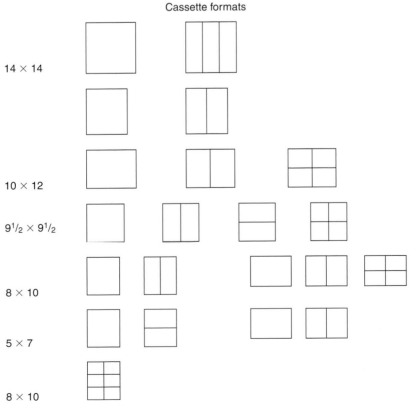

Cassette formats

14 × 14

10 × 12

9½ × 9½

8 × 10

5 × 7

8 × 10

FIGURE 8-9 Film/screen spot film formats.

placed between the patient and any personnel in the fluoroscopic room. This curtain must contain at least 0.25-mm lead equivalent, which should be verified on acceptance. This can be accomplished by exposing the lead curtain to 100-kVp x-rays and taking radiation measurements on either side. The reading behind the lead curtain should be about 50% of the input reading (because the HVL of lead at 100 kVp is 0.24 mm).

- *Bucky slot cover.* When the Potter-Bucky diaphragm is moved to the far end of the examination table, a metal cover should move in place and must attenuate to the equivalent of at least one tenth value layer (TVL) (about 0.5 mm of lead). Radiation readings should be taken on either side of the cover, with the amount outside of the cover being 10% of the input exposure, and should be verified on acceptance. Operation of the cover should be verified on each inspection.

- *Exposure switch.* Every fluoroscopic system exposure switch must be a dead-man type of switch, which requires continuous pressure for activation, and should be verified on acceptance. Subsequent visual inspections should focus on sticking or malfunction of this switch.

- *Fluoroscopic timer.* A 5-minute reset timer is required for monitoring the length of time that the fluoroscopic x-ray tube is energized. An audible signal should sound at the end of 5 minutes. The timer accuracy can be verified with a stopwatch.

- *Lights/meter function.* All indicator lights and meters should function as specified by the manufacturer.

- *Compression device, or spoon, observation.* The compression device, or spoon, should move easily and be free of any splatters of contrast media.

- *Park position interrupt.* When the tower is in the parked position, it should not be possible to energize the x-ray tube. This may be checked while wearing a lead apron and depressing the fluoroscopic exposure switch to see if the system is activated.

- *Primary protective barrier.* The entire cross section of the useful beam should be intercepted by a primary protective barrier at all source-to-image distances (SIDs). This is usually built into the tower assembly for units in which the image intensifier is above the x-ray table. ❻ *With the tower at the maximum SID and the shutters wide open, the exposure rate above the tower should not exceed 2 milliroentgen (mR)/hr (measured at 10 cm from any accessible surface of the fluoroscopic imaging assembly beyond the plane of the image receptor for every roentgen [R] per minute measured at tabletop [1020.32(a), 21 CFR Subchapter J]).* This can be evaluated by the use of a dosimeter with a homogenous phantom made of 15 cm of acrylic in place or with the shutters completely closed to protect the image intensifier. Moveable grids and

compression devices shall be removed from the useful beam during measurement.

- *Collimation shutters.* ❻ *When the adjustable collimators are fully open, the primary beam should be restricted to the diameter of the input phosphor and must be accurate to within ± 3% of the SID (1020.32 (b), 21 CFR Subchapter J).* For rectangular x-ray fields used with circular image receptors, the error alignment shall be determined along the length and width dimensions of the x-ray field that pass through the center of the visible area of the image receptor. Means shall be provided to permit further limitation of the field. Beam limiting devices manufactured after May 22, 1979, and incorporated in equipment with a variable SID and/or visible area of greater than 300 cm^2 shall be provided with means for stepless adjustment of the x-ray field. Equipment with a fixed SID and a visible area of 300 cm^2 or less shall be provided with either stepless adjustment of the x-ray field or with means to further limit the x-ray field size at the plane of the image receptor to 125 cm^2 or less. Stepless adjustment shall, at the greatest SID, provide continuous field sizes from the maximum obtainable to a field size of $5 \times 5 \text{ cm}$ or less. In addition, the primary beam should be aligned to the center of the image intensifier to within 2% of the SID. This can be verified with a commercially available fluoroscopic beam alignment test tool, consisting of ruler increments or a series of equally spaced holes, which is placed on the face of the image intensifier (Fig. 8-10). When the image is observed, the ruler markings or holes should indicate the size of the input phosphor that is being irradiated. If this is not available, a phantom can be imaged under the fluoroscope with the shutters fully open. When viewing the image on the monitor, a shutter tangent must be seen at all edges of the monitor at both the lowest and highest SID positions. For spot image devices, the total misalignment of the edges of the x-ray field with the respective edges of the selected portion of the image receptor along the length

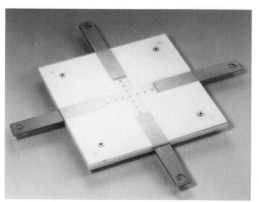

FIGURE 8-10 Fluoroscopic beam alignment device. (*Courtesy Nuclear Associates, Carle Place, N.Y.*)

or width dimensions of the x-ray field in the plane of the image receptor shall not exceed 3% of the SID when adjusted for full coverage of the selected portion of the image receptor. The sum without regard to sign of the misalignment along any two orthogonal dimensions shall not exceed 4% of the SID. It shall be possible to adjust the x-ray field size in the plane of the image receptor to a size smaller than the selected portion of the image receptor. The minimum field size, at the greatest SID, shall be equal to or less than 5×5 centimeters. The center of the x-ray field in the plane of the image receptor shall be aligned with the center of the selected portion of the image receptor to within 2% of the SID.

- *Monitor brightness.* A penetrometer should be placed on a homogenous phantom (6 to 10 inches of water in a plastic bucket, 15 cm of acrylic plastic [Lucite], or 1.5-inch-thick block of aluminum). The brightness and contrast controls on the monitor should be adjusted to show as many of the steps as possible.
- *Table angulation and motion.* The table should move freely to the upright position and stop at the appropriate spot. The table angle indicator and the actual table angle should coincide within 2 degrees.
- *Lead aprons and gloves.* Lead apparel should be exposed during remote fluoroscopy at 100 kVp, with the image observed on the television monitor for the presence of any cracks or irregularities. Otherwise, radiographs of the apron should be made to reduce operator exposure. This was discussed in detail in Chapter 7.

Environmental Inspection

Environmental inspections are essentially the same in fluoroscopic units as in radiographic units and should be performed at least every 6 months. Generally, these can be performed at the same time as the visual inspection of many of the items included on the checklist. The condition of high-tension cables and the mechanical condition of the image intensifier tower and table are especially important.

Performance Testing

As with radiographic units, performance testing of fluoroscopic units is critical to avoid variation in system performance. Many states have strict guidelines for fluoroscopic systems and mandate performance testing as a condition for granting the license to operate such equipment. Because of the potentially high patient dose in fluoroscopic procedures, these tests should be performed at least every 6 months (semiannually) or as indicated by state law. The fluoroscopic system should be tested in both the vertical and horizontal position if the system is capable of operation in both positions.

Reproducibility of Exposure

PROCEDURE

1. Place a homogenous phantom on the fluoroscopic tabletop and place a dosimeter between the phantom and the image intensifier input phosphor. Select the maximum mA and kVp available on the fluoroscopic unit.
2. Center the dosimeter probe to the center of the fluoroscopic x-ray beam. Depress the expose button for 10 seconds (use a stopwatch) and record the reading.
3. Clear the dosimeter and repeat this procedure twice.
4. Determine the mR/milliampere-second (mAs) ratio for each 10-second exposure of the dosimeter. Compare the readings and calculate the reproducibility variance using the equation from Chapter 7. **G** *The reproducibility variance must be less than 0.05 (5%).* Reproducibility outside of the accepted variance can result in fluctuations in image quality and patient dose and is most likely caused by problems with the x-ray generator or fluoroscopic x-ray tube.

Focal Spot Size

PROCEDURE

1. Place any one of the focal spot test tools described in Chapter 7 on top of a homogenous phantom that is on the tabletop and center to the fluoroscopic x-ray field. Set the fluoroscopic mA and kVp to the most commonly used settings.
2. Tape a nonscreen film to the bottom of the image intensifier tower and expose (you will probably need about 10 seconds of fluoroscopic exposure). If one is not available, use a high resolution computed radiography (CR) cassette with the preprocessing image data recognition set to fixed mode (CR acts like a film/screen cassette) and print a hard copy using a dry laser printer.
3. After the film is processed, calculate the focal spot size according to the instructions with the test tool. Focal spot blooming should conform to the guidelines of the National Electrical Manufacturers Association (NEMA) discussed in Chapter 7.

Filtration Check

PROCEDURE

1. Use the aluminum plates and a dosimeter to measure the HVL, using the same procedure described in Chapter 7 for radiographic systems. The dosimeter probe should be placed in a support stand that holds it halfway between the tabletop and the bottom of the image intensifier tower. Be sure to collimate to an area that is slightly smaller than the aluminum plates.
2. Because fluoroscopic kVp values are usually higher than those in radiography, the HVL should be determined with the most common kVp used for that unit. For example, if a particular fluoroscopic unit is used mostly for upper GI examinations at 100 kVp, then calculate the HVL for 100 kVp. Table 8-1 contains the HVL values for common fluoroscopic kVp. Filtration that is less than adequate increases the patient skin dose.

TABLE 8-1	Half-Value Layer Valves for Common Fluoroscopic Kilovolts (Peak)
Fluoroscopic kVp	Minimum HVL in mm of Aluminum
80	2.3
90	2.5
100	2.7
110	3
120	3.2
130	3.5
140	3.8
150	4.1

HVL, Half-value layer; *kVp*, kilovolt (peak).

Kilovolt (Peak) Accuracy

PROCEDURE

1. The digital kVp meter can be used as described in Chapter 7.
2. Place the kVp meter on the tabletop facing the direction of the x-ray tube and center to the fluoroscopic x-ray field. Set the fluoroscopic kVp to 80.
3. Expose the kVp meter for 2 seconds and record the reading. Repeat two more times.
4. Repeat the first two steps for the 90-, 100-, 110-, and 120-kVp stations.
5. Average the three meter readings for each kVp station and compare with the value selected on the control panel.
6. Calculate the kVp variance using the following equation:

$$kVp\ variance = \frac{(kVp_{max} - kVp_{min})}{(kVp_{max} + kVp_{min})}$$

7. The kVp variance should be less than or equal to 0.05. **ⓖ** *The measured* **kVp** *and the value indicated on the control should coincide within 65%.*

Milliampere Linearity. A dosimeter and stopwatch are used with a homogenous phantom in place.

PROCEDURE

1. With the dosimeter placed between the phantom and the image intensifier and centered to the fluoroscopic x-ray field, make a 10-second exposure at 0.5 mA.
2. Record the reading and calculate the mR/mAs values.
3. Repeat at 1 mA and then 2 mA (or all other fluoroscopic mA stations available on your particular fluoroscopic unit).
4. Determine the mR/mAs values for each mA station tested and then calculate the linearity variance from the following equation:

$$Linearity\ variance = \frac{(mR/mAs_{max} - mR/mAs_{min})}{(mR/mAs_{average})} \div 2$$

ⓖ *The linearity variance should be within 0.1 (10%).*

X-Ray Tube Heat Sensors. X-ray tube heat sensors can be tested with the same basic procedure used in Chapter 7, but with a stopwatch and a homogenous phantom to determine the exposure time.

PROCEDURE

1. Calculate the heat units for a 30-second exposure at the maximum fluoroscopic kilovolt (peak) and mA and compare these with the maximum tube limit stated in the manufacturer's specifications.
2. Now look at the light-emitting diode (LED) readout on the sensor to see if the values coincide. If necessary, continue fluoroscopy until 75% of the maximum is achieved to see if an alarm is activated. If the alarm is not activated, contact a service engineer.

Grid Uniformity and Alignment

PROCEDURE

Follow the same procedure as discussed in Chapter 7 for grid uniformity, using a spot film for evaluation.
1. For grid alignment, tape the test tool to the bottom of the image intensifier and image with a homogenous phantom in place.
2. Alignment is then determined according to the instructions with the test tool.

Voltage Waveform. An x-ray output detector can be attached to an oscilloscope, and the voltage waveform of the x-ray generator can be displayed, as discussed in Chapter 7.

Automatic Brightness Stabilization Systems. The automatic brightness stabilization (ABS) system should automatically adjust the technical parameters (kVp, mA, and pulse width) for changes in part thickness. A dosimeter and homogenous phantom of varying thickness should be in place.

PROCEDURE

1. Place the dosimeter between the phantom and the x-ray source, using a phantom of 7.5-cm-thick acrylic plastic (Lucite).
2. Expose for 10 seconds and record the reading.
3. Add another 7.5-cm thickness (15-cm total) and repeat. The dosimeter reading should be approximately double the 7.5-cm reading, if the system is functioning properly.

Automatic Gain Control. Some fluoroscopic systems are equipped with **automatic gain control** to maintain image brightness. These systems vary the gain of the video system rather than adjust the technical factors.

PROCEDURE

1. Place a dosimeter under the 7.5-cm homogenous phantom and expose for 10 seconds, watching the monitor for image brightness.
2. Repeat the procedure for a 15-cm thickness. The radiation readings and the image brightness should be the same for both exposures.

Maximum Entrance Exposure Rate. The maximum entrance exposure rate is the highest possible exposure rate that the fluoroscope system can deliver to the patient measured at tabletop for fluoroscopic tubes that are mounted under the table or where the beam enters the patient for fluoroscopic tubes mounted above the tabletop. ❻ *The intensity of the x-ray beam at tabletop should not exceed 10 R/min (2.6 mC $kg^{-1}min^{-1}$) for units equipped with ABS and 5 R/min (1.3 mC $kg^{-1}min^{-1}$) for units without ABS (1020.32(d), 21 CFR Subchapter J).*

The radiology departments in some states use a value known as air kerma rather than exposure or intensity to measure the amount of radiation entering the patient. **Kerma** is an acronym for **k**inetic **e**nergy **r**eleased in **matter,** and it measures the amount of kinetic energy that is released into particles of matter (such as electrons created during Compton and photoelectric interactions) from exposure to x-rays. Kerma may be measured in either rad or the SI unit gray (Gy). Air kerma is the kinetic energy released per unit mass of air. An exposure of 1 R corresponds to an air kerma of about 8.7 milligrays (mGy). For fluoroscopic systems, the air kerma rate is measured in air at the position where the center of the useful beam enters the patient (the probe position on the phantom of the Centers for Devices and Radiological Health [CDRH] is placed for air kerma measurement). According to standards of the Food and Drug Administration (FDA), the air kerma rate for all fluoroscopic units *should* be less than 5 centigray (cGy)/min or 5 rad/min and *shall* be less than 10 cGy/min (10 rad/min) unless a high level control is provided. For photofluorographic spot film cameras, the entrance kerma to the image intensifier at maximum tube potential and mA *should not* be greater than 0.0003 cGy (0.3 rad) per exposure. This limits the entrance kerma to the patient to about 0.1 cGy (0.1 rad) per exposure. For cinefluorography, the entrance kerma to the image intensifier *should not* be more than 0.3 microgray (μGy) (0.03 rad) per frame.

Magnification studies in which multifield image intensifiers (specially activated fluoroscopy) and high-level-control (HLC) fluoroscopy (also known as boost fluoroscopy), limit the maximum entrance exposure rate to 20 R/min when acquiring images without recording devices. The HLC fluoroscopy is an operating mode for fluoroscopic equipment where a higher exposure rate is produced. This allows for visualization of smaller and lower contrast objects that may not be seen during conventional fluoroscopy. The FDA and the CRCPD are investigating these studies, and possible limits may be forthcoming. These fluoroscopic units are required to have a separate exposure switch or pedal, and an audible sound must be emitted by the system when high-intensity fluoroscopy is delivered.

PROCEDURE

1. Place a dosimeter on the tabletop along with two, 3-mm-thick lead sheets that are placed in front of the image intensifier. For units in which the image intensifier is under the table and the x-ray tube is over the table (Fig. 8-11), the dosimeter should be placed 30 cm above the tabletop.
2. Expose for 30 seconds using the maximum kilovolt (peak) and mA available.
3. Record the dosimeter reading in roentgens (or C kg^{-1}) and multiply by 2 to obtain the roentgen per minute (or C $kg^{-1}min^{-1}$) value; compare with the previously mentioned limits.

Standard Entrance Exposure Rates. The Joint Commission (TJC) requires that standard or typical exposure rates be monitored because the maximum values do not represent typical usage. For this information to be obtained, a dosimeter, along with a CDRH fluoroscopic phantom, is recommended by both the ACR and the AAPM (Fig. 8-12). This phantom contains a 7-inch acrylic block to simulate tissue equivalence, along with lead and copper attenuators for air kerma measurement. It also contains an optional high- and low-contrast test pattern (discussed in the next section).

For photofluorospot cameras, the entrance exposure should be monitored with a dosimeter and a homogenous phantom at an exposure that creates an optical density between 0.8 and 1.2 on the resulting film. The exposure should be in the range of 50 to 200 microroentgens (μR) per image (13 to 52 nC kg^{-1} per image). For cine film exposures, the Inter-Society Commission for Heart Disease Resources (ICHD) recommends a minimum entrance exposure of 15 μR per frame (4 nC kg^{-1} frame^{-1}) for 9-inch-diameter (23-cm-diameter) image intensifiers and 35 μR per frame (9 nC kg^{-1} frame^{-1}) with the 6-inch (15-cm) mode.

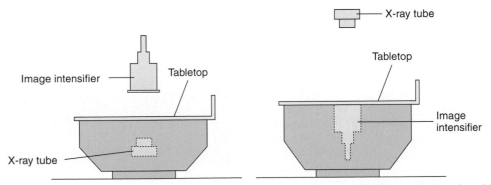

FIGURE 8-11 Diagram of fluoroscopic units with the image intensifier mounted above or below the tabletop.

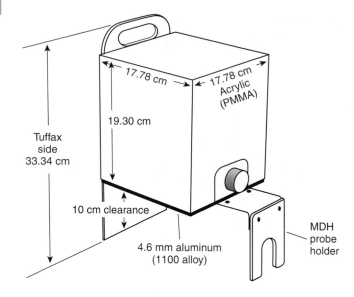

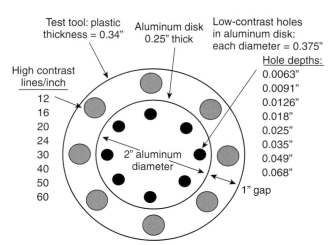

FIGURE 8-12 Fluoroscopic phantom of the Centers for Devices and Radiological Health (CDRH). *(Courtesy Centers for Devices and Radiological Health, Rockville, Md.)*

The standard entrance exposure rate should remain constant for a single room each time this test is performed (every 6 months). When different rooms are compared, any variation exceeding ± 25% should be investigated.

PROCEDURE

1. Place the phantom on the tabletop for tower image intensifiers or at 30 cm above the tabletop for image intensifiers mounted under the tabletop (Fig. 8-11). Be sure that the dosimeter probe is placed in the appropriate slot on the phantom.
2. The exposure should be made at the standard kilovolt (peak) and mA levels for that unit, for 30 seconds.
3. Record the reading in roentgen or mC kg^{-1} and multiply by 2 to determine the roentgen per minute or mC kg^{-1} min^{-1} value. Exposure values should range from 1 to 3 R/min (0.3 to 0.5 mC kg^{-1}min^{-1}) for typical use. Air kerma equivalent values are 8.7 to 26 mGy/min (0.87 to 2.6 rad/min). Grid exposures may be 1.5 to 2 times greater. With multifield image intensifiers, this procedure should be performed for each mode.

High-Contrast Resolution. **High-contrast resolution** is the ability to resolve small, thin, black-and-white areas and is a measure of spatial resolution. A test tool for high-contrast resolution consists of copper mesh patterns of 16, 20, 24, 30, 35, 40, 50, and 60 holes per inch (Fig. 8-13).

- Center and tape the test tool to the bottom of the image intensifier.
- Set the kVp to the lowest possible setting.
- Collimate the fluoroscopic x-ray beam to the size of the test tool and observe the image on the monitor.

An image intensifier with a 9-inch input phosphor should be able to resolve at least 20 to 24 holes per inch in the center of the image and 20 holes per inch at the edge when monitored with a CCTV system. With a 6-inch image intensifier, the center of the image should resolve a pattern of at least 30 holes per inch and at least 24 holes per inch at the edges. If a mirror optic system is present, rather than a CCTV system, the 9-inch mode should image at least 40 holes per inch in the center and 30 holes per inch at the edges; 6-inch systems should resolve at least 40 holes per inch in the center and 35 holes per inch at the edges.

The evaluation of high-contrast resolution of images created with spot film systems also can be performed with the same test tool.

- Follow steps 1 and 2 in the previous list.
- Obtain a spot film image with the spot film device present in your fluoroscopic system (e.g., cassette spot film, photofluorospot, cine).
- Process the image and evaluate the image of the test tool from the hard copy obtained.

Spot film images should demonstrate at least 40 holes per inch at the center and 30 holes per inch at the edge of the image. The Image Quality Test Object that is a

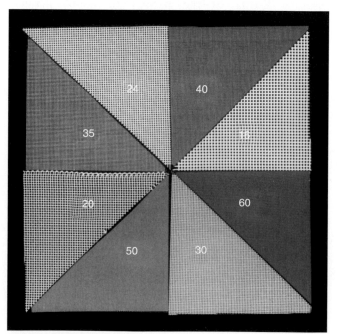

FIGURE 8-13 Image of fluoroscopic high-contrast resolution test tool.

part of the CDRH fluoroscopic phantom contains a high-contrast resolution test pattern that can be used with the listed procedures.

Low-Contrast Resolution. **Low-contrast resolution** is the ability to resolve relatively large objects that differ slightly in radiolucency from the surrounding area. A low-contrast resolution tool consists of two 1.9-cm-thick aluminum plates and a 0.8-mm aluminum sheet with two sets of holes of 1.5 mm, 3.1 mm, 4.7 mm, and 6.3 mm (Fig. 8-14). The Image Quality Test Object that is a part of the CDRH fluoroscopic phantom contains a low-contrast resolution test pattern consisting of a series of 0.375-inch-diameter holes in an aluminum disk. These holes range in depth from 0.0063 to 0.068 inch. This should create a subtle shade of gray beneath each hole in the resulting image.

> **PROCEDURE**
>
> 1. Place the low-contrast resolution test tool or CDRH fluoroscopic phantom between the focal spot and the image intensifier.
> 2. Expose at 100 kVp and observe the image on the monitor. With the low-contrast resolution test tool, the contrast between the holes and the surrounding area is 2%. All fluoroscopic systems should image the two largest holes clearly, and the third largest (3.1-mm) holes should just barely be visible. With the CDRH phantom, the three deepest holes should be visible. Better systems are able to visualize the smaller holes on the test tool or the shallower holes on the CDRH phantom.

Source–Skin Distance. The following are the minimum source–skin distances (SSD's) for fluoroscopic units established by the FDA (1020.31(i), 1020.32(g), 21 CFR Subchapter J):

Fixed or stationary units: 38 cm or 15 inches
Mobile units: 30 cm or 12 inches
Specialized units*: 20 cm or 8 inches

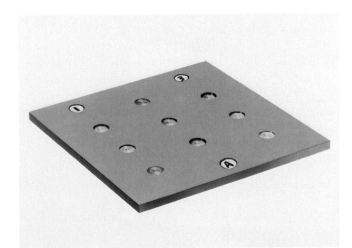

FIGURE 8-14 Low-contrast resolution rest tool. *(Courtesy Nuclear Associates, Carle Place, N.Y.)*

*An example is a handheld fluoroscopic unit of fluoroscopes intended for specific surgical application that would be prohibited at the source-skin distance specified.

In units in which the fluoroscopic x-ray tube is above the tabletop, a simple tape measure can be used to measure the SSD. For units in which the x-ray tube is under the table, two metal plates can be used, one 4 inches long and the other 2 inches long.

> **PROCEDURE**
>
> 1. The 4-inch plate is taped to the bottom of the image intensifier, and the 2-inch plate is placed on the tabletop. A homogenous phantom of 15-cm acrylic plastic (Lucite) is placed on top of the 2-inch plate to protect the image intensifier. The long axis of the two plates should be in the same direction, with both centered to the central ray of the x-ray beam.
> 2. During fluoroscopy, the height of the image intensifier should be adjusted until the outer edges of the plates coincide. Under these conditions, the distance between the tabletop and the 4-inch strip is equal to the target-to-tabletop distance (and therefore the SSD). An alternative is to use the similar triangle method discussed in Chapter 7. For mobile C-arm fluoroscopic units, a cone or spacer frame should be permanently attached to maintain a 12-inch or 30-cm SSD.

Distortion. A wire mesh pattern (similar to that used for film/screen contact) is taped to the bottom of the image intensifier, and a homogenous phantom is placed on the x-ray table. During fluoroscopy, the image of the wire mesh is observed for any signs of pincushion or S distortion (see Fig. 8-4). If any signs are present, consult a service engineer.

Image Lag. **Image lag** is defined as a continuation or persistence of the image and can blur objects as the image intensifier is moved over the patient. This can be evaluated by the following procedure.

> **PROCEDURE**
>
> 1. Place a metal washer with a ¼-inch (6-mm) hole (or lead diaphragm with a similar-sized hole) in the center of a homogenous phantom.
> 2. Perform fluoroscopy on the phantom while moving the image intensifier back and forth and observe the image for lag. Some amount of lag is inherent in the system, with vidicon camera tubes demonstrating more than the other types of cameras. *The maximum amount of lag should be less than 10% for cardiac, vascular, and interventional studies because a 0.014-inch moving guidewire must be visualized. For GI studies, lag times up to 20% are acceptable.* If excessive lag is present, a service engineer should be consulted to adjust the system or possibly replace the camera.

Image Noise. Most noise in fluoroscopic images results from either quantum mottle or electronic noise. To determine the specific nature of the noise, first observe the monitor with no fluoroscopic image. If noise is present, it is electronic in nature, and a service engineer should be contacted to correct the problem, usually by reducing the gain of the video amplifier. Once this is corrected, use the following procedure.

Relative Conversion Factor. The **relative conversion factor** measures the amount of light produced by the output phosphor per unit of x-radiation incident on the input phosphor. This can be measured in the following units:

$$\frac{Candela/m^2}{mR/sec} \quad or \quad \frac{Nit}{\mu C\ kg^{-1}sec^{-1}}$$

A dosimeter measures the amount of x-radiation at the entrance to the input phosphor, and a photographic light meter measures the light emitted from the output phosphor. This should be measured at 80 kVp and the same fluoroscopic mA each time. A homogenous phantom should be placed in the beam path to protect the image intensifier. This value should be recorded and compared with all future values. Image intensifiers can potentially deteriorate at a rate of 10% per year, which is reflected by the resultant values. Once the values have degraded by more than 50% from the value at acceptance, a service engineer should be consulted because image quality becomes poor and patient dose significantly increases.

Veiling Glare, or Flare. As previously mentioned, veiling glare, or flare, is defined as scattered or reflected light, usually within the linkage between the output phosphor and the television camera, which reduces image contrast. Two methods may be used to evaluate for flare. The first involves a homogenous phantom and a small lead disk of 1 to 2 cm in diameter. A photofluorospot or cine film image should be obtained, along with optical density values of the center of the disk area and the area outside the disk. These optical density values can then be used to calculate the contrast modulation of the system with the following equation:

$$Contrast\ modulation = \frac{(OD_{max} - OD_{min})}{(OD_{max} + OD_{min})} \times 100$$

OD_{max} is the optical density of the film outside the image of the lead disk, and OD_{min} is the optical density in the center of the lead disk. This value should be at least 70% for most fluoroscopic applications.

Another method of measuring flare involves a video waveform monitor attached to the camera output video cable (most easily accessed by disconnecting it from the back of the television monitor). The same setup with the lead disk and homogenous phantom is used, but no spot films are taken. Instead, the disk is imaged during fluoroscopy, and the voltage waveform pattern is observed on the waveform monitor, which plots voltage versus time (Fig. 8-15). The voltage measurements from the area behind the disk and outside of the disk are compared and used to calculate the contrast with the following equation:

$$\%Contrast = \frac{1 - Voltage\ behind\ lead\ strip}{Peak\ white\ voltage} \times 100\%$$

❻ *Video signal levels should be within ± 5% of those specified in the RS 170 standards.* This procedure is described in detail elsewhere.*

Fluoroscopic Systems for Cardiac Catheterization and Interventional Procedures. Fluoroscopic systems used during cardiac catheterization and interventional procedures must demonstrate a type of resolution known as *temporal resolution*. This is the ability of the imaging system to display events in time (temporal refers to "time") that are occurring close together as separate events. With these procedures, a physician guides various catheters and guidewires through blood vessels to a desired location. The fluoroscopic system must be able to capture the motion of these guidewires precisely (with minimal motion blur) so that the physician can place them in the correct location at the correct time. This requires a high (fast) frame rate for the fluoroscopic system. The ability of these fluoroscopic systems to display clear images of moving guidewires can be evaluated with a rotatable spoke test pattern (Fig. 8-16). This test object consists of six 5-inch-long

---

*Gray J, Winkler N, Stears J, et al: *Quality control in diagnostic imaging*, Baltimore, 1983, University Park Press.

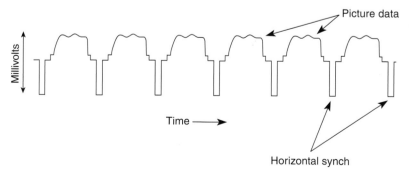

FIGURE 8-15 Video waveforms.

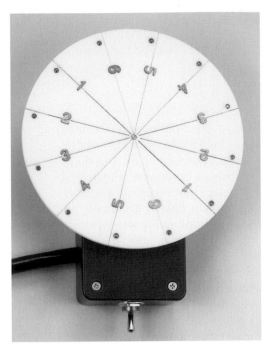

FIGURE 8-16 Rotatable spoke test pattern. *(Courtesy Nuclear Associates, Carle Place, N.Y.)*

steel wires of varying diameters (ranging in size from 0.005 to 0.022 inch) arranged at 30-degree intervals like spokes in a wheel. The wheel is attached to an electric motor with a rotation speed of 30 rpm. The image of this moving pattern is displayed on the monitor, and the ability to visualize the moving wire is evaluated.

These fluoroscopic systems should be able to visualize the wire's diameter, which is 0.013 inch or smaller, for optimum performance. This test pattern also should be visualized with cine cameras and digital recorders to ensure that these systems are delivering optimal image quality.

Video Monitor Performance. The final fluoroscopic image is usually displayed on a television monitor, even though this is the weakest link in the imaging chain in terms of loss of resolution. Over time, monitors are subject to defocusing, which reduces the spatial resolution of the observed image. Newer computer monitors used for viewing digital images also can develop unique problems. These monitors contain video cards that "drive them" (allow them to display the digital information). Sometimes these cards can generate enough heat to "pop" out of their slots, and there is a loss of operation. A test pattern created by a multiformat test generator or downloaded from a computer is required for the evaluation of proper monitor performance. These test patterns vary according to the manufacturer of the pattern, but the most common pattern is that designed by the Society of Motion Picture and Television Engineers (SMPTE), in accordance with SMPTE Recommended Practice RP 133-1986, "Medical Diagnostic Imaging Test Pattern for Television Monitors and Hard Copy Recording Cameras" (Fig. 8-17). An alternative test pattern is the AAPM TG 18-QC test pattern, created by the American Association of Physicists in Medicine.

A more in-depth discussion of video monitors and their performance takes place in the next chapter.

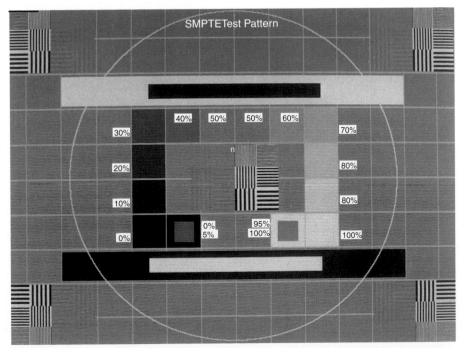

FIGURE 8-17 Test pattern of the Society of Motion Picture and Television Engineers (SMPTE).

SUMMARY

Fluoroscopic examinations can potentially administer high doses of x-radiation, particularly if the equipment is not functioning within accepted guidelines. For this risk to be minimized, quality control protocols for this equipment are essential for diagnostic radiology departments.

Refer to the Evolve website at https://evolve.elsevier. com for Student Experiments 8.1: Fluoroscopic Visual Inspection; 8.2: Fluoroscopic Exposure Levels; 8.3: Image Resolution of a Fluoroscopic System; 8.4: Fluoroscopic Image Noise; and 8.5: Fluoroscopic Automatic Brightness Control.

REVIEW QUESTIONS

1. Which of the following is not normally part of an image intensifier tube?
   a. Filament
   b. Photocathode
   c. Anode
   d. Output phosphor
2. Which material is most often used in the input phosphor of an image intensifier?
   a. Calcium tungstate
   b. Cesium iodide
   c. Zinc cadmium sulfide
   d. Lanthanum oxybromide
3. Which of the following terms best describes the increase in image brightness resulting from the difference in size between the input and output phosphors?
   a. Brightness gain
   b. Flux gain
   c. Minification gain
   d. Resolution gain

4. Which of the following increases the brightness of a fluoroscopic image: (1) an increase in kVp, (2) an increase in mA, or (3) an increase in pulse width?
   a. 1 and 2
   b. 2 and 3
   c. 1 and 3
   d. 1, 2, and 3
5. Which of the following is the main advantage of using a multifield image intensifier?
   a. The field of view is increased.
   b. The image brightness is increased.
   c. Magnification option is available.
   d. The patient dose is decreased.
6. Which of the following terms best describes the type of image intensifier artifact that results from projecting an image onto a flat surface?
   a. Veiling glare
   b. Pincushion distortion
   c. Vignetting
   d. S distortion
7. Which of the following is not a "tube" type of television camera?
   a. Orthicon
   b. Plumbicon
   c. Vidicon
   d. CCD
8. The primary beam should be restricted to the diameter of the input phosphor to within ± _____ % of the SID.
   a. 2
   b. 3
   c. 4
   d. 5
9. The video monitor of a fluoroscopic system should be evaluated with a test pattern created by which of the following organizations?
   a. NEMA
   b. ACR
   c. The SMPTE
   d. The American Society of Radiologic Technologists (ASRT)
10. The intensity of the x-ray beam at tabletop should not exceed _____ R/min for units that are equipped with ABS.
    a. 3
    b. 5
    c. 10
    d. 20

Digital and Advanced Imaging Equipment

KEY TERMS

active matrix array
amorphous
analog-to-digital converter
aspect ratio
cinefluorography
computed radiography
detective quantum efficiency
Digital Imaging and Communications
   in Medicine group
digital fluoroscopy
digital radiography
digital subtraction angiography
digital x-ray radiogrammetry

direct-to-digital radiographic systems
dual-energy x-ray absorptiometry
F-center
fill factor
frame rate
image contrast
image enhancement
image management and
   communication system
image restoration
interpolation
liquid crystal display
Nyquist frequency

photostimulated luminescence
picture archiving and communication
   system
preprocessing
postprocessing
refresh rate
special procedures laboratory
specular reflection
teleradiology
thin-film transistor
window level
window width

OBJECTIVES

At the completion of this chapter the reader should be able to do the following:

- Describe the basic methods of obtaining digital radiographs
- State the advantages and disadvantages of digital radiography versus conventional film/screen radiography
- Discuss the quality control procedures for evaluating digital radiographic systems
- Describe the basic methods of obtaining digital fluoroscopic images
- Explain how digital subtraction angiography is performed
- Discuss the quality control procedures for evaluating digital fluoroscopy
- Describe the basic principle of image production from multiformat cameras, laser cameras, dry laser printers,

cathode-ray tube cameras, videotape and videodisc recorders, and cinefluorographic equipment and discuss the quality control procedures for each
- Describe the various types of electronic display devices and discuss the applicable quality control procedures
- Explain the basic image archiving and management networks and discuss the applicable quality control procedures
- Describe the basic quality control process for special procedures equipment
- Explain the various methods for obtaining bone mineral density measurements

OUTLINE

In recent years, diagnostic imaging has undergone an explosion in technology with the advent of computerized imaging, magnetic resonance imaging (MRI), and digital archiving and retrieval systems. All of these technologies are now commonplace in diagnostic imaging departments and can be subject to variations with age and use; therefore, quality control protocols should be in place to monitor for these variations so that they can be kept to a minimum.

DIGITAL RADIOGRAPHIC IMAGING SYSTEMS

Virtually all diagnostic imaging systems can be considered to have three key components: image acquisition, image processing, and image display. Since the late 1890s, radiographic images were acquired by exposing a screen/film combination that required chemical processing and was displayed on a viewbox illuminator. In digital imaging, an image acquisition system obtains image data in the form of an electronic signal, which is processed electronically in a computer memory whereby the image exists as electronic values in a computer matrix (rather than as grains of silver on a sheet of polyester plastic), and displayed on an electronic display device (computer monitor). The computer matrix is made up of tiny squares called pixels (a contraction of the term *picture element*). The more pixels in a matrix, the smaller each pixel becomes, thereby increasing spatial resolution (Fig. 9-1). The production of digital radiographic images is rapidly replacing this method of film/screen radiography. Creating radiographic images in a digital format has many advantages over the analog format (film/screen images), including:

- the reduction of repeat images due to technique error (Most overexposures and slight underexposure can be corrected with software and not have to be repeated, but gross underexposure cannot.),
- simplification in the filing of images (They can be stored electronically rather than in hard copy.),
- reduction in the number of lost images (Digital images are stored electronically and can be retrieved as long as it has been correctly entered and saved in the computer system.),
- **postprocessing** of the image (Detail and contrast can be enhanced by the computer software.),
- and electronic transmission of images (This allows quick access to images by referring physicians and for consultation over large distances.).

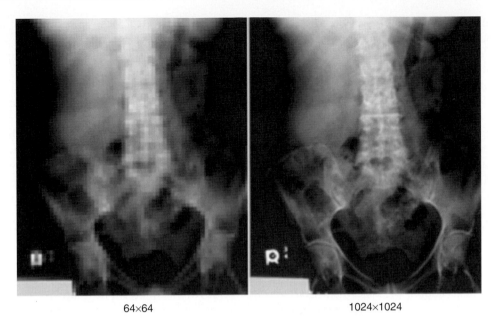

64×64   1024×1024

FIGURE 9-1 Images showing the difference in spatial resolution as the size of the matrix increases.

Currently, digital images can be acquired by using one of three methods: secondary capture, **computed radiography** (CR), or digital radiography (DR).

Secondary Capture

This method of creating digital images involves the initial creation of an analog image (on film) and then its conversion into a digital format. One method of accomplishing this conversion would involve taking a photograph of a film radiograph with a digital camera. This method has been used for years by diagnostic imaging educators (like myself) to obtain digital images. However, there is considerable loss of resolution even with a large matrix (>3-megapixel) camera. Therefore, it may be acceptable for teaching files or professional meeting presentations but should never be used to make a diagnosis. More acceptable conversion of analog film images to digital format can be accomplished by a laser scanning digitizer or a charge-coupled device (CCD) scanner. Common uses of secondary capture devices include:

- Film radiographs are archived into a **picture archiving and communication system** (PACS).
- Computer-aided diagnosis is a software program whereby the computer can look for abnormalities in mammography and chest radiographs.
- **Teleradiology** is the process of sending digitized images to distant locations for interpretation and consultation.
- Duplicate Images allows the original film-based radiograph to remain at the original clinical site while an electronic copy made by the digitizer can be burned onto a CD or DVD and given to the patient.

Laser Scanning Digitizer. The laser scanning digitizer is used to convert an existing radiographic image that is recorded on film into a digital format that can be stored and transmitted electronically (Fig. 9-2). It is similar in function to a scanner that is used with a personal computer to scan photographic images into the computer data storage. The existing radiograph is placed in the digitizer, where it is scanned by a laser and then detected by photosensors on the other side. The signals sent by the photosensors are then sent through analog-to-digital converters (ADCs) and into the computer memory. The higher optical density areas of the film image attenuate a higher percentage of the laser light

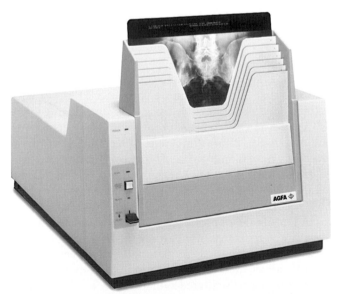

FIGURE 9-2 Laser scanning digitizer. *(Courtesy Agfa in Bushong SC: Radiologic Science for Technologists, ed 9, St Louis, 2008, Mosby.)*

than the areas with a lower optical density. The differences in the amount of laser light transmitted through the various areas are used to convert the analog image information into a digital image. The shade values are then displayed on a computer monitor based on a look-up table (LUT) that indicates which shade of gray is associated with each value (see Figure 9-9 later in this chapter). Scanning takes about 25 seconds, depending on the scanning resolution. These systems currently have a resolution capability of about 5 megapixels. They have been around since about 1990 and are considered the gold standard for film digitization. Like the scanner for a personal computer, it is important to keep the scanning surface clean and free of any dirt or dust. Otherwise, artifacts that are not present in the original film image can appear in the digital version of the image.

Charge-Coupled Device Scanner. The CCD scanner is similar to a document copier or a scanner that you would use with your personal computer, whereby the CCD captures reflected light from the image, creates an electrical signal, and then sends it into a computer for processing. This device is smaller and less expensive than the laser scanning digitizer, but it has poorer contrast resolution. They are also slower than laser scanning digitizers (up to 80 seconds per scan) and can have problems accurately reproducing extreme light and dark areas on the original film radiograph.

Computed Radiography (CR)

Computed radiography (CR) is a digital image acquisition and processing system for producing static radiographs. It was developed in 1981 by the Fuji Corporation, with the first clinical application in 1983. This system uses standard x-ray tubes and generators but requires specialized image receptors and processing. CR systems consist of the image receptors, an image reader device, and a workstation.

The image receptor resembles a traditional film/screen cassette but does not contain intensifying screens and film. The outside is made of carbon fiber and has a bar code that is scanned into a computer to link it with patient data. Inside of the cassette is an imaging plate (IP) made of either metal or plastic and is coated on one side with photostimulable phosphors (PSP) in a layer less than 1 mm thick. The phosphor material can be either (Ba Fb R:Eu^{2+}) barium fluorobromide doped with europium (an activator or impurity) or (CsBr: Eu^{2+}) cesium bromide doped with europium. The cesium bromide phosphor yields better resolution due to light divergence as compared with barium fluorobromide. The K-edge of these materials is between 35 and 50 keV (lower than rare earth phosphors), making them more sensitive to scattered radiation.

When these crystals are exposed to x-rays, they are energized until they are exposed to light from a laser. This is known as **photostimulated luminescence** (PSL).

The crystal electrons (after x-ray absorption) are trapped in empty lattice sites called F-centers. When laser light hits the **F-centers**, the trapped electrons are released, causing the emission of visible light (which is blue in color), which is then detected by photosensors and sent through ADCs and into the computer for processing. The standard plate has a relative speed of between 200 and 400, while the high resolution plate is between 50 and 100 (comparable to film/screen systems). Once an IP is exposed to x-rays, a latent image is present and can remain on the IP for up to 24 hours but will gradually weaken through a process called *fading*. This fading process will occur exponentially over time. A typical IP will lose about 25% of its stored energy within 8 hours of exposure.

The exposed image receptor is placed into a slot in the front of an image reader device (IRD) (Fig. 9-3) that removes the plate. The plate is then stimulated by a scanning helium-neon laser (emitting a red light with a wavelength of 633 nanometers) or a solid state laser (670 nm), which causes the crystals to release blue-violet light (390-400 nanometer wavelength). The F-centers in the IP respond best to red light having a wavelength of about 600 nm. A rotating polygon or an oscillating

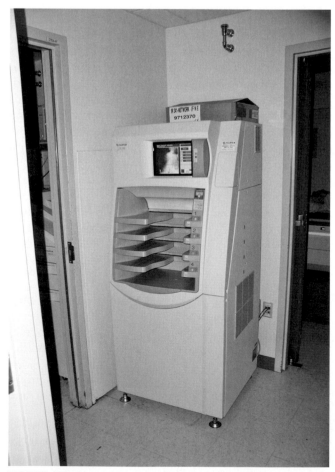

FIGURE 9-3 The computed radiography (CR) Image Reader Device (IRD). *(Courtesy Good Samaritan Hospital, Downers Grove, Ill.)*

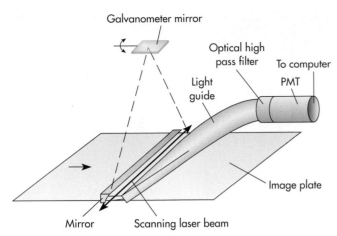

FIGURE 9-4 Schematic diagram of a computed radiography (CR) reader system. *PMT,* Photomultiplier tube.

mirror deflects the laser beam back and forth across the IP as it is moving. This is known as the "fast scan" mode. The light emitted by the PSP's is then detected by photosensors that converts the amount of light detected to an electronic signal value that is then sent through an ADC (analog-to-digital converter) and then to the computer for processing (Fig. 9-4). The IP must be moved at a constant, slow speed (known as slow scan) along the long axis of the IP. Any fluctuations in velocity can result in banding artifacts.

After the image is obtained from the IP, it is transferred to another part of the IRD, where a high-intensity sodium discharge lamp erases any residual image so that it can be reused. These plates are kept in a storage bin until needed, at which time they can be transferred back into the image receptor. Most current systems can process about 200 IPs per hour and take about 30 to 60 seconds to process. There are also x-ray tables and upright Bucky units that contain multiple PSP plates and a reader in the unit so that no cassette handling is required. The units will move and process the IPs after each exposure, which allows the radiographer to view the images on a monitor in the control booth area.

The IRD is responsible for all **preprocessing** functions (preprocessing is anything done to the image data before they are entered into the computer memory) such as the average value of a signal, which data are clinically useful, the orientation of the part(s) on the IP, the number of projections present on the IP, and histogram generation. A histogram is a graph of signal intensity values that corresponds to a spectrum of pixel values (Fig. 9-5). The IRD generates a histogram from the data in the scanned area and compares it with an existing histogram for the programmed body part. This histogram is selected by body part by the radiographer when the IP is loaded into the IRD. The correct algorithm must be selected before processing the IP or the image will not process the correct brightness and contrast levels. With older CR systems, if the algorithm is wrong, and the IP is placed in the IRD and read, the plate could not be processed again, and any information on the plate would have been lost (necessitating a repeat radiograph). Newer systems now allow the algorithm to be corrected once the image is displayed on the quality control (QC) workstation so the exam would not have to be repeated.

A workstation consisting of a computer console, whereby the manifest image can be manipulated through postprocessing (everything done to the data after they have been entered into the computer memory), is the final component (Fig. 9-6). The workstation functions can include the following:

- Gradational enhancement (contrast) is also known as G setting, contrast enhancement, contrast rescaling, contrast processing, tone scaling, or multiscale image contrast algorithm (MUSICA) by various equipment manufacturers. Figure 9-7 shows the effect of gradational enhancement on the radiographic image.
- Spatial frequency enhancement (recorded detail) is also known as R setting, edge enhancement, unsharp masking, or frequency processing. This postprocessing function allows enhancement of spatial resolution at the expense of increased noise and artifacts.

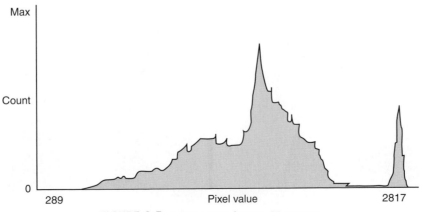

FIGURE 9-5 A histogram from a CR system.

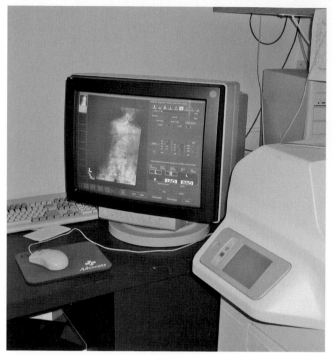

FIGURE 9-6 The computed radiography (CR) system workstation. *(Courtesy Good Samaritan Hospital, Downers Grove, Ill.)*

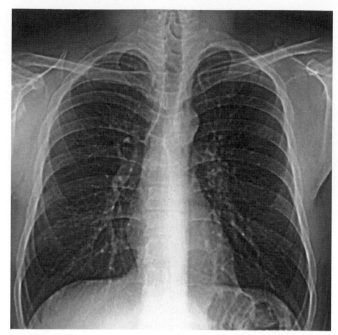

FIGURE 9-8 Effect of edge enhancement on a radiographic image.

Figure 9-8 shows the effect of contrast enhancement on the radiographic image.

- Histogram equalization eliminates black and white pixels that contribute little diagnostic information and expands the remaining image data in order to use the full dynamic range.
- Look-up tables are used to alter the tonal qualities of an image by mapping the values of exposure intensity to a desired brightness level (Fig. 9-9). These are similar to an H & D curve used for film/screen images.
- Subtraction/addition option isused to remove bony structures or reduce the effect of scatter in order to increase image contrast.

- Image magnification electronically magnifies or zooms into specific areas.
- Region of interest display allows viewing of specific areas of interest.
- Statistical analysis is used for calculating surface areas and estimating volumes or changes in tissue density.
- Windowing is the manipulation of window width and level to adjust image brightness and contrast.
- Energy subtraction is based on subtracting projection radiographs obtained at two different photon energies. These are often used for chest radiography to diminish bony rib structures in order to better visualize lung and soft tissue. Figure 9-10 shows the effect of energy subtraction on the radiographic image.

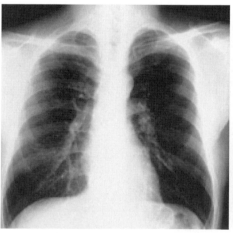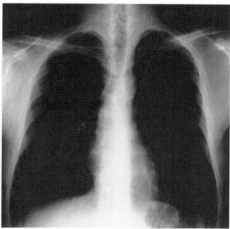

FIGURE 9-7 Effect of contrast enhancement on a radiographic image.

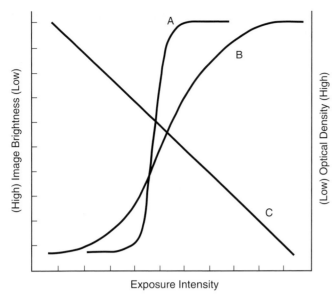

FIGURE 9-9 Look-up tables for digital image processing. The curve shape defines the relationship between the intensity of exposure and image brightness (comparable to optical density in film images). **(A)** High contrast curve. **(B)** Low-contrast (wide latitude) curve. **(C)** Linear response curve with a reversed grayscale.

- Image stitching is the formation of a long body part image (such as a complete spine during a scoliosis study) from a series of overlapping subimages.
- Database functions are used for image storage and display and for printing hard copy images.

The image is usually created with a 2560 × 2048 matrix. Hard-copy images are created with a dry laser printer.

Advantages of Computed Radiography versus Conventional Radiography. CR has several advantages over conventional film/screen radiography including the following:

1. A lower patient dose is incurred as a result of the higher quantum detection efficiency (up to 50%) of the IP phosphors (in some systems only). Table 9-1 lists the percentage dose reduction for various radiographic examinations. Some CR systems may require an increase in exposure of the IP, in which case the dose reduction would occur due to a lower repeat rate.
2. The repeat rate is lower because of improper technical factors.
3. Higher-contrast resolution and wider exposure latitude are possible than with radiographic film emulsion. These can be demonstrated with a sensitometric curve (Fig. 9-11). The response of the CR imaging plate is linear over an x-ray exposure range of four orders of magnitude between 5 milliroentgen (mR) and 50 mR. The film/screen combination is limited to about two orders of magnitude and a sigmoidal response. This means that at high and low exposures, the contrast is greatly reduced; a linear response exists only for about one order of magnitude in exposure.
4. No darkroom or film costs are incurred (unless hard copy images are desired).
5. The images can be postprocessed to improve quality.
6. Image storage is easy through either hard-copy or electronic storage.
7. Easy interface is possible with the **picture archiving and communication system** (PACS) or the **image management and communication system** (IMACS).

TABLE 9-1	Percentage Dose Reduction for Various Radiographic Examinations
Examination	**Decrease in Patient Dose (%)**
Upper GI tract	5
Pelvis	12
Chest	14–20
IVP or IVU	50

GI, Gastrointestinal; *IVP/IVU,* intravenous pyelogram/urography.

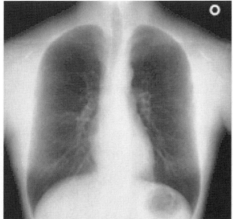
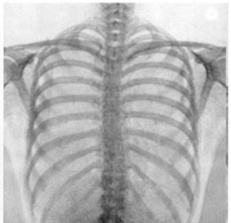

FIGURE 9-10 Effect of energy subtraction on a chest examination. The image on the left has bony structures subtracted while the image on the right shows soft tissue subtraction.

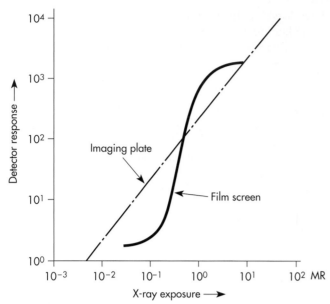

FIGURE 9-11 Plot of system response of film/screen imaging system and digital radiographic imaging plate.

Disadvantages of Computed Radiography versus Conventional Radiography. The disadvantages of CR include the following:

1. Capital costs are high for image receptors, CR reader unit, and workstation hardware and software.
2. Spatial resolution is lower. Spatial resolution is controlled by the dimension of the crystals in the IP, the size of the laser beam in the CR reader unit, and the matrix size. Film/screen combinations can resolve more than 5 line pairs per millimeter (lp/mm) compared with 4 to 5 lp/mm for CR systems. This can make visualization of linear fractures in bone difficult. CR systems with spatial frequencies of 10 lp/mm are available for mammographic imaging, and are discussed in Chapter 11.
3. Collimation and centering of the part are critical for the computer to determine the proper pixel shade brightness (optical density) and contrast.
4. The patient could potentially be overexposed to radiation. With film/screen systems, the correct amount of radiation exposure is necessary to obtain an acceptable radiographic image. With CR systems, the computer can compensate overexposure of up to 2 times the necessary amount of milliampere-second (mAs), which can cause radiographers to routinely overexpose the patient to unnecessary radiation (sometimes referred to as dose creep). Various CR system manufacturers use a numeric system to monitor the amount of exposure to the IP (and therefore the patient). Unfortunately, these systems vary by manufacturer and are not standardized (unlike the relative system speed value that all radiographers can use with film/screen systems). For example, the Fuji CR system uses

a value known as the sensitivity (or "S" value), which is inversely proportional to the amount of exposure reaching the IP. These values are calibrated so that an exposure of 1 mR from an 80 kVp beam to a standard IP will yield an "S"-number of 200 in the semiautomatic mode. Therefore an exposure of 0.1 mR to the same plate would yield an "S"-number of 2000, while 10 mR would yield a value of 20. In the normal mode, cutting the exposure in half would double the S-number and vice versa. Proper exposure to IPs should produce S-values of between 150 and 250. An S value of greater than 250 for non-Bucky exposure or 400 for Bucky exposures indicates underexposure while a value of less than 100 would indicate overexposure. In comparison, Carestream Health (formerly known as Kodak) uses a value known as Exposure Index, which is directly proportional to the amount of radiation that strikes the IP. This index is the average pixel value calculated within the defined anatomic region. It is calibrated so that an exposure of 1 mR from an 80 kVp beam on a standard plate would yield a value of 2000. Thus, an exposure of 0.1 mR results in an exposure index of 1000, while 10 mR would produce a value of 3000. Doubling the exposure will cause an increase in the exposure index of 300, while cutting the exposure in half causes it to drop by 300. IPs should produce Exposure Index values between 1800 and 2200 when properly exposed. Agfa uses a value know as the log of the median exposure (logM). It is calibrated with a beam of 75 kVp for a 20 mR exposure and the plate is scanned using a speed class setting of 100 to yield a logM value of 2.6. For a given speed class setting, the value of logM varies according to the log of the radiation dose to the IP. A doubling of the exposure should result in an increase in the value of logM by 0.301. The typical range of logM values is between 1.95 and 2.6. Regardless of the system manufacturer, it is important for the radiographer to keep these values within the manufacturer's specifications. An underexposed IP can create an image that will demonstrate quantum mottle, even though the brightness level is acceptable (see Fig. 10-17 in the next chapter). Overexposed IPs can create images that may suffer from low contrast (even though most software can produce a diagnostic image with up to a 500% overexposure). Automatic exposure control (AEC) systems can be calibrated to work with CR systems and should be used.

5. Image artifacts may occur with the use of grids. A Moire' or zebra pattern artifact (discussed in the next chapter) can occur if the grid frequency and the scan frequency of the IRD are similar and oriented in the same direction (grid lines should run perpendicular to the plate reader's scan lines to avoid this problem). These artifacts also can be caused by the sampling rate of the Analog-to-Digital Convertor (ADC) in the reader unit having a sampling rate that is too

TABLE 9-2	List of CR Manufacturers (Selling in the United States)
Manufacturer	**Web Address**
Agfa Healthcare	www.agfa.com/healthcare
Alara	www.alara.com
AllPro Imaging	www.allproimaging.com
Carestream Health (formerly Kodak)	www.carestreamhealth.com
FujiFilm Medical Systems USA	www.fujimed.com
Konica Minolta Medical Imaging	www.medical.konicaminolta.us
Philips Medical Systems	www.medical.philips.com
iCRco Inc.	www.icrcompany.com

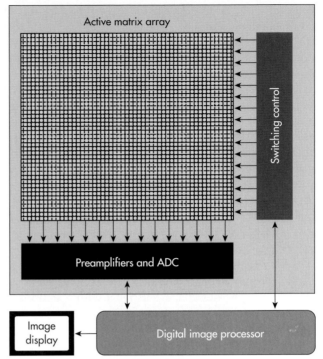

FIGURE 9-12 Flat-panel x-ray image receptor. *ADC,* Analog-to-digital converter.

slow. Thus, grid frequency should be about 85/inch (33 to 34/cm) for a 14" × 17" image receptor and 103/inch (40 to 43/cm) for a 10" × 12" image receptor. Because IPs are especially sensitive to scatter, grids should be used for all exposures greater than 80 kVp. The IPs also are very sensitive to background radiation (even more than film/screen systems). Most plates can respond to radiation exposures as low as 10 μR, while background radiation can vary between 40 and 80 μR/day in many areas. It is therefore recommended that the plates be erased daily, if they have not been used, to eliminate unwanted noise. They also will need to be routinely cleaned just like intensifying screens in film/screen cassettes. A listing of manufacturers selling CR imaging equipment in the United States (complete as of the writing of this edition) can be found in Table 9-2.

Digital Radiography

This method of creating digital radiographic images, also known as either **digital radiography** (DR) or *flat-panel* or *flat-plate* imaging, appeared in the late 1990s. They also have been referred to as **direct-to-digital radiographic** (DDR) **systems**. This method involves the installation of a flat-panel image receptor in the Bucky of a radiographic table or upright Bucky; the receptor sends an electronic signal directly to a digital image processor. The flat-panel image receptor is a large-area (the size of conventional film/screen image receptors) integrated circuit called an **active matrix array** (AMA) that consists of millions of identical semiconductor elements deposited on a glass base (Fig. 9-12).

The active matrix array is similar to a CCD camera (used in digital cameras, digital video camcorders, and television cameras in fluoroscopic systems), but much larger in size. These flat-panel image receptors also can be used for fluoroscopic imaging, as well as radiographic imaging. Each element in the AMA is known as a *pixel*. Each pixel of the array has a switch made from a **thin-film transistor** (TFT). These TFT switches

are connected to switching control circuitry that allows all switches in a row of the array to be operated simultaneously (Fig. 9-13). For radiographic imaging, all of the TFT switches are kept in the "off" position during the x-ray exposure. Once the exposure is complete, the switches in the first row are turned on, and the signal

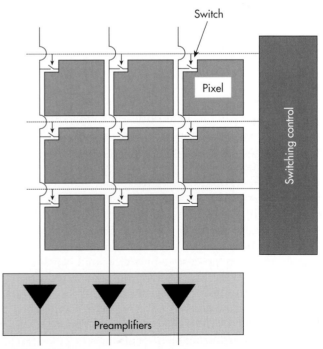

FIGURE 9-13 Illustration of a section of the active matrix array *(AMA)* showing the switch associated with each pixel.

from each pixel is amplified, converted into digital form by an **analog-to-digital converter** (ADC), and then stored in the memory of the digital image processor. These switches are then turned off, and the switches in the second row are turned on, then the third, and so on, until the image from the entire array is acquired. For fluoroscopic exposures, the array is scanned continuously. The active matrix array can get signal data immediately to the computer for processing, so the image will appear on the monitor quickly. Two different types of flat-panel devices have been developed: indirect-conversion and direct-conversion image receptors.

Indirect-conversion or Scintillator Digital Radiography System. This type of system involves converting x-ray energy into light energy, and then converting that light energy into an electronic signal (hence the term *indirect* because the x-ray energy is not converted directly into an electric signal). These systems are available in two basic designs, a flat panel with a scintillator or a charge-coupled detector.

The flat panel with a scintillator system involves coupling the scintillator (usually cesium iodide or terbium doped gadolinium dioxide sulfide) with **amorphous** silicon (a-Si). The term *amorphous* means "without form." In this context, it means that silicon (which normally exists in a crystalline state) is in a noncrystalline state. Since the atomic number of silicon is 14, it will not absorb x-rays well. Therefore, a phosphor layer of cesium iodide (used by Phillips, Siemens, General Electric, and Carestream Health, among others) or a rare earth intensifying screen composed of lanthanum and gadolinium oxysulfides (currently used by Canon), which emits light when struck by x-rays, is used. This light then activates the a-Si photodetectors (of which there are millions in the active matrix array). This interaction results in the creation of an electric signal that is stored by a TFT assembly until readout, at which time the signal is sent to the computer. A disadvantage to this design is decreased spatial resolution due to light divergence from the scintillator. These detectors are manufactured in columns to minimize this light diffusion and increase spatial resolution. This system is currently used by Phillips, Siemens, General Electric, and many other manufacturers.

The charge-coupled detector system couples (by lenses or fiber optics) an intensifying screen made of rare earth phosphors such as gadolinium oxysulfide (Gd_2O_2S:Tb) or cesium iodide to a CCD or CMOS (complimentary metallic oxide semiconductor) device. Both types of imagers will convert light into an electric charge and then process it into electronic signals. In a CCD sensor, every pixel's charge is transferred through a very limited number of output nodes to be converted into a voltage, buffered, and sent off from the chip as an analog signal. All of the pixel can be devoted to light capture, and the output signal's uniformity (a key factor in image quality) is high. In a CMOS sensor, each pixel has its own charge-to-voltage conversion, and the sensor often includes amplifiers, noise correction, and digitization circuits, so that the chip can output a digital signal. However, these other functions increase the design complexity and reduce the area available for light capture. This system works in much the same way as the output phosphor of a fluoroscopic image intensifier being coupled to a CCD camera. This design is marketed by Swiss Ray.

Direct-conversion or Photoconductor Digital Radiography System. This type of system involves the use of the photoconducting material amorphous selenium (a-Se) rather than a phosphor material. The silicon used in indirect-conversion image receptors has an atomic number of 14, so x-rays do not interact to a significant degree unless thick amounts are used. Selenium has an atomic number of 34 and therefore interacts more readily with x-rays to create an electronic signal (so no phosphor material is necessary). The electric charge produced after x-ray interaction is detected by an array of pixels that consists of an electrode and a capacitor, which store the charge until switched by a TFT. This system is utilized in some General Electric DR systems as well as those sold by DEL Medical.

The advantage of the direct-conversion method over the indirect-conversion method is that there is no spreading of light from the phosphor material (similar to the effect in conventional intensifying screens) and the loss of spatial resolution that occurs as a result. However, the phosphor used in the indirect-conversion system possesses a higher DQE or detective quantum efficiency (it can absorb more x-rays) and therefore results in a lower patient dose. The relatively low DQE of selenium also means that it is not quite suitable for higher kVp exposures due to its relatively low K-edge. Photoconductors such as lead iodide (PbI) and mercury iodide (HgI) are being introduced to replace selenium for higher kVp studies.

The spatial resolution of direct-conversion systems is determined primarily by the detector size (also known as aperture size) and the sampling pitch (which is the length of an array divided by the number of detectors along that length). For example, if there are 2000 detectors on a line that is 35 cm long, the sampling pitch is 175 µm (35 divided by 2000). The sampling pitch determines the limiting spatial resolution that is achievable by the digital imaging system. The limiting spatial resolution, also known as the **Nyquist frequency,** is given by the reciprocal of twice the sampling pitch or 1/ (2 × sampling pitch). If we use the sampling pitch of 175 µm (175 mm) from earlier, the limiting spatial resolution would be 2.9 lp/mm 1/ (2 × 0.175 mm). Systems currently available have pixels as small as 85 µm, which yield a spatial resolution of approximately 5 lp/mm (comparable to CR systems).

Another feature that can influence spatial resolution and patient dose with direct-conversion image receptors is the **fill factor.** The **fill factor** is the percentage of pixel area that is sensitive to the image signal (contains the x-ray detector). The fill factor for most current systems is approximately 80% because some of the pixel area must be devoted to electronic conductors and the TFT.

Comparison of Computed Radiography with Digital Radiography. Both the CR and DR methods create digital images that have many advantages over the analog images created by film/screen radiography. But how do they compare with each other? Both methods produce spatial resolution that is comparable to that of film/screen systems (about 5 lp/mm). They also have superior contrast resolution compared with film/screen systems. To make a better comparison of image quality among digital systems, many physicists recommend using a new parameter known as **detective quantum efficiency** (DQE). DQE is a measure of the information transfer efficiency of a detector and is defined as the signal-to-noise ratio squared coming out of a detector divided by the signal-to-noise ratio squared going into a detector (SNR^2_{out}/SNR^2_{in}). Like modulation transfer function (MTF) values, DQE values will always range from 0 to 1. A DQE value of 1 would be a perfect detector because no information is lost between the detector input and detector output. Therefore the greater the DQE, the better the digital detector system at displaying image quality.

The advantage of DQE is that it is a measure of the combined effect of the noise and contrast performance of an imaging system, expressed as a function of object detail. Greater DQE values will increase one's ability to view small, low-contrast objects (such as in mammography). Direct-conversion DR systems tend to have the highest DQE values, followed by indirect-conversion DR systems, CR systems, and film/screen systems. However, the CR method has had an advantage of being portable because the image receptor can be taken anywhere for exposure to x-rays. This means that they also can be used for non-Bucky examinations such as extremities.

The majority of DR systems are built into the Bucky assembly and are therefore confined to Bucky use. However, there are now portable DR systems that can be used in table and upright Bucky assemblies or during mobile radiography. The image data can be downloaded from the portable DR active matrix array via a cable or through a wireless connection being introduced that also can be used for non-Bucky use. The DR systems also have a higher capital cost because the image receptor panels must be installed in the Bucky assembly of each radiographic room (unless a portable DR system is utilized). The cost per room for DR systems built into the Bucky assembly is approximately 3 to 4 times greater than CR systems (however, portable DR systems are comparable in cost to CR systems). However, DR systems are less labor intensive because image receptor plates do not have to be physically moved and handled by the radiographer. This also reduces examination time, which can increase patient satisfaction. It also

TABLE 9-3	List of DR Manufacturers (Selling in the United States)
Manufacturer	**Web Address**
Canon USA, Inc.	www.usa.canon.com/dr
Carestream Health (formerly Kodak)	www.carestreamhealth.com
DEL Medical	www.delmedical.com
Dinamik Rontgen	www.dynamicx-ray.com
EVI Medical Systems	www.vieworks.com
FujiFilm Medical Systems USA	www.fujimed.com
GE Healthcare	www.gehealthcare.com
IDC (Imaging Dynamics)	www.imagingdynamics.com
IMIX Americas	www.imixadr.com
Konica Minolta Medical Imaging	www.medical.konicaminolta.us
Lodox Systems NA LLC	www.lodox.com
Philips Medical Systems	www.medical.philips.com
Siemens Medical Solutions	www.siemensmedical.com
Swissray International	www.swissray.com
Toshiba America Medical Systems	www.medical.toshiba.com
ZAO PONI	www.poni.com

can allow for more patients to be served in a given period of time, especially with high-volume examinations such as chest radiography. Indirect-conversion DR systems with cesium iodide phosphors have achieved U.S. Food and Drug Administration (FDA) approval for mammographic procedures (discussed in Chapter 11). Time will tell which system is more popular. A listing of manufacturers selling DR imaging equipment in the United States (complete as of the writing of this edition) can be found in Table 9-3.

Quality Control of Digital Radiographic Imaging Systems

Because the image is created digitally, variation in system performance is less than with film/screen systems. However, digital imaging can create a host of new problems that require a quality management program that must take into consideration the entire imaging chain (and the people involved within it). For example, a misidentified conventional film image can be fixed rather easily with an adhesive label containing the correct information taped over the incorrect information. With digital imaging, several copies of the image may have been created, archived, and transmitted electronically within a PACS, making correction more difficult. In addition, new versions of system software might cause changes in image quality when added to existing systems. Three levels of system performance for quality control and system maintenance exist:

1. Routine—performed by QC technologists
2. Full inspection—performed by medical physicist and involves radiation measurements and noninvasive adjustments

3. System adjustment—performed by vendor service personnel and involves hardware and software maintenance

Unfortunately, many different types of digital systems exist, and there is no standard quality control process that can be used by all systems. This means that quality control technologists must rely on the manufacturer's guidelines for specific quality control procedures. However, some basic quality control procedures are common to all systems:

- Check the CR systems. The IP loading and unloading mechanisms in the CR reader unit must be cleaned and lubricated regularly (at least weekly). Care must be taken to avoid dirt or dust on the IPs to prevent artifacts on the final image, which can mimic pathologic conditions (Fig. 9-14). CR plates also can yellow over time, which can reduce their efficiency. It is important to use a dry cloth or a cleaning solution that is specified by the manufacturer and is not water based. The IPs also should be inspected for hairline cracks at least monthly, as these cracks also can cause artifacts on the image that can mimic pathology. The IPs also should be erased daily to reduce image noise. They are especially sensitive to exposure from fluorescent lighting, so they should be stored in the IRD or erased before use.

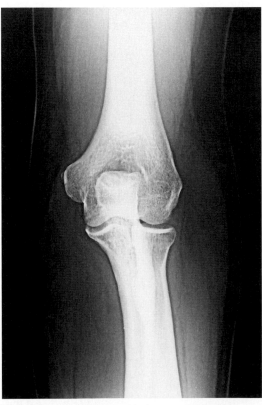

FIGURE 9-14 Digital radiographic image with artifact caused by dirt on plate.

- Laser scanning digitizers must be kept clean and free of dirt and debris, as previously mentioned.
- The image receptors used with DR systems also must be kept clean and free of dirt, debris, blood, contrast media, and other items.
- Check the performance of the display monitors at least monthly, as recommended by the American College of Radiology (ACR). A high-resolution monitor is used for all types of digital radiographic systems to display the final image. These monitors are available with either a cathode-ray tube (CRT) display or a **liquid crystal display** (LCD) flat-panel display. Many radiologists are making their diagnoses according to the images from these monitors rather than hard-copy film images, and they may perform operations 24 hours a day, 7 days a week. The CRT monitors can defocus over time and lose image brightness and contrast. They are the weakest link in terms of the variability in the quality of digital image display. The LCD flat-panel displays have a disadvantage of limited viewing angle (you have to look straight at them to see the image clearly). They also require periodic replacement of their light source after approximately 30,000 hours of operation. However, LCD displays are subject to far less variability than CRT display monitors. Procedures for checking video monitor performance are discussed later in this chapter.
- A resolution test tool indicating lp/mm should be imaged upon acceptance and then every six months, and compared with previous test images and the manufacturers' specifications. Changes in image quality should be brought to the attention of a service engineer. Phantom images using a special test phantom (Fig. 9-15) should be obtained as suggested by the manufacturer (Box 9-1). If a phantom or test tool is unavailable, the following options may be used as an alternative for CR systems:

(A) Uniformity—expose the CR cassette to a uniform dose of radiation by using a 72" SID (to eliminate heel effect variation) and a technique of 80 kVp and enough mAs to produce about 10 mR of radiation to the plate. Process the plate and examine the image for uniformity. One way to accomplish this is to print the image with a dry laser printer and take optical density readings across the surface of the image. These should be within a value of ± 0.2 of each other. To evaluate uniformity of the soft-image on the monitor, you can use the region of interest to check brightness at various points throughout the image. These should be within 10% of each other.

(B) Spatial accuracy—the wire mesh test tool used for evaluating film/screen contact can be used to evaluate this parameter by placing it on a

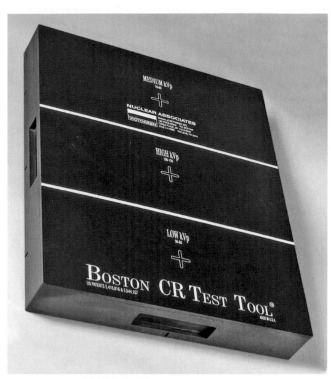

FIGURE 9-15 Boston CR Test Tool.

CR cassette and making an exposure at 72" SID, 60 kVp, and enough mAs to produce about 5 mR to the plate. After processing, the image should appear uniform in brightness and resolution, with no geometric distortions. If any appear, inspect the plate for any defects. If these appear across multiple plates, the cause is probably the laser in the reader unit.

(C) Erasure test—use a knee or other phantom and make an extreme overexposure. After processing, verify that the image has been completely erased from the plate.

(D) Laser function—a metal ruler can be imaged on a CR cassette using 80 kVp, 72" SID, and enough mAs to yield about 5 mR to the IP. Be sure that the ruler is placed perpendicular to the laser scan lines. After processing the image, view it on the monitor and verify that the edges of the ruler appear as straight lines. If not, there is a problem with the laser in the reader unit and a service engineer should be called.

The American Association of Physicists in Medicine (AAPM) suggests the following QC program for digital radiographic systems:

Acceptance Tests are performed by a medical physicist. You may recall from Chapter 1 that acceptance testing is done on brand new equipment or equipment

---

BOX 9-1 | Digital Radiography Phantom Image Testing

Because CR and DR systems are relatively new, federal quality control standards that are uniform for all manufacturers have yet to be implemented. Each system manufacturer has quality control protocols described in the operating manual provided to each user. Many equipment vendors, as well as private organizations, have developed evaluation phantoms for CR and DR systems (see Fig. 9-15). The phantom image can evaluate the performance of the IRD, IP, detector array function (in DR systems), workstations, hard-copy printer, and the x-ray exposure room. Most manufacturers recommend that these phantom images be taken on acceptance and then at least once a month (can be performed by QC technologist or medical physicist) or when problems are suspected. Information obtained from the phantom includes the following:

- Relative sensitivity test—used to confirm that the CR reader system sensitivity calibration is consistent with the baseline test. The sensitivity of a CR system affects patient dose. This same test also can provide information on the x-ray generator output and consistency. A CR system should display a consistent sensitivity index number when a cassette with the same dose is digitized. Each CR manufacturer should provide an acceptable standard deviation.

- Shading or uniformity test—evaluates the uniformity of the image brightness (comparable to optical density in film/screen imaging) across the scanning width. It also confirms the CR reader system's light guide position and optics. If a laser is not performing uniformly, low contrast light and dark bands may appear running either horizontally or vertically.

- Contrast evaluation—measures the contrast resolution capability of the image processor, workstation monitors, and hard-copy printers.

- Spatial accuracy or sharpness test—measures the spatial resolution capability of the CR reader optics, x-ray tube, and hard-copy printer. It also will demonstrate whether the CR system is presenting images with the correct geometric relationships.

- Laser jitter test—evaluates the horizontal and vertical performance of the laser optic and transport systems of the CR reader and hard-copy printer.

- Image noise test—evaluates the image for noise or artifacts (usually caused by dirt on the IP), as well as monitor degradation.

- Erasure test—used to confirm that the CR reader system has completely erased the previous image. Incomplete erasure creates an artifact known as dark noise. This can be checked by running a newly erased plate through the IRD of a CR system. The exposure guide indicator numbers should show no exposure to the IP. Any exposure guide number that is not within the manufacturer's recommended values may indicate a damaged IP or erasure lamps in the IRD that are not functioning properly.

- Accuracy of measurement tools—ensures the accuracy of workstation measurement tools and hard-copy printer software.

- System linearity test—measures CR reader system linearity. Linearity is also an important factor regarding patient dose. For example, if exposures of 0.1 mR, 1.0 mR, and 10 mR are digitized, the systems exposure guide indicator numbers should track linearly within 10 % changes.

CR, Computed radiography; *DR*, digital radiography.

that has undergone a major repair to make sure that it is performing at manufacturer's specification.

1. Erasure thoroughness evaluates the ability of the sodium discharge lamp in IRD to completely erase previous data (especially those from extreme overexposure. If not completely erased, ghosting artifacts can appear on subsequent images that can mimic disease processes. Testing involves creating an image at extreme overexposure (about 50 mR exposure to an IP), processing the plate (including erasure) and then taking a second image of the same plate with about 1 mR exposure. The image created by this second exposure of the IP is then analyzed for the presence of the previous image taken at 50 mR.

2. Phantom image testing is discussed in Box 9-1, which includes specific phantom image data.

Daily Tests are performed by a technologist.

1. As part of the general inspection, inspect the CR cassettes for cleanliness (surfaces should be free of dirt and debris to avoid image artifacts or processing problems in the IRD), barcode labels (make sure that they are clean and free of any surface dirt), and that hinges and latches are in good condition. Also make sure that IRD removes IPs smoothly and easily and that they are read and replaced in the cassette properly. Once these tasks are completed, a system walk-through should be performed to verify general equipment operation and network transmission.

2. Check the laser printer to make sure it is functioning properly to obtain hard-copy images. If paper printers are used, make sure that they are working properly.

3. Erase all IPs before use.

4. Verify that the reader unit and workstation/s are communicating properly with each other. Also make sure that the barcode readers are working properly.

5. Perform processor QC if the laser camera is used for obtaining hard-copy images.

Weekly Tests are performed by a technologist.

1. Verify monitor calibration (CRT only).

2. Test phantom images by performing phantom image analysis as suggested by the manufacturer and compare with previous images and look for any variation.

3. Clean and inspect all image receptors.
   - CR—clean and inspect all CR cassettes.
   - DR—clean and inspect the active matrix array area of the DR unit for dirt and scratches. Also inspect any visible cables leading to the DR image receptor for any cracks in the insulation or plastic connectors or any exposed or bare wires.

4. Clean the air intake ports on the CR system IRD. This will prevent damage to the IRD and minimize artifacts that may be caused by dirt on the reader mirrors or on the lens of the scanning laser.

5. Clean the computer keyboard and mouse according to the manufacturer's guidelines. This will prolong the life of the computer components and also reduce the transmission of illness among the department staff.

6. Clean the screen of CRT monitors according to the manufacturer's guidelines. CRT monitors attract dirt and dust due to electrostatic attraction. In addition, many monitors utilize touch-screen technology, which can cause dirt to build up quickly. LCD monitors are less likely to attract dirt and debris, but should still be inspected. Care must be taken in cleaning LCD screens, as it is easy to damage the plastic face and the LCD crystals underneath the face. Closely follow manufacturer's guidelines.

Monthly Tests are performed by a technologist.

1. Film processor maintenance is necessary only if the laser camera is used instead of a dry laser printer for hard copies.

2. Inspect and clean all image receptors.
   - CR—remove the IPs from each cassette and clean them according to manufacturer's specifications. Generally, a lint free cloth (photographic lens cloth) or a camel hair brush should be used to gently wipe any loose debris from the IP. Most manufacturers have a special cleaning solution that can be used for IPs that have any dirt that is more difficult to remove. IPs that can no longer be cleaned effectively will have to be replaced. Since the PSP material contains some barium, they cannot be disposed of in the standard trash and must be disposed of according to Environmental Protection Agency (EPA) regulations. A licensed disposal company should be contacted to properly dispose of these IPs, and the proper paperwork must be kept on file.
   - DR—clean and inspect the active matrix array area of the DR unit for dirt and scratches. Also inspect any visible cables leading to the DR image receptor for any cracks in the insulation or plastic connectors or any exposed or bare wires. A thorough cleaning of the DR image receptor should be performed by a qualified service technician and scheduled accordingly.

3. Perform a repeat analysis and review the data to correct any ongoing issues. A repeat or reject analysis looks at images that were not acceptable diagnostically and determines why they occurred in order to minimize the chance of recurrence in the future. This generally involves looking at these images and using a repeat analysis form to classify the rejects according to cause. This procedure is discussed in detail in Chapter 10.

4. Service logs of digital equipment should be reviewed to see if a specific problem is reoccurring. If so, possible solutions should be explored to minimize down time.

Semiannual/Annual tests are performed by a medical physicist.

1. X-ray generator testing involves testing the x-ray generator, tube, and accessories according to the procedures discussed in Chapter 7. This type of testing is done to make sure that any errors discovered are caused by the digital imaging components and not by the x-ray generator.
2. Evaluate image quality by reviewing actual patient images as well as phantom images. Phantom images should be obtained and analyzed in both automatic and nonautomatic modes.
3. Image processing evaluation are conducted to make sure that all of the preprocessing (histogram analysis, LUT, etc.) and postprocessing functions are operating properly.
4. Repeat acceptance tests to reestablish baseline values.
5. Review patient exposure trends, repeat analysis data, QC records, and service history.
6. Evaluate exposure indicator accuracy using a dosimeter to record exposure to image receptors.
7. Determine the necessity for system adjustment by vendor service personnel.

A summary of these tests are listed in Box 9-2.

Digital Fluoroscopy

Digital fluoroscopy (DF), or computerized fluoroscopy (CF), was developed during the 1970s at the University of Wisconsin and the University of Arizona. The concept involves taking the fluoroscopic image (whether from the television camera or a flat panel system), digitizing the electronic signal carrying the image information, and sending this digital signal into a computer for real-time processing. Advantages of digital fluoroscopy include *last frame–hold*, *road mapping*, *digital temporal filtering*, *image enhancement*, and *image restoration*.

Last Frame–Hold. One of the many advantages of digital fluoroscopy includes a *last frame–hold* feature that allows the last image in the computer memory to be displayed on the monitor, even though the x-ray beam is off.

Road Mapping. Another advantage is a feature known as *road mapping*, which can permit an image to be captured and displayed on a monitor, while a second monitor shows a real-time image. Road mapping also can be used to record an image with contrast material that can then be overlaid onto a live fluoroscopic image.

Digital Temporal Filtering. Still another advantage is a feature known as *digital temporal filtering* (also known as *frame averaging*), which can add together different image pixel values and then average the values during display of successive images. This process is used to reduce the effect of random noise (quantum mottle) but does cause a noticeable increase in image lag due to a lower image frame rate.

BOX 9-2 Summary of QC Tests for CR and DR Systems

Acceptance Tests—performed by medical physicist
1. Erasure thoroughness
2. Phantom imaging testing

Daily Tests—performed by technologist
1. General inspection
2. Laser printer
3. Erasure thoroughness
4. IRD and workstation communication
5. Processor QC (laser cameras only)

Weekly Tests—performed by technologist
1. Verify monitor calibration (CRT monitors only)
2. Phantom image testing
3. Clean and inspect all image receptors
4. Clean air intake ports on CR system IRD
5. Clean computer keyboard and mouse
6. Clean monitor screen

Monthly Tests—performed by technologist
1. Film processor maintenance (laser cameras only)
2. Clean and inspect all image receptors
3. Perform repeat analysis
4. Service log review

Semiannual/Annual Tests—performed by medical physicist
1. X-ray generator testing
2. Image quality evaluation
3. Image processing evaluation
4. Repeat acceptance tests to reestablish baseline values
5. Review patient exposure trends, repeat analysis data, QC records, and service history
6. Evaluate exposure indicator accuracy
7. Determine necessity for system adjustment by service personnel

---

Image Enhancement. The computer allows **image improvement** or **image enhancement** of structures of interest in the image through various means. The image contrast can be manipulated by controlling window width and the image brightness can be manipulated by controlling **window level. Window width** selects the width of the band of values in the digital signal, which can be represented as gray tones in the image. This provides a means of compressing or expanding **image contrast.** The window level selects the level of the displayed band of values within the complete range. This allows for the manipulation of the pixel brightness in different parts of the image to optimize image quality.

Image Restoration. The computer allows **image restoration** to correct for distortion and vignetting that may occur in the image intensifier.

Currently, two methods are used for performing DF: with an analog image intensifier tube or with a flat-panel or flat-plate image receptor.

Image Intensifier Tube Digital Fluoroscopy Systems. Standard fluoroscopic units feed the image from the television camera (which is focused onto the output phosphor of an image intensifier tube) directly to the

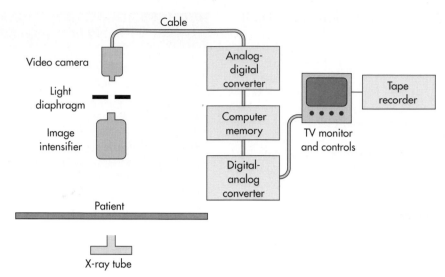

FIGURE 9-16 Block diagram of digital fluoroscopic system.

monitor for immediate viewing. In this method of DF, the analog signal from the camera is first sent through an ADC and then through a microprocessor circuit that processes the image (Fig. 9-16).

Flat-panel Digital Fluoroscopy Systems. This method of DF uses similar flat-panel image receptors such as those in direct-conversion radiographic systems. This flat-panel image receptor replaces the image intensifier and television camera combination and feeds the image information directly into an image processor, which is essentially the same as that used in DF with an image intensifier tube. The rows of pixels in the AMA are switched continuously, rather than in sequential rows (used in DR radiographic systems). This allows continuous updating of the image to obtain a real-time image.

The digitally generated image can be displayed on the monitor either with monochrome gray-scale images, in which each pixel produces a certain gray tone (most common), or with bi-stable images, in which the pixel is either black or white with no intermediate gray tones. This is generally used in radionuclide imaging. The monitor can use several scan modes for image display, including continuous fluoroscopy mode, pulsed interlaced scan mode, pulsed progressive scan mode, and slow scan mode.

Continuous Fluoroscopy Mode. A standard 525-line monitor is used with continuous fluoroscopy at a low milliampere (mA) value (<5 mA). With this lower mA value, quantum mottle and low signal-to-noise ratio are problems; therefore, the computer uses as many as 20 to 30 separate frames to produce a single image.

Pulsed Interlaced Scan Mode. In the pulsed interlaced scan mode, the x-ray tube delivers radiation in short, high-intensity pulses at about one per second. This reduces quantum mottle and increases resolution and

signal-to-noise ratio. This pulsed mode also can reduce patient dose and is more commonly used than continuous fluoroscopy.

Pulsed Progressive Scan Mode. In the pulsed progressive scan mode, the x-ray beam is pulsed but the monitor scans the lines in natural order rather than in an interlaced manner. This reduces image flicker and improves resolution but requires a 1023-line monitor.

Slow Scan Mode. In slow scan mode, 7.5, 1050-line frames are scanned per second, which doubles image resolution.

All modes have freeze-frame and last-image recall options that allow the image to remain on the monitor even though no fluoroscopy is currently taking place. This function reduces patient dose.

Digital Subtraction Angiography

The main application for DF systems is for **digital subtraction angiography** (DSA). This involves removing or subtracting background structures from an image so that only contrast media-filled structures remain (Fig. 9-17). Before DSA, radiographs were taken before the administration of contrast media. Because a standard radiograph is a photographic negative, a positive of this image, called a *mask film*, is then created. When a second radiograph is taken with contrast media present (again, a photographic negative), it is combined with the mask film to create the subtraction image. This method is time consuming and cumbersome. DSA involves imaging the patient before the arrival of contrast media; the computer stores the image as the mask. When the image with the contrast media is created, the computer stores it in a separate area and then combines it with the mask to create the subtracted image. Figure 9-18 shows a block diagram of this process.

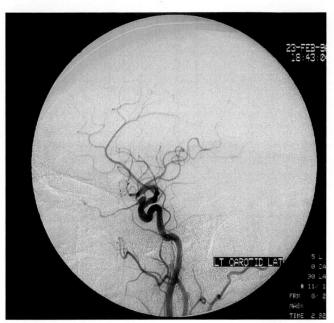

FIGURE 9-17 Image obtained during digital subtraction angiography (DSA).

The advantages of DSA over the film method include wider exposure latitude, computerized enhancement of image contrast (contrast differences of <1% can be visualized), and quick image acquisition. The main disadvantages are small field of view (because it is limited by the input phosphor size) and lower spatial resolution (because of pixel size and the limitation of the monitor). A laser camera should be used to create hard-copy images. DSA is of several types including temporal mask subtraction, time-interval difference subtraction, and dual-energy subtraction.

Temporal Mask Subtraction. Temporal mask subtraction is the standard type of DSA described earlier, in which the computer uses a noncontrast mask with the contrast media image to create the subtracted image. Patient motion must be avoided between the two images, or image noise and degradation result (Fig. 9-19).

Time-Interval Difference Subtraction. In the process of time-interval difference subtraction, a series of images are obtained at equally spaced times after injection of

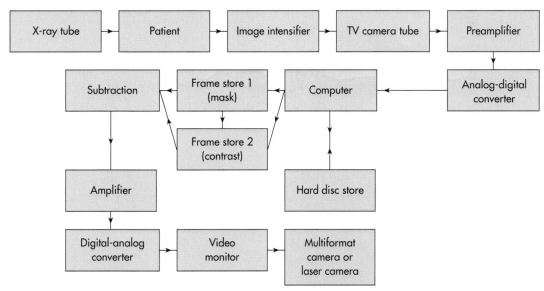

FIGURE 9-18 Block diagram of DSA.

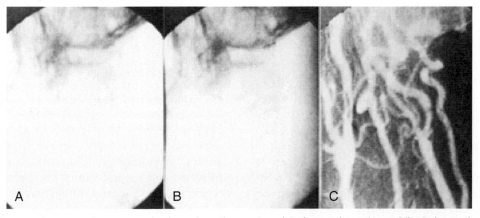

FIGURE 9-19 Images demonstrating temporal subtraction. Figures **A** and **B** show subtraction, while **C** shows the original image.

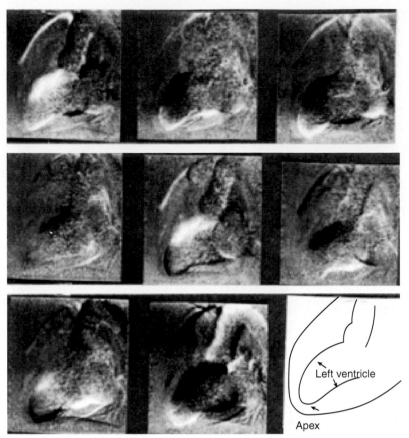

FIGURE 9-20 Images showing the effect of TID subtraction process.

contrast media. Each image is subtracted from the next to form new subtraction images. This helps identify certain pathologic conditions in the vasculature that inhibit the flow of contrast media over time (Fig. 9-20).

Dual-Energy Subtraction. In dual-energy subtraction, two different qualities (energies) of x-ray beam are used, one at just below 33 kiloelectron volts (keV) and one at just above this value. This is because the K-edge of iodine is at 33 keV, so the images created at each different energy level are compared by the computer to create the subtracted image.

Quality Control of Digital Fluoroscopy Units

The non-digital functions of DF units should be checked with the use of the conventional fluoroscopic methods described in Chapter 8. Once these have been evaluated and are performing within specified parameters, then the DF functions should be checked on acceptance and then every 6 months or when service is performed on the system. This requires a phantom that conforms to the recommendations found in Report No. 15 by the AAPM Digital Radiography/Fluorography Task Group of the Diagnostic Imaging Committee (Fig. 9-21). The phantom evaluates the variables of high- and low-

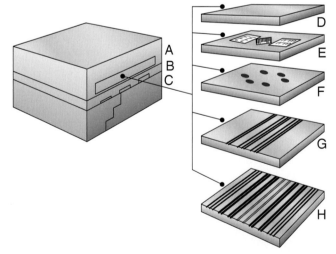

FIGURE 9-21 Digital subtraction angiography (DSA) phantom. **A,** Slot block. **B,** Bone block. **C,** Step wedge. **D,** Block insert. **E,** High-contrast resolution pattern insert. **F,** Linearity insert. **G,** Low-contrast artery insert. **H,** Low-contrast iodine line pair insert. *(Courtesy Nuclear Associates, Carle Place, N.Y.)*

contrast resolution, spatial resolution, subtraction effectiveness, image uniformity, amplifier dynamic range, registration (to detect any changes in pixel position between the test image and the mask image), and linearity. Linearity in this context refers to changes in iodine content (measured in milligram per square centimeter) within a specific area, which should change the pixel shade or tone accordingly. For example, if an image is obtained of two iodine-filled vessels, one with an iodine content of 1 mg/cm^2 and the other 2 mg/cm^2, then the shade or tone of the pixel should differ by a factor of 2. Some phantoms also have components that simulate blood vessels and aneurysms of various sizes.

ELECTRONIC DISPLAY DEVICES

All digital diagnostic imaging modalities must display the final image on some type of electronic display device such as a television or computer monitor. This is sometimes referred to as "soft-copy" viewing (as opposed to "hard-copy" viewing, such as a film image on a conventional viewbox). The obvious advantage of soft-copy viewing is the ability to postprocess the image while viewing. However, disadvantages include limited luminance range; poor resolution; reflection of ambient light; veiling glare (a light-spreading phenomenon caused by internal light scattering; light leakage; or electron backscattering, causing a degradation of image contrast); and degradation over time. Often times, these devices can be the weakest link in the imaging chain in terms of image resolution. This means that the quality of the display device can have a direct bearing on the quality of the image and therefore the accuracy of the diagnosis obtained from this image.

The American College of Radiology (ACR) and the FDA classify electronic display devices as being either primary or secondary. Primary display devices are those that will be used for the interpretation of diagnostic images by radiologists and other physicians. The recommended matrix size for primary display devices used to view radiographic images is 2048 × 2560 (5 megapixels). The active pixel size is about 0.15 mm. Secondary systems would be those used for viewing diagnostic images for purposes other than for providing medical interpretation (such as operators' console monitors and QC workstations, PACS workstations, and workstations used by general medical staff). Secondary matrix sizes can range from 1024 × 1280 (1.3 megapixels) to 1200 × 1600 (2 megapixels). The active pixel size is about 0.3 mm. Monitors for viewing digital mammographic images have a matrix size of 4096 × 6144 with an active pixel size of 40 to 50 μm. This is necessary for proper display of spatial resolution but can cost up to $40,000. Care must be taken when viewing an image of a certain matrix size to a display device of another size because information can be lost from the image. **Interpolation** refers to the mapping of an image of one matrix size to a display of another size. For example, if an image created in a computer with a matrix size of 2 k × 2 k is displayed on a 1 k × 1 k monitor, 4 pixels from the original image will have to be mapped to each single pixel in the monitor, causing a loss of image data.

An important characteristic of an electronic display device is a value known as the **aspect ratio**. This is the ratio of the width of the display to the height of the display. Most standard CRT computer monitors have an aspect ratio of 4:3 while flat screen LCD and plasma monitors have a ratio of 16:9. Primary display monitors for viewing radiographic images are generally 5 megapixel displays and have an aspect ratio of 5:4. The software settings of the computer controlling the display device must be adjusted to match the aspect ratio of the monitor or geometric distortions will occur in the image. Another important monitor characteristic is the **refresh rate** (also known as the **frame rate** or vertical scan frequency) of the monitor. This refers to how many times each second that the monitor rewrites or updates the image on the display. A refresh rate that is too low can cause a flickering effect that can cause eye strain and fatigue for the viewer. The refresh rate for viewing monitors can range from 55 Hz to 150 Hz (in this context, a Hertz refers to a frame per second). A minimum refresh rate of 70 Hz is recommended for primary class CRT displays. LCD and plasma displays take longer to switch from one image to the next, so less flicker is visible.

In the past, high-resolution monochrome (black and white) cathode-ray tubes (CRTs) have been the most common displays for viewing digital radiographic and fluoroscopic images. Currently, flat-panel active matrix liquid crystal displays have become more commonplace as their capital cost continues to decline. Flat panel plasma displays are beginning to appear as image display devices. Figure 9-22 shows the various classifications of electronic display devices.

Cathode-Ray Tube Displays

The cathode ray tube has been around since the late 1870s (the Crooke's tube that Roentgen was experimenting with when he discovered x-rays was a cathode ray tube, as is the fluoroscopic image intensifier tube) and is still used today for both image display, as well as television camera tubes to acquire the initial image. The basic components (Fig. 9-23) include a cathode (which will release electrons through thermionic emission); control grids; accelerating electrodes; electrostatic focusing lenses (to accelerate and focus the electrons toward the front screen); deflection coils (to move the electron beam back and forth and up and down, in order to create scan lines and pixels); an anode (to attract the electrons from the cathode); and the front screen (which is a glass plate coated with crystals that will emit light when struck by the electron beam). An antireflection layer is placed on the faceplate of the screen to reduce ambient light reflection and veiling glare. Phosphor materials that are used in the screens are designated by a P-number system created by the U.S. Electronics Industry Association. A higher P-number

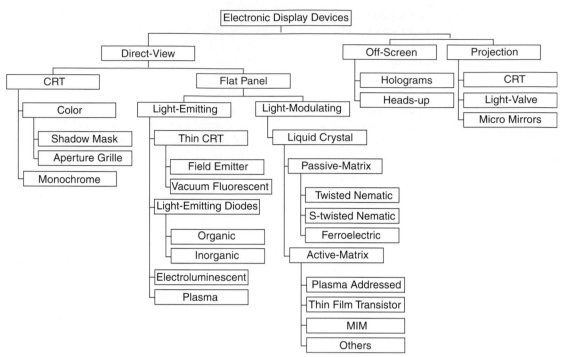

FIGURE 9-22 Block diagram showing various classifications of electronic display devices. *(Samei E, et al: Assessment of Display Performance for Medical Imaging Systems. Draft Report of the American Association of Physicists in Medicine (AAPM) Task Group 18, Version 10.0, August 2004.)*

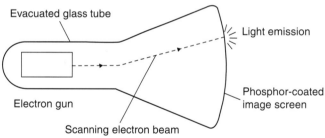

FIGURE 9-23 Basic components of a cathode-ray tube display device.

indicates that it will create a greater degree of luminance for a given amount of current in the electron beam (i.e., a P45 phosphor will emit more light for a given tube current than a P11). Currently, P4, P45, and P104 phosphors have all been used successfully in high-resolution monitors used in diagnostic imaging. The P45 phosphor is the most commonly used because it is more stable than the others at high beam currents, exhibits a slower loss of efficiency due to aging, and has less noise. Monochrome monitors produce a luminance level of 300 to 500 nit, as compared with 2000 (general radiography) to 3500 (mammographic) nit for film images on a viewbox. To obtain a higher brightness level with a CRT, a larger beam current would be necessary; however, this would tend to increase the size of the beam and therefore reduce spatial resolution, as well as reduce the life of the tube.

Liquid Crystal Displays

Flat-panel liquid crystal displays have become more and more popular as display devices in diagnostic imaging, much as they are with home desktop computers (laptop computers have used LCDs from the beginning). LCDs consist of a large array of LC cells (each of which will represent a single pixel in the image), polarizer filters, and a backlight (Fig. 9-24). The liquid crystals will change their molecular orientation when an electrical field is applied to them. This in turn will change the light transmission capability of the liquid crystal, thereby causing more or less light to be transmitted through it, thus controlling the brightness value of the pixel. Filter materials are added for color displays. LCDs have many advantages over CRT monitors in that they do not defocus over time because no electron beam is used to create the image, they have better grayscale definition than CRTs, and they better reduce the effect of ambient light on image contrast. LCDs also produce a higher level of luminance than CRTs (up to 700 nit). They also give the appearance of greater resolution and contrast due to the light emission being emitted perpendicular to the faceplate (caused by the passage of light through the polarizing filters). This also leads to a significant disadvantage in that they have a limited viewing angle (usually 40 degrees either side of a line that is perpendicular to the center of the faceplate). This is known as angular dependence of viewing. LCDs used for diagnostic imaging should have at least an 80-degree or higher viewing angle in the horizontal direction and 50 degrees in the vertical direction.

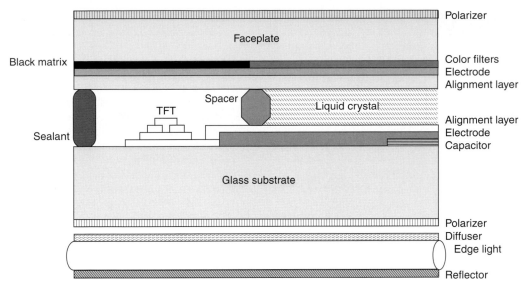

FIGURE 9-24 Basic components of a liquid crystal display device. *(Courtesy Nuclear Associates, Carle Place, N.Y.)*

Plasma Displays

Flat panel plasma displays consist of an active matrix of tiny fluorescent bulbs that will emit light from each pixel location. An advantage of this type of display device is that they are thinner than LCD panels but have a higher luminance output than CRT or LCD displays and have a wide angle of viewing capability. However, they are much more expensive than LCD monitors and have a shorter life span.

Quality Control of Electronic Display Devices

Because electronic display devices are responsible for image display in all digital imaging, it is imperative that they be evaluated for optimum performance on a regular basis. Many groups have published guidelines for QC procedures including the National Electronics Manufacturer's Association (NEMA), the Society of Motion Picture and Television Engineers (SMPTE), the **Digital Imaging and Communications in Medicine** (DICOM) group, and the AAPM, as well as the various manufacturers of these devices. As of the writing of this edition, no one set of recommendations has been endorsed by the medical community. Medical physicists and radiologists should be consulted for setting the performance standards at facilities until universal standards are adopted.

Virtually all display device manufacturers recommend that they be operated between 0° and 40° C with a relative humidity range of between 10% and 70% (to avoid condensation). LCD monitors are especially sensitive to changes in temperature. The American College of Radiology recommends evaluating performance at least monthly. The AAPM is more rigorous in its recommendations, suggesting evaluation on acceptance, daily, monthly/quarterly, and annually. Acceptance and annual evaluation should be performed by a physicist, while daily and monthly/quarterly evaluation can be performed by either a physicist or a trained QC technologist. Daily QC should take less than 1 minute to complete and involves imaging either an SMPTE test pattern (Fig. 9-28) or the AAPM TG18-QC (Fig. 9-25) test pattern. Parameters to evaluate during daily QC include the following:

1. Turn on the monitor and execute the normal boot-up procedure. Allow CRT monitors to warm up for 30 minutes.
2. Cleanliness of front screen—clean the front screen using manufacturer's guidelines if dirty.
3. Geometric distortion—involves verification that all lines and borders in the pattern are visible and straight and centered within the active area of the display device.
4. General image quality and appearance—involves evaluating the overall appearance of the pattern for any non-uniformities or artifacts such as dropped pixels.
5. Luminance—involves verification that all 16 luminance patches are distinctly visible, especially the 5% and 95% patches.
6. Resolution—involves verification that all letters and numbers within the pattern are visible.

Monthly or quarterly inspections should take about 20 minutes, and the following procedure should be used:

PROCEDURE

Monthly/Quarterly

1. Turn on the monitor and execute the normal boot-up procedure. Allow CRT monitors to warm up for 30 minutes.
2. Inspect the front screen of the monitor for cleanliness. If dirty, clean using the manufacturer's instructions.
3. Determine if specular reflection of light sources (e.g., lights, other monitors, viewboxes, and windows) are present on the monitor from a normal viewing direction. Reduce or eliminate if possible.
4. Assess the following image quality parameters while viewing the appropriate SMPTE or AAPM-TG 18 test pattern:
   a) Luminance response—Luminance response refers to the relationship between displayed luminance (luminance values obtained during testing) and the input values of a standardized display system (test pattern brightness). Use a photometer and AAPM TG18-LN test patterns (Figs. 9-26 to 9-28) to measure luminance at the center of the monitor. Primary display monitors (those used by physicians to diagnose images) should have a luminance greater than 170 nit (50 foot-lamberts), while secondary display monitors (those used by technologists) should have a luminance greater than 100 nit (30 foot-lamberts). These luminance values should not vary by more than 10% from values that were previously obtained. Also, workstations with multiple monitors should not vary by more than 10%. The monitor brightness control can be readjusted if the luminance is not within limits. In addition, the luminance readings from the center of the TG18-LN01 pattern (L_{min}) and the TG18-LN18 pattern (L_{max}) should be used to determine the contrast ratio of the monitor. The photometer to measure the luminance of the minimum black level (L_{min}) and the maximum white level (L_{max}) displayed on the monitor. The contrast ratio is the ratio of the maximum white level (L_{max}) to the minimum black level (L_{min}), OR L_{max} / L_{min}, and should be greater than 250. As a comparison, this corresponds to optical density values in film screen imaging of between 0.1 and 2.5, which is where most diagnostically useful structures would typically be found. If a photometer is not available, luminance response can be evaluated visually using the TG18-CT test pattern (Fig. 9-29). This pattern should be evaluated for visibility of the central half-moon targets and the four low-contrast objects at the corners of each of 16 different luminance regions. The low contrast targets in all 16 regions should be visible (a common failure is not being able to see the targets in one or two of the dark regions). In addition, the bit depth resolution of the display (the maximum number of gray scales that can be displayed simultaneously) should be evaluated using the TG18-MP test pattern (Fig. 9-30). The relative location of contouring bands and any luminance levels should not be further than the distance between the 8-bit markers (long markers). No contrast reversal (bright areas appearing dark and dark areas appearing bright) should be visible.
   b) Luminance dependencies—refer to the luminance response mentioned above, but it is how this value is dependent on the nonuniformity across the entire display and the viewing angle between the observer and the center of the display. Nonuniformity refers to the maximum variation in luminance across the display area when a uniform pattern is displayed. This is a common characteristic in CRT displays, with the luminance typically decreasing from the center to the edges and corners of the display, due to differences in the path length and beam landing angle of the electron beam (because the glass front is curved). This effect is less pronounced in LCD displayed but must still be evaluated. Use the photometer to measure the luminance of the TG18-UNL10 (relatively dark image) and TG18-UNL80 relatively bright image) test patterns (Figs. 9-31 and 9-32) in the center of the display, as well each of the four corners. The five luminance readings from each of the same test pattern should be within 20% of each other. If not, the monitor controls can be adjusted or a physicist or biomedical engineer should be consulted. If a photometer is not available, luminance nonuniformity can be evaluated visually using the TG18-UN10 and TG18-UN80 test patterns. When viewing, each pattern should be free of gross nonuniformities from the center to the edges. No luminance variations with dimensions on the order of 1 cm or larger should be observed. Angular dependence is how bright the image appears from each viewing angle between the observer and the center of the display. Ideally, luminance and viewing angle should be independent of each other. However, this can vary considerably depending on the type of monitor used. Flat panel LCD monitors tend to suffer severe variation due to viewing angle changes, even suffering from contrast reversal (light areas appearing dark and dark areas appearing bright). Angular response can be evaluated using the TG18-CT test pattern (see Fig. 9-29). Begin by viewing the pattern straight-on and determine the visibility of the half-moon targets. Then move to the right and left of center to see when or if the patterns disappear (they probably won't with CRT or plasma displays but will with LCD displays). Any viewing angle limits should be clearly labeled on the front of the monitor and these limits should not change from one test to the next.
   c) Spatial or geometric distortion—view the large squares of the SMPTE or AAPM TG18-QC pattern throughout the image using a viewing distance of 30 cm. They should appear as perfect squares over the entire screen. A flexible ruler can be used to measure the width and height of each square. This should be done in each quadrant, as well as the center of the image. The difference between expected and measured lengths within the pattern should not exceed 2% for primary class displays or 5% for secondary class displays. Monitor controls can be adjusted if they are beyond these limits. Also make sure that there are no magnetic fields present, as these can cause geometric distortions in CRT monitors.
   d) Spatial resolution—view high-contrast boundaries (such as white text on a dark background) and verify that they are well defined. Adjust monitor controls if they are not visible. A more detailed test involves assessing the appearance of the Cx patterns in either the TG18-QC or TG18-CX (Fig. 9-33) test patterns. Examine the displayed Cx patterns at the center and at the four corners of the image using a magnifying glass. Note any differences in the visibility of the test patterns between the horizontal and vertical lines (they should all be the same whether they are in the center or at the edges). CRT displays may show less resolution at the edges than at the center.
   e) Low-contrast resolution—verify that the 5% contrast patches are visible in both the 100% video (white) and 0% video (black) squares from either the SMPTE or the AAPM TG18-QC test pattern.
   f) Gray scale uniformity—verify that the gray background of the SMPTE or AAPM TG18-QC pattern is uniformly gray across the entire display.
   g) Display artifacts—verify that the display does not contain streaks, lines, or dark/light patches. Also look for any small black dots, which indicate nonfunctioning (dropped) pixels.

PROCEDURE—CONT'D

h) Display Reflection—verify that all light coming from the display surface has been generated by the display device only and not contain any reflected light. Generally, reflection from the face of the display comes in two basic forms: specular and diffuse. Specular reflection produces a mirror image of the light source creating it while diffuse reflection produces a more uniform luminance on the display with no detectable patterns of the source creating it. Antireflective coatings on the faceplate of the display and reduction of ambient light in the viewing area should reduce these reflections. With the display in the power-save mode or turned off, observe the display with the ambient light at normal levels at a distance of about 30 to 60 cm and a viewing angle of ± 15 degrees. Look for the presence of specularly reflected light sources or illuminated objects. Reflections from white lab coats and other bright clothing are common sources of specular reflection. If present, reduce ambient light levels. To test for diffuse reflection, observe the low contrast patterns in the TG18-AD test pattern (Fig. 9-34) in both near total darkness and in normal ambient lighting. The low contrast patterns should appear the same whether viewed in total darkness or normal light conditions. If the patterns are not visible in normal light conditions, ambient light must be reduced as this is causing a reduction in contrast within the image.

A checklist for documentation of this procedure is provided on the accompanying Evolve website.

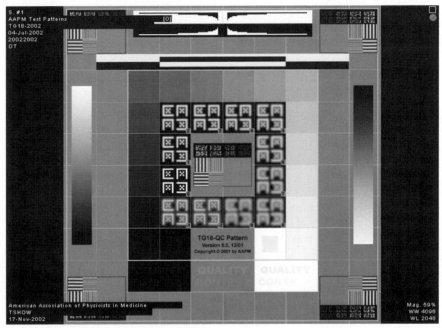

FIGURE 9-25 AAPM TG-18 QC Test Pattern. *(From Samei E, et al: Assessment of Display Performance for Medical Imaging Systems. Draft Report of the American Association of Physicists in Medicine (AAPM) Task Group 18, Version 10.0, August 2004.)*

Annual inspections should only be performed by a medical physicist using the procedures described by the AAPM, Task Group 18. The procedures are extensive and beyond the scope of this book, but can be downloaded from the following website: www.aapm.org.

A more detailed procedure for evaluating electronic display devices is listed below, and summarized in Box 9-3.

MULTIFORMAT CAMERAS

Most diagnostic imaging modalities (with the exception of conventional radiography, fluoroscopy, **cinefluorography,** and photofluorography) do not automatically create a hard copy of the final image. Instead, the image is stored in computer hardware or created on some form of video display. Therefore, an electronic device is required to transfer the image onto film or other storage medium. One such device is the multiformat camera, so-called because each film can be formatted or divided up into as many as 25 separate images (Fig. 9-36). This is a useful and cost-effective method of recording hard copy images from computed tomography (CT), MRI, ultrasound, and DSA.

Components

The video signal from the respective modality is fed into the camera, where it is displayed on a CRT. The front of the CRT is flat, as opposed to the curved face on standard television monitors, to avoid pincushion distortion.

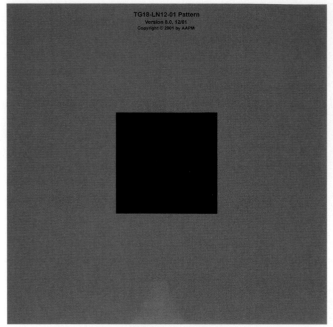

FIGURE 9-26 AAPM TG18-LN01 Test Pattern.

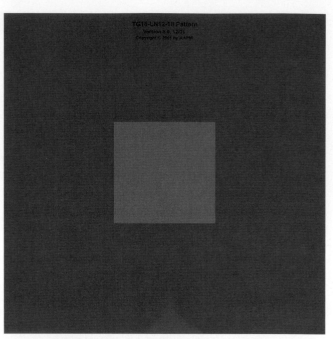

FIGURE 9-28 AAPM TG18-LN18 Test Pattern.

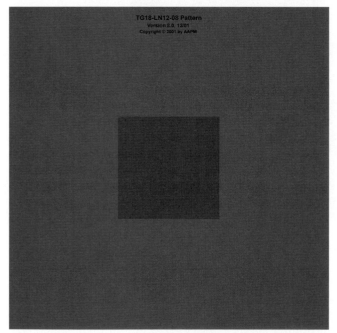

FIGURE 9-27 AAPM TG18-LN08 Test Pattern.

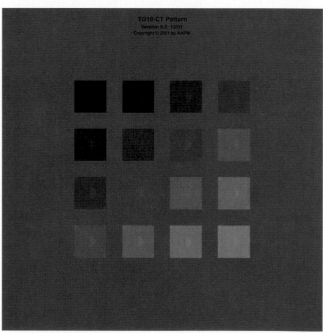

FIGURE 9-29 AAPM TG18-CT Test Pattern.

These tubes use a 525- or 1023-line raster, and the screen phosphors are commonly P11 (blue emitting) or P45 (blue-green emitting). Standard fluoroscopic monitors (and black-and-white televisions) use P4 phosphors, which emit white light. The image from the screen is reflected through a series of mirrors and lenses onto a film platform (Fig. 9-37). Depending on the manufacturer, the CRT, the film platform, the optical system, or combinations of these will move in order to format the film. Most multiformat cameras have three parameters on the unit control panel to control image quality: brightness, contrast, and exposure time.

Brightness. When the brightness level of the CRT increases, the optical density of the resulting image increases, especially in images with an optical density of less than 1.0.

Contrast. If the CRT's contrast level increases, the maximum optical density values (those above 2.0) in

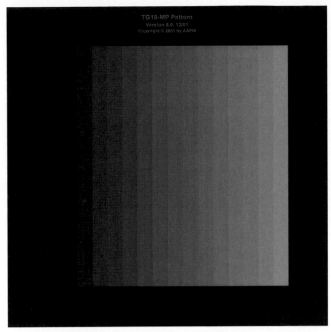

FIGURE 9-30 AAPM TG18-MP Test Pattern.

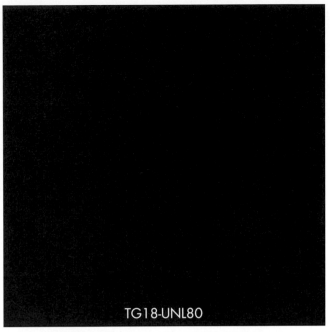

FIGURE 9-32 AAPM TG18-UNL80 Test Pattern.

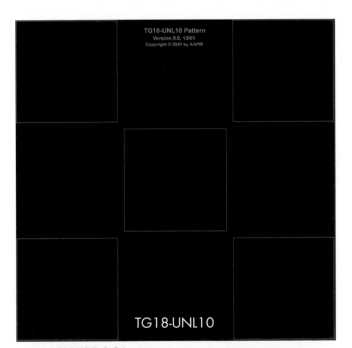

FIGURE 9-31 AAPM TG18-UNL10 Test Pattern.

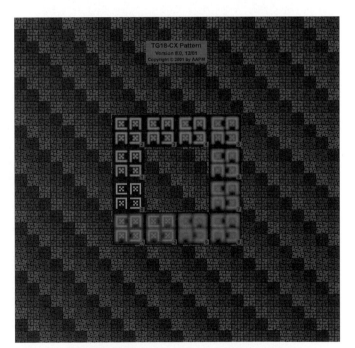

FIGURE 9-33 AAPM TG18-CX Test Pattern.

the image increase as well. Very little difference is seen in the lower values. Conversely, reducing the contrast level decreases maximum density.

Exposure Time. When the amount of time that the film is being exposed increases, the optical densities of the resulting image increase in all regions.

Quality Control of Multiformat Cameras

To evaluate the performance of a multiformat camera, use a multiformat test-pattern generator that creates a test pattern of the Society of Motion Picture and Television Engineers (SMPTE) (described in Chapter 8), as shown in Figure 9-38.

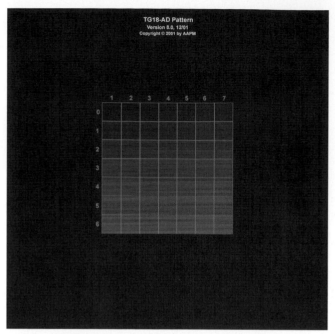

FIGURE 9-34 AAPM TG18-AD Test Pattern.

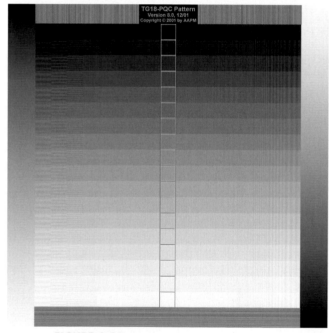

FIGURE 9-35 AAPM TG18 PQC Test Pattern.

BOX 9-3	Summary of Viewing Monitor QC

Monthly/Quarterly

Test Parameter	Variance allowed (if applicable)
Monitor cleanliness	
Specular reflection	
Luminance response	> 170 nit for primary and > 100 nit for secondary
Contrast ratio	> 250
Luminance dependencies	± 20%
Spatial or geometric distortion	± 2% for primary and ± 5% for secondary
Spatial resolution	
Low contrast resolution	5% and 95% patches must be visible
Gray scale uniformity	
Display artifacts	None should be visible
Display reflection	Reduce or eliminate if possible

Annual

Test Parameter	Variance allowed (if applicable)
Monitor cleanliness	
Specular reflection	
Luminance response	> 170 nit for primary and > 100 nit for secondary
Display noise	
Luminance dependencies	± 20%
Spatial or geometric distortion	± 2% for primary and ± 5% for secondary
Spatial resolution	
Low contrast resolution	5% and 95% patches must be visible
Gray scale uniformity	
Veiling glare	GR ≥ 400 for primary and ≥ 150 for secondary
Chromacity	

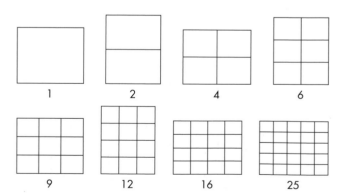

FIGURE 9-36 Format patterns for multiformat cameras.

LASER CAMERAS

Also known as a *laser imager*, the laser camera was first introduced in 1983 and can be used for providing hard-copy images from CT, MRI, CR, DR, and DSA (Fig. 9-39).

Components

Instead of a CRT, a thin (85-μm) laser beam rapidly scans the film (at about 600 lines per second). The intensity of the laser beam light modulates in proportion to the intensity of the signal received from the original image to regulate the optical density of the final image. Because the laser used in most of these units emits light in the red portion (7500 to 8500 angstroms [Å]) of the visible light spectrum, special film is required (red

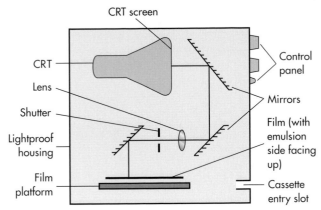

FIGURE 9-37 Schematic diagram of multiformat camera. *CRT,* Cathode-ray tube.

sensitive, silver halide based). An optical system composed of a rotating polygonal mirror and lenses focuses the laser onto the film. Because the laser produces a coherent light source that is intense and not divergent (light photons are perfectly parallel), image resolution is high (about 20 times better than a 1023-line CRT monitor). Usually, no phosphor or electronic noise is associated with laser cameras. Other advantages include multiple inputs (so that many modalities can interface with the same unit), improved contrast or gray scale, clear or black border option, positive or negative images, 20 image formats, and remote control.

PROCEDURE

1. With the image of the SMPTE of AAPM TG18-QC test pattern on the CRT, the brightness, contrast, and exposure time should be adjusted to optimum levels, and a hard copy image should be created. This image is used to evaluate such parameters as resolution and contrast gray scale.

2. A densitometer should be used to record the following areas of the hard-copy SMPTE film:
   40% patch: This value determines the level of the middensity or speed indicator, which should be approximately 1.15.
   10% and 70% patches: The optical densities of these two regions are subtracted from each other to yield the contrast indicator, which should be approximately 1.2.
   90% patch: This value is just above the base + fog and should be about ± 0.1 of 0.25.

3. The brightness, contrast, and exposure time settings should be recorded on the film for future reference. This test should be performed on acceptance and then should be performed daily if possible (or at least weekly). The films created each time should be compared with the original for signs of variation. The image screen of the CRT has an electrostatic charge that attracts dust particles. The screen should be cleaned at least monthly to prevent dust from producing artifacts on the recorded image. A regular preventive maintenance program should be established with a qualified service engineer and should include proper lubrication of moving parts, the cleaning of mirrors and optical lenses, and verification of proper alignment of all internal components. A checklist should be used to verify completion of the preventive maintenance program.

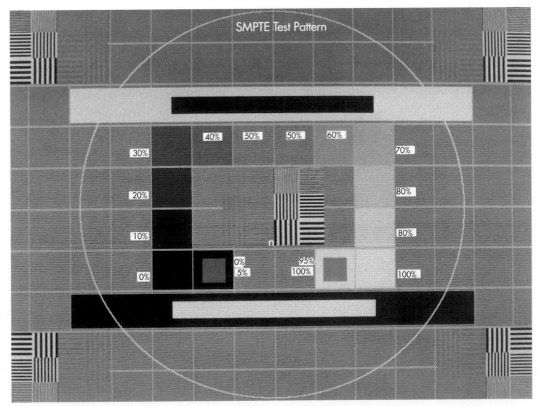

FIGURE 9-38 Society of Motion Picture and Television Engineers (SMPTE) test pattern.

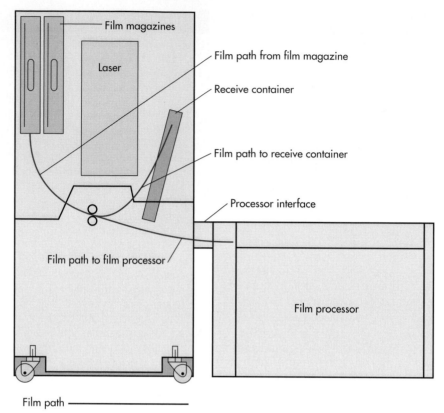

FIGURE 9-39 Schematic diagram of a laser camera.

The main disadvantages of laser cameras are higher cost compared with multiformat cameras, longer exposure time (20 to 30 seconds vs. 1 to 5 seconds for multiformat cameras), and lower resolution when small size images are multiformatted. In this case, each individual small image is created with the same number of scan lines as in a full-size image. With multiformat cameras, the optical system changes the image size, whereas the CRT uses the same number of scan lines as for a full-size image to form the smaller image. An automatic processor is usually directly linked to the laser camera for direct access to images. For this reason, the laser camera is also known as a wet imager. The film processing component of this unit also requires all of the standards for automatic film processors (well ventilated area, proper drainage and plumbing, chemical cost and disposal, quality control monitoring, etc.). For this reason, dry laser printers (covered later in this chapter) have become a more popular option for making hard copies of digital images.

Quality Control of Laser Cameras

Evaluation of laser cameras or printers is similar to that of multiformat cameras.

PROCEDURE

1. A multiformat test generator should be used to create either an SMPTE, TG18-QC or a TG18-PQC test pattern.
2. Hard-copy images should be produced and analyzed with the same standards that are used for multiformat camera images.
3. If an automatic processor is linked to the unit, it should be evaluated and serviced the same way as a standard film processor. Regular preventive maintenance is critical, and the maintenance program should include cleaning and lubricating of the internal components and the assessment of laser function.

DRY LASER PRINTERS

Most imaging departments have replaced multiformat cameras and laser cameras with dry laser printers to produce hard copies of digital images. These devices were introduced in 1996 and require specialized film (photothermographic) that uses silver behenate rather than silver halide to produce the image and is processed thermally rather than with liquid developer and fixer. Silver behenate is a crystalline long-chain silver carboxylate ($AgC_{22}H_{43}O_2$) that has been used in x-ray diffraction, as well as microfilms, for many years. The silver metal image formation is based on the heat-induced reduction of the silver behenate. The film is exposed

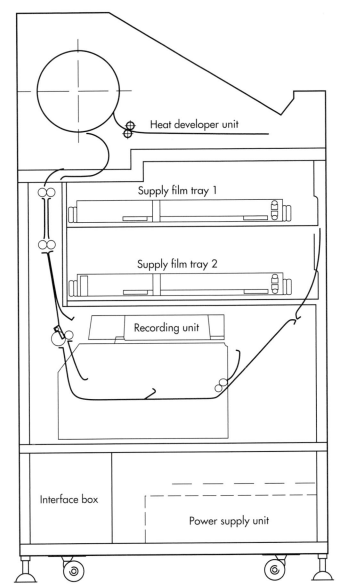

FIGURE 9-40 Schematic diagram of a dry laser printer.

Density Step 0
Density Step 1
Density Step 2
Density Step 3
Density Step 4
Density Step 5
Density Step 6
Density Step 7
Density Step 8
Density Step 9
Density Step 10
Density Step 11
Density Step 12
Density Step 13
Density Step 14
Density Step 15
Density Step 16
Density Step 17
Density Step 18
Density Step 19
Density Step 20
Density Step 21
Density Step 22
Density Step 23
Density Step 24
Density Step 25
Density Step 26
Density Step 27
Density Step 28
Density Step 29
Density Step 30
Density Step 31

FIGURE 9-41 Demonstration of step test pattern for evaluation of dry laser printer.

For quality control, dry laser printers can be evaluated in much the same way as the laser camera. Most newer models of dry laser printers have a built-in test pattern generator programmed into the unit that can be printed and evaluated according to the manufacturer's guidelines (Fig. 9-41). This usually involves the creation of a characteristic curve from this pattern and comparing it with those obtained on previous days. If this option is unavailable on a particular system, an external test pattern generator can be used and the procedure for evaluation of the laser camera followed.

CATHODE-RAY TUBE CAMERAS

Components

The CRT cameras consist of a single lens that connects to the front of a CRT screen and a "back" to hold the film. The most common back is called the *Shackman*; it holds an 8- × 10-inch cassette. Up to six images can be formatted on one sheet of film at a much lower cost compared with a laser or multiformat camera. The CRT cameras are often found in nuclear medicine and ultrasound equipment. Operation of a CRT camera requires focusing of the camera lens, setting the aperture size (measured in f-numbers ranging from 1.9 to 11; the smaller the value, the larger the aperture opening), and setting the exposure time. The exposure time should be

with a scanning laser, much the same as with a laser camera. After laser exposure, the film is heated to a temperature of 120° C for 24 seconds to process the image (Fig. 9-40).

After an image has been recorded, the film, immediately after it is ejected from the machine, is still in the process of image development, and the room illumination or light emanating from a viewbox illuminator can cause slight changes in the optical density. This can cause traces of overlapped films or transferred images to appear temporarily, but they disappear when those films are left under the normal light condition. The images recorded on these films can experience an increase in optical density over time if stored at temperatures above 30° C; however, because the images originally existed in digital form, they can be recalled in soft form (if stored properly) and then reprinted in hard copy at the desired future date.

longer than $^1/_{30}$ second because of the interlacing in a 525-line CRT monitor. The screen material found on the CRT monitor is usually a P11 (blue emitting), P24, or P31 (green emitting).

Quality Control of Cathode-Ray Tube Cameras

CRT cameras have fewer moving parts than multiformat or laser cameras, but they still require maintenance. The CRT screen should be cleaned weekly, and the back also should be cleaned regularly. Evaluation should occur on acceptance and then daily. An image should be created with a test pattern generator or special imaging phantom specific to the modality in which the camera is used. The resulting image should be analyzed for variation in image quality from the manufacturer's specifications.

VIDEOTAPE, VIDEODISC, AND DIGITAL RECORDERS

Videotape and videodisc recorders are used in certain applications to record fluoroscopic images, especially in gastrointestinal (GI) studies and cardiac imaging.

Components

Videotape units involve recording the image on magnetic tape contained inside of a plastic cassette. Video-cassettes for home units use either 8-mm (used in video cameras) or 13-mm ($^1/_2$-inch VHS or Beta) tape. These smaller tape sizes are inadequate for most diagnostic imaging because of excessive noise and a bandwidth that is too narrow. At least a 20-mm ($^3/_4$ inch U-matic) or, preferably, a 25-mm (1-inch) tape size should be used for proper image quality. Analog videodisc recorders use a disk (similar to a computer disk) to record images and yield superior quality "stop action" or "freeze-frame" images compared with videotape. This makes them useful for mobile C-arm fluoroscopic units, in which a "last-image-hold" feature often is incorporated. When the fluoroscopic switch is released, the last image is frozen and remains on the screen until the switch is again depressed. Framing rates for videodisc units vary from one image per second to 30 frames per second.

Videotape and videodisc recorders have many advantages over cinefluorography, including immediate playback, no separate film processor, no special viewer or projector, reusable tape, and contrast and brightness adjustment on the video monitor. Perhaps the greatest advantage is lower patient dose. The entrance skin dose is approximately 0.01 to 0.04 rad per frame (0.1 to 0.4 milligray [mGy]) for cinefluorography, whereas video recording delivers only 0.025 to 0.1 rad (0.25 to 1 mGy) per second. A 10-second image recording time for each delivers about 10 rad (100 mGy) with cinefluorography compared with only 1 rad (10 mGy) with video recording. The disadvantages of video recording include a lower image resolution than in cine film images and poor-quality still frame images with videotape recording.

Digital image recorders (also known as *digital photospot imaging*) have replaced videotape and videodisc recorders, as well as spot film and photospot imaging in many newer applications. These systems will obtain static spot images by having a short exposure of the image intensifier made with a high mA, while the real-time video is inactivated. The fluoroscopic television camera will instead send the signal through an ADC and then into a computer memory for later retrieval and processing. The images are usually 1024 × 1024 pixels, although some newer systems have 2048 × 2048 pixels. These units store the image in a digital form through computer hardware and software until needed. They are essentially computer "hard drives." The image can then be recalled onto a video monitor, or hard copies may be generated with a laser camera or dry laser printer. Images can be stored on computer disks. Digital image recorders also allow images to be enhanced or manipulated for better visualization of anatomic structures, but currently they record only a few frames in their memory circuits.

Quality Control of Analog and Digital Recorders

Analog videotape and videodisc recorders should be evaluated on acceptance and then at least every 6 months. Variation in performance is usually caused by the buildup of dirt on the recording heads, tape guides, and drive system, which can alter tape or disk speed and image quality

---

PROCEDURE

1. A multiformat test generator that creates an SMPTE or TG18-QC test pattern should be used for evaluation of these units. If this is unavailable, a videotape or videodisc of the test pattern is available from various distributors at a much lower cost.
2. When the test pattern image is recorded and evaluated, the image should display all of the 10% patches, and distortion should be minimal. The contrast or gray scale on the recorded image should be the same as on the original image.

A regular preventive maintenance program should be in place to ensure that the internal components are cleaned and evaluated. Digital recorders have fewer moving parts and are not subject to as much variation as analog units. The SMPTE test pattern can be used to evaluate the performance of these units in the same way as with analog units. Digital units generally perform correctly or not at all because of the solid-state nature of the equipment.

CINEFLUOROGRAPHY AND PHOTOFLUOROGRAPHY

As discussed in Chapter 8, the camera used for cinefluorography uses black-and-white motion picture film to record the motion of fast-moving objects, such as in cardiac catheterization studies. When framing rates in excess of 16 frames per second are used, the human eye perceives the successive images as continuous. In addition to a lens, shutter, and aperture, the camera also contains a variable-speed motor to advance the film and control the framing rate, along with a film magazine containing a film supply spool and a take-up spool (Fig. 9-42). The x-ray generator and camera are synchronized so that x-rays are emitted only when the film frame is in place. This pulsed operation greatly reduces patient dose. Photofluorographic cameras create static images at slower framing rates than cine cameras that use larger-format film.

Cinefluorography produces a relatively high patient dose under normal operating conditions. These units are also susceptible to variations in performance, which can degrade image quality and increase patient dose. Therefore periodic evaluation (at least every 6 months) of these units should occur, along with a preventive maintenance program to clean the optical system. High- and low-contrast resolution can be evaluated with test tools similar to those used for evaluating image intensifiers. The high-contrast tool should have a fine copper mesh pattern ranging from 60 to 150 holes per inch. A special cine-video quality control phantom is available from various distributors. This phantom contains a high-resolution test pattern, a step wedge for optical density and contrast measurement, and a mesh screen to test uniformity of focus (Fig. 9-43). Some of these

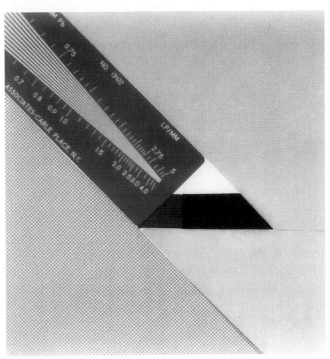

FIGURE 9-43 Cine-video quality control phantom. *(Courtesy Nuclear Associates, Carle Place, N.Y.)*

phantoms also provide patient identification information so that they may be imaged at the beginning of the study, before the patient is placed on the table. In this way, quality control is continuous and provides immediate feedback on system performance. Photofluorospot cameras can be evaluated with the same phantom.

Films recorded on cine film require an automatic processor to convert the latent image into a manifest image (Fig. 9-44). These processors are equipped with a processor-loading cassette that removes the exposed film from its magazine. The film is then advanced through

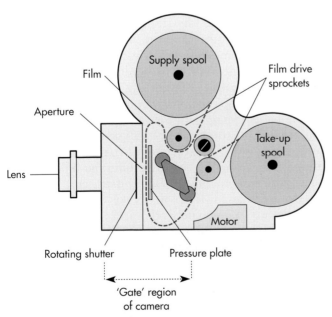

FIGURE 9-42 Diagram of a cine camera.

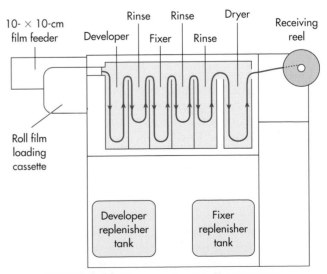

FIGURE 9-44 Diagram of a cine film processor.

the processor onto a take-up spool, where it is ready for viewing. These processors should be monitored in the same way as standard processors, with the sensitometric tests and procedures discussed in Chapter 5. The film advance drive motor requires a few drops of light machine oil in the gear case every 6 months.

After the processing, the cine film is viewed on a cine projector, which must function according to manufacturers' specifications to demonstrate proper image quality. Most units use a 500-watt quartz-iodine lamp to project the image onto a viewing screen. The light output should be at least 16 foot-candles (ft-cd) or 170 lux at the viewing screen and should be checked periodically with a photometer. Routine maintenance should include cleaning of the film advance claw and optical elements. Projector image quality is evaluated with a cine image of the SMPTE test pattern, which should demonstrate all of the resolution elements in the test film. Maintenance and test strip evaluation should occur at least every 6 months.

IMAGE ARCHIVING AND MANAGEMENT NETWORKS

With digital imaging becoming the dominant acquisition mode for diagnostic imaging, the storage of these images into a central computer system for retrieval at a later date has become an essential component of imaging departments. This reduces the space required for film storage in analog departments and increases the speed and accuracy of retrieval. The computer system allows remote access of patient images and other pertinent information from within the hospital itself and from physicians' offices and clinics several miles away and even around the world as a result of satellite transmission of digital data. Digital images can be easily downloaded into these systems from their original units. Conventional film images (which are analog in nature) must be converted to digital data by means of film digitization scanners that are similar to scanners used with personal computers to enter pictures or data (discussed earlier in this chapter). Most scanners use a CCD digitizer or a laser to scan the image and convert it to digital form. The resolution created by these scanners is less than the original film image because the pixel size used is larger than the silver grains found in the film.

The most common system for storing and retrieving digital images is the PACS, which stores digital images and allows access from remote locations. Most PACS systems use the DICOM standard, which is a system of computer software standards that allows different digital imaging programs to understand one another. For example, a digital radiographic system, a digital fluoroscopic system, CT scanners, and MRI scanners in a healthcare organization can all share the same PACS, even though they are different systems and may have been made by different manufacturers. The ACR and the National Electrical Manufacturers Association (NEMA) formed a committee to develop a standard for digital imaging and communications in 1983. The DICOM version 3 is the current standard developed by this committee and has become the de facto global standard. As the field of digital imaging continues to evolve, the DICOM-3 standard is subject to continuous revision, with supplements issued by the committee at various times. PACS systems contain four main components: image acquisition, image display and interpretation, image storage and retrieval, and a communications network.

1. Image acquisition is achieved by downloading the image from a CR, DR, MR, CT, etc. or from a film digitizer.
2. Image display and interpretation are the workstations for viewing images. Each workstation in the system is called a node or a client.
3. Image storage and retrieval is controlled by an archive server (PACS file room). It is composed of a database server or image manager, short-term and long-term storage, and a computer that controls the PACS workflow (known as a workflow manager).
4. The communications network allows images to be transmitted to remote workstations. The networks can be either a local area network (LAN) or a wide area network (WAN). A LAN is a network confined to one facility and usually connected by cable, optical fiber, or a wireless system. A WAN would include remote facilities and uses telecommunication devices such as the Internet. **Teleradiology** is the term given when images are transmitted over a WAN from one location to another for the purposes of interpretation and consultation.

The PACS is gradually being upgraded into the IMACS (Image Management and Communication System), which includes the storage and transmission of images and all other patient medical records. The IMACS is sometimes referred to as the *picture and paper archiving system* (PPACS). Traditionally, healthcare institutions have had a Radiology Information System (RIS) and a Hospital Information System (HIS). RIS's contain patient imaging history and scheduling information but do not store images. HIS's track patient admission, diagnostics, treatment, discharge and billing information, as well as employee information and pharmaceutical and equipment supply data, but, again, do not store images. IMACS networks can merge all of these systems into one network.

A problem with developing IMACS's is that the DICOM-3 standard used for transmission of images is not designed for transmission of other patient data such as laboratory reports. The current standard for transmission of medical record data is the Health Level 7 (HL7) standard, developed by the Healthcare Information and Management Systems Society (HIMSS).

The Radiological Society of North America (RSNA) has formed a joint committee with the HIMSS that has completed work to integrate the DICOM-3 and HL7 standards to allow for a universal format for the IMACS of the PACS. This is known as the Integrating Healthcare Enterprise (IHE) and the latest information can be found on their website at www.ihe.net. Other concerns with the digital transmission of image data are the privacy and security of the information. The Health Insurance Portability and Accountability Act (HIPAA) required that security standards for electronic transactions of patient information be implemented by October 2002 (October 2003 for small health plans) and are now in place. Similar legislation has been created by the European Community (EC Data Protection Directive 95/46/EC) and in Japan (HPB 517).

A main concern for instituting the PACS or the IMACS is the amount of computer hardware and data storage required. A digital chest image is about 8 megabytes in size, while a digital mammogram is 32 to 48 megabytes, so a typical diagnostic imaging department could generate enough image data to require a total memory of 20 terabytes (20 billion bytes) or more. Another problem is the network capacity, since most hospital-based PACS systems must share the LAN and its bandwidth with the rest of the healthcare organization, which can slow the speed of image transmission. The large data sets can benefit from image compression, which reduces the size of data files by removing and encoding redundant information. Lossless compression is completely reversible with compression up to 5 times. Lossy compression is not reversible and can introduce some degree of data loss, but can compress data size from 5 to 50 times. A widely used lossy compression standard is JPEG (Joint Photographic Export Group), which breaks the digital image into 8×8 pixel blocks and then compresses these blocks. Compression also can exaggerate original image errors and archival image errors. A new storage protocol called the storage area network (SAN) is being introduced to PACS's that can transfer large data files much more quickly. SANs use fiber channels, which can carry five times more bandwidth than the more commonly used small computer system interface (SCSI). Because this is a considerable amount of hardware to maintain, many healthcare organizations have turned to application software providers (ASPs). These are independent storage contractors outside of the healthcare organization who maintain the hardware and software necessary for a successful archiving system.

Because archiving systems are digital, variation in system performance is relatively rare. However, a quality control mechanism should be in place to guarantee optimum performance (see procedure box). Documentation of other characteristics such as System Down-Time and System Training for department employees also should be included in QC/CQI program. This can be

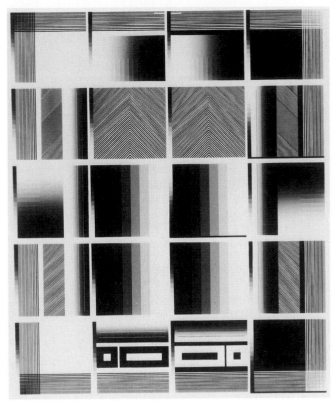

FIGURE 9-45 Picture archiving and communication system (PACS) test pattern. *(Courtesy Nuclear Associates, Carle Place, N.Y.)*

accomplished through the use of a log noting the details (name, dates, reason for problem, what was done to fix the problem, etc.).

For imaging departments that are transferring analog (film/screen) images into a PACS or IMACS system using film digitization scanners, these devices should be kept clean and free of dust or debris to avoid artifacts on the downloaded images (Fig. 9-45).

MISCELLANEOUS SPECIAL PROCEDURES EQUIPMENT

Many diagnostic imaging departments contain a so-called **special procedures laboratory**, or area in which angiographic, cardiac, and interventional procedures are performed. These types of procedures require additional equipment that is not normally found in standard radiographic and fluoroscopic suites including pressure injectors for administration of contrast media, film changers, electrocardiographic units, physiologic monitors, and recorders. Proper functioning of this equipment is critical to a successful procedure and patient well-being; therefore, proper quality control testing should be performed at least semiannually. However, this equipment varies greatly, and there are currently no uniform national protocols for quality control testing. The operating manual for the equipment supplied by the manufacturer should be consulted for this testing, or a procedure should be developed by a medical physicist and the service representative for the equipment. Some suggested guidelines follow.

PROCEDURE

1. An image of an SMPTE test pattern, AAPM TG18-QC or a special PACS test pattern (see Fig. 9-35) consisting of horizontal, vertical, and diagonal lines should be digitized and displayed on the monitor.
2. The test pattern image should be captured, transmitted, archived, retrieved, and displayed by the PACS system and compared with the original image for any changes in quality. This should be performed at least weekly.
3. Image resolution should conform to the manufacturer's specifications. This test should be performed at least monthly to test the overall operation of the system under conditions that simulate the normal operation of the system. No change should be observed from one month to the next.
4. Compression recall should be evaluated quarterly by saving the following versions of the test patterns mentioned in step one of this procedure: a) no compression, b) lossless compression (usually a 2:1 ratio), and c) lossy compression (if used by your department). Examine the images of the test patterns in each of the above versions and determine whether any information, image quality, or significant spatial resolution has been lost.
5. Laser printers, which are used to make hard-copy images from a PACS system, and electronic display devices (both primary and secondary) should be evaluated as previously discussed.
6. Additional testing specified by the system's manufacturer should be performed.

Film Changers

Film changers are available in many different formats, but most transport the film through a pair of intensifying screens, where it is exposed and the image is recorded. Film-to-screen contact is critical for proper image resolution, just as it is in standard screen cassettes. This can be tested with the wire mesh test tool described in Chapter 3. Images of the test tool should be obtained during dynamic conditions (when rapid filming is taking place) and compared with an image obtained during static conditions (when just a single exposure is made). These images should demonstrate no significant differences in a properly functioning film changer.

Another variable that should be tested with film changers is the uniformity of optical density during dynamic imaging. Because film changers produce a series of images in rapid sequence, each image should not vary in optical density from the others obtained during the same run. An anthropomorphic phantom or high-contrast resolution fluoroscopic test phantom should be imaged during rapid filming with technical factors that create optical densities in the diagnostic range of 0.25 to 2.5. The optical densities of these images should be compared for uniformity. These values should not vary by more than an optical density of ± 0.2.

Film changers also should be evaluated for low- and high-contrast resolution, similar to fluoroscopic x-ray units. A low- and high-contrast fluoroscopic test tool (discussed in Chapter 8) can be used for this evaluation. Each type of test tool should be imaged during static and dynamic imaging and the images compared. They should not vary significantly in a properly functioning film changer.

Pressure Injectors

Pressure injectors are used to administer contrast media into vascular or lymphatic vessels during many diagnostic procedures. Variables such as injected volume and injection time should be tested so that what is selected on the programmer is exactly what is administered to the patient. This usually involves the selection of a specific catheter and contrast media (usually the type most commonly used by the facility) and the injector's administration of the material into a beaker or other graduated container. The volume in this container can then be compared with the control panel for variation. This procedure also can be timed with a stopwatch so that the administration time can be compared with the value set on the unit.

BONE DENSITOMETRY SYSTEMS

The ability to obtain accurate measurements of bone mineral density can help identify patients with osteoporosis and other atrophic diseases of the bone and minimize their risks for the development of painful and debilitating fractures. Various methods for the measurement of bone mineral density have been developed and marketed.

Single-Photon Absorptiometry

This method of measuring bone mineral density was first described in the early 1960s and uses a radioactive source and a detector (most often a sodium iodide scintillation detector). The radioactive source is most often iodine-125, which emits a gamma ray with an energy of 35 keV. Because this is a relatively low-energy photon, bone measurement is most often performed in small, distal areas of the body, such as the distal forearm or lateral calcaneus. Radiation measurements are performed with and without the anatomic structure in the path of the gamma ray beam. Because of the difference in the radiation readings, the degree of attenuation of the beam allows for estimation of bone mineral density (i.e., a greater bone mineral density absorbs more of the radiation beam). The accuracy rate for this method approaches 98% if performed correctly. Because ^{125}I has a half-life of about 60 days, periodic replacement and recalibration of the equipment are required. This method is rarely used in clinical practice because of the cost of replacement and disposal of radioactive waste.

Single-Energy X-Ray Absorptiometry

Single-energy x-ray absorptiometry (SXA) is similar to single-photon absorptiometry (SPA), except that an x-ray source replaces the radioactive source. This eliminates the replacement cost of the radioactive material. The x-ray beam is heavily filtered so that it is monoenergetic. The amount of x-ray attenuation is used to estimate the bone mineral density.

Dual-Photon Absorptiometry

This method of bone mineral density measurement was introduced in the early 1970s. Like SPA, dual-photon absorptiometry (DPA) uses a radioactive source, but two different energy photons are released. The most common source is gadolinium-153, which emits gamma ray photons with energies of 44 keV and 100 keV. The higher energies allow for bone density measurement of thicker areas of the body including lumbar and thoracic vertebrae. Using photons with two separate energies also allows the DPA technique to withdraw the absorption by soft tissues, which results in a more accurate measurement of bone mineral density than that obtainable with SPA or SXA. The detector assembly also could be made larger and be scanned back and forth over the patient to create an image, similar to a nuclear medicine scan. As with SPA, DPA uses a radioactive source with a finite half-life; periodic replacement is required. Because of this, DPA has been abandoned in most clinical sites in favor of **dual-energy x-ray absorptiometry** (DEXA).

Dual-Energy X-Ray Absorptiometry

DEXA was introduced clinically in 1987. The premise is similar to that of DPA, except that an x-ray tube is used as the source of radiation, rather than a radioactive source. As its name implies, x-rays with two separate energies are used to obtain the bone density data. Obtaining these different energies depends on the manufacturer; they can be obtained by either varying the amount of filtration in the x-ray beam or varying the x-ray generator output (kilovolt [peak] [kVp]). Early versions of the unit emitted a single pencil beam of radiation and required 5 minutes or more to scan an area of interest. More advanced systems use a fan-shaped beam with an array of detectors, which drop scan time to as little as 5 seconds. Models are available for either peripheral scanning, known as *peripheral DEXA* (pDEXA) *units* (distal extremities), or central body scanning (vertebra or hip). Both types of units have precision error rates of only 1% to 2%. In addition to bone mineral density measurements of virtually any body part, DEXA scanners also allow for measurement of the total body calcium content and body composition (with a whole body scan). The DEXA scanners also are

TABLE 9-4	World Health Organization Definitions of Bone Density Levels
Category	**T Score**
Normal	≥ -1
Osteopenia	< -1 and > -2.5
Osteoporosis	≤ -2.5
Established osteoporosis	≤ -2.5 with one or more osteoporosis-related fractures

Courtesy World Health Organization.

programmed to include a value known as the "T" score, which is a comparison with the young adult peak bone mass. It is determined by the number of standard deviations above or below the mean bone mineral density for a healthy 30-year-old adult. The diagnosis of normal, osteopenia, or osteoporosis can be made with the T score according to criteria developed by the World Health Organization (WHO). Table 9-4 contains the WHO criteria.

Quantitative Computed Tomography

Quantitative computed tomography (QCT) uses a CT scanner with the patient placed in the gantry in the supine position. However, a phantom containing reference densities is placed under the patient that allows the computer in the CT scanner to compare the Hounsfield units (mathematical numbers indicating the mass density of the particular structure in the patient) of the vertebral bodies with the values in the phantom to obtain bone density information. This method results in relatively accurate bone density information (especially in the measurement of highly metabolic active trabecular bone in the spine), but the units are relatively large and considerably more expensive than DEXA scanners.

Quantitative Ultrasound

This method of obtaining bone density information has been performed since the mid-1960s. This method uses ultrasound with a relatively low frequency range (200 to 600 kHz) and measures the amount of attenuation of the ultrasound beam by a portion of bone (most often the calcaneus). Because normal bone generally attenuates more of the ultrasound beam than osteoporotic bone does, the approximate bone mineral density can be calculated. The precision error for measurement of these units is not as good as that of DEXA scanners. However, they are relatively low in cost and small in size, and they do not expose the patient to ionizing radiation. Their main application is their use as a screening tool in physicians' offices, with a follow-up DEXA scan for patients who may have osteoporosis.

Digital X-Ray Radiogrammetry

Digital x-ray radiogrammetry (DXR) is a relatively new method of estimating bone density whereby an x-ray image of the hand is obtained and analyzed by computer software. For film-based images, a digitizer is used to scan the image into the computer. Images obtained with CR and DR can be called up from a PACS for analysis. The DXR technology is based on a radiogrammetry and texture analysis and is insensitive to the relevant variations affecting the quality of the x-ray image. The term, radiogrammetry, is the measure of distances on the image and the computer software calculates bone volume based on measurements of the cortical bone thickness, bone width and texture analysis. Texture analysis provides information on the microstructure of the bone, specifically the fraction of holes in the cortical bone. Specific regions of interest are automatically selected by the computer software to minimize error.

Quality Control of Bone Densitometry Equipment

Currently, DEXA scanning is the primary method of evaluating bone mineral density, followed by quantitative ultrasound (QU) and QCT. Regardless of the equipment that is being used, careful quality control procedures are required to ensure accurate bone mineral density measurements. Because of the variety of equipment in use, no uniform set of quality control guidelines is in place for these systems. Technologists who perform these studies have to rely on the quality control procedures specified by the manufacturer. These most often involve daily phantom scans, those either supplied by the manufacturer or commercially available from various vendors (Fig. 9-46). The accepted densities of the phantoms are then compared with what is obtained on the equipment during the phantom scan to determine if the equipment is performing properly. The values from these daily scans should fall to within ± 1.5% of the accepted value (± 2.5% for pDEXA systems). The daily values also should be plotted on a control chart with the 1.5% value used as the upper and lower limit. Some manufacturers will provide two phantoms for quality control purposes, one for testing the mechanical operation and calibration of the system and the other to mimic bone density to detect a shift in bone mineral density values. Many equipment manufacturers have installed automated quality control hardware and software to monitor performance (they will even create a control chart for documentation).

SUMMARY

Advanced imaging systems are commonplace in most diagnostic imaging departments. A current trend in diagnostic imaging is an emphasis toward digital imaging and away from conventional film images to reduce department costs. This should increase the use of these devices in the future; therefore, proper quality control protocols must be in place to ensure that this equipment is operating within accepted guidelines.

Refer to the Evolve website at https://evolve.elsevier. com for Student Experiments 9.1: Digital Image Display Monitor Evaluation and 9.2: Computed Radiography (CR) Quality Control

REVIEW QUESTIONS

1. Which of the following is found inside the image receptor used for a CR system?
   a. Intensifying screen
   b. Duplitized film
   c. Imaging plate
   d. All of the above
2. Which of the following is an advantage of CR versus conventional radiography?
   a. Lower patient dose
   b. Higher-contrast resolution
   c. Edge enhancement
   d. All of the above
3. Which of the following is true in comparing CR versus conventional radiography?
   a. CR has greater spatial resolution than conventional radiography.
   b. CR has a lower capital cost than conventional radiography.
   c. Collimation and part centering are critical for CR images.
   d. CR demonstrates larger image size than conventional radiography.

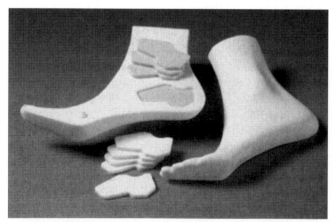

FIGURE 9-46 Dual-energy x-ray absorptiometry (DEXA) phantom used for determining the accuracy of bone density measurements. *(Courtesy Nuclear Associates, Carle Place, N.Y.)*

4. Which of the following identifies the fluoroscopic scan mode by which the x-ray tube delivers radiation in short, high-intensity pulses?
   a. Continuous fluoroscopic mode
   b. Pulsed, interlaced scan mode
   c. Slow scan mode
   d. All of the above

5. The standard black-and-white television monitor scans _____ horizontal lines per frame.
   a. 125
   b. 325
   c. 525
   d. 1025

6. Types of DSA include (1) temporal mask subtraction, (2) time-interval difference subtraction, and (3) dual-energy subtraction.
   a. 1 and 2
   b. 2 and 3
   c. 1 and 3
   d. 1, 2, and 3

7. Which of the following devices transfers a hard-copy image from a CRT onto a hard-copy film?
   a. Laser camera
   b. Multiformat camera
   c. Photofluorospot
   d. Cine camera

8. When the framing rate of a cine camera exceeds _____ frames per second, the human eye perceives the images as continuous.
   a. 4
   b. 8
   c. 12
   d. 16

9. The laser used in most CR reader units emits light in this portion of the color spectrum:
   a. Red
   b. Green
   c. Blue-violet
   d. All of the above

10. Which of the following are components of a CR system: (1) image receptors, (2) reader unit, or (3) workstation?
    a. 1 and 3
    b. 2 and 3
    c. 1 and 3
    d. 1, 2, and 3

Outcomes Assessment of Radiographic Images

OBJECTIVES

At the completion of this chapter the reader should be able to do the following:
- Explain the importance of repeat analysis studies in quality management
- Determine the causal repeat rate of a diagnostic imaging department
- Determine the total repeat rate of a diagnostic imaging department

- Identify artifacts that may appear in radiographic images
- Explain the corrective action required for elimination of the appearance of image artifacts
- Explain the difference between the concepts of accuracy, sensitivity, and specificity

The desired outcome of a diagnostic x-ray study is the creation of an acceptable diagnostic image, a correct diagnosis by the interpreting physician, and the satisfaction of all internal and external customers (e.g., the patient, referring physician, and third-party payer). Most of the material in the previous chapters has involved a discussion of quality control testing to ensure that the equipment delivers optimal image quality. However, quality control testing can only minimize the risk of obtaining subquality images but cannot prevent them entirely; therefore, a quality management program also must include looking at the final outcome of a diagnostic x-ray procedure (e.g., image quality and correct diagnostic) and determining the quality of the outcome to see if further improvement can be achieved. Steps involved in this outcome assessment include a **repeat analysis** of images (to avoid future repeats); an artifact analysis of images (to identify the cause and prevent future occurrence); and an **accuracy, sensitivity,** and **specificity** analysis of the diagnosis (to measure the combination of image quality and correct diagnosis of the interpreting physician).

REPEAT ANALYSIS

An important aspect of a quality management program is a retake, or repeat analysis, procedure. This is a systematic process of cataloging rejected images and determining the nature of the repeat so that repeat images can be minimized or eliminated in the future. Repeat analysis provides important data about equipment and accessory performance, departmental procedures, and the skill level of the technical staff. With this knowledge, solutions can be found to minimize repeats and also document the effectiveness (or lack thereof) of quality control and quality assurance protocols. Even departments that have switched to digital imaging can benefit greatly by using a repeat analysis program.

Advantages

The main advantages of lower department repeat rates are improved department efficiency, lower department costs, and lower patient doses.

Improved Department Efficiency. With the number of repeats kept low, the amount of time that patients must spend undergoing diagnostic procedures decreases. This increases patient (customer) satisfaction and allows the department to service more patients in the same period.

Lower Department Costs. When the number of repeat images is reduced, the costs associated with film, processing, labor, and depreciation of the equipment decrease significantly. Studies by the Food and Drug Administration (FDA) estimate the average cost of a repeat radiograph in a film/screen department to be about $25 per image (on the basis of a 14- × 17-inch sheet of film at a unit cost of $2) when the previously mentioned factors are considered. If a diagnostic imaging department averages 20 repeats per day for 1 year, the department wastes more than $182,000 (which would pay the annual salaries of six technologists or equip an x-ray room with a new x-ray tube and generator). Film and processing costs are considerably less in digital departments, but labor and depreciation of equipment costs are still significantly reduced with a lower repeat rate.

Lower Patient Doses. A diagnostic image that is unacceptable results in the repeat of that particular view, which means that the patient must be re-exposed to ionizing radiation. As an example, a lumbar spine series performed on a 200-speed imaging system yields an entrance skin exposure of approximately 600 millirad (6 milligray [mGy]). A repeat of this study would obviously double this amount of radiation.

Causal Repeat Rate

In repeat analysis studies performed on departments without quality control procedures for the darkroom, processor, and equipment, 75% of all repeats were caused by improper optical density of the radiographic images. With quality control protocols in place, studies have demonstrated that most repeats are results of positioning errors. Digital departments with quality control procedures also show positioning errors as the number one cause of repeat exposures. Table 10-1 indicates

TABLE 10-1	Nationwide Averages of Repeat Causes for Departments with Quality Control Procedures
Category	**% Repeat**
Positioning	35
Overexposure	15
Miscellaneous (e.g., artifacts)	14
Underexposure	13
Patient motion	9
Mechanical problems	8
Darkrooms	6

nationwide averages of repeat causes for departments with quality control procedures.

For a repeat analysis study to be done, a worksheet such as the one included in Figure 10-1 (for film/screen departments) or Figure 10-2 (for CR or DR departments) should be used so that the proper statistical information is obtained and recorded. Because reject film images are saved for silver reclamation purposes in film/screen departments, sorting them daily and recording the data on the worksheet are the easiest methods. In digital departments, the database of many CR and DR systems can be accessed to yield repeat analysis data. Most departments tabulate the data monthly to obtain a large enough statistical sample (at least 250 patients) for reliability. It is recommended that the same individual be responsible for performing the analysis, as image viewer differences can affect the outcome of the repeat analysis study. The worksheet should include the radiographic procedures performed in the department, along with the possible causes of rejection such as positioning, overexposure, underexposure, motion, **artifacts,** and miscellaneous causes. Once the data have been recorded for the specified period, the causal repeat rate and the total department rate should be determined. The causal repeat rate is the percentage of repeats from a specific cause such as positioning error or technique error and is calculated with the following equation:

$$\text{Casual Repeat Rate} = \frac{\text{Number of repeats for a specific cause}}{\text{Total number of repeats}} \times 100$$

For example, if a radiology department has a total of 185 repeat images during a 1-month period and 67 of the 185 are the result of positioning errors, then the percent of repeats caused by positioning error is 36%. Many radiology information systems (RIS's) can calculate the causal repeat rate when department staff enter the number and cause of repeat images into the system.

Total Repeat Rate

The total department repeat rate is determined with the following equation:

$$\text{Total repeat rate} = \frac{\text{Number of repeat images}}{\text{Total number of views taken}} \times 100$$

For example, if a department performs a total of 1160 views during a 1-month period and 132 are rejected and must be repeated, then the total department repeat rate is 11.4%. Some automatic film processors have a counting device recording the total number of images processed that can be used as the total number of views taken in the equation (most CR and DR systems have software that can access the total number of images processed during a given period of time to obtain the same information). Many factors influence this rate,

such as the quality of the equipment, the competence of the technical staff, the patient population, data collection method, shift (weekend, evening, or day shift), and the number of images accepted by radiologists to diagnose.

Data from the repeat analysis are used to identify which of these factors is a major contributor to the overall repeat rate. If a particular piece of equipment is often identified as being at fault for repeat images, data from the repeat analysis can be used to justify repair or replacement costs. If certain employees demonstrate an abnormally high number of repeats, additional in-service education or other corrective action can be used to help alleviate the problem. *Repeat rates for radiographic procedures should not exceed 4% to 6% and should be less than 5% for mammographic procedures. Mammographic repeat rates cannot change by more than ± 2% each quarter.* However, this may not be practical in all departments, when the amount of variation that may be present in imaging equipment, technologist experience level, institutional image quality acceptance standards, and patient population is considered. Any departments with repeat rates exceeding 10% to 12% should be examined seriously because these departments are inefficient and contribute to a high patient dose.

ARTIFACT ANALYSIS

One cause of rejected images listed in the repeat analysis worksheet is the presence of image artifacts. An artifact is anything on a finished radiograph that is not part of the patient's anatomy. Artifacts can contribute significantly to the total repeat rate; therefore, a thorough knowledge of artifacts and their possible causes is necessary so that corrective action can be taken.

Film/Screen Radiography

Image artifacts found in film/screen radiography can be placed into one of three categories: processing artifacts, exposure artifacts, and handling and storage artifacts.

Processing Artifacts

Processing artifacts are caused by or occur during the processing of diagnostic images.

Emulsion Pickoff. In emulsion pickoff, the emulsion is removed from or "picked off" of the film base. This occurs when two images are stuck together before or during processing and then pulled apart afterward. It also occurs with single sheets of film that are processed in underreplenished developer that results in glutaraldehyde failure. Since glutaraldehyde is the weak hardener added to the developer solution that keeps the film from sticking to the rollers, failure of this ingredient will cause the emulsion to be removed from the film and deposited on the rollers.

REPEAT ANALYSIS WORKSHEET

SURVEY PERIOD _____ to _____   LOCATION _____

REPEAT CATEGORY EXAMINATION	POSITION	OVER-EXPOSED	UNDER-EXPOSED	MOTION	ARTI-FACTS	OTHER	TOTAL	%
Chest								
Ribs								
Shoulder								
Humerus								
Elbow								
Forearm								
Wrist								
Hand								
C-Spine								
T-Spine								
L-Spine								
Skull								
Facial								
Sinuses								
Abdomen								
Pelvis								
Hip								
Femur								
Knee								
Lower leg								
Ankle								
Foot								
UGI								
LGI								
IVP								
Other								
Total								
%								

FIGURE 10-1 Repeat analysis worksheet (Film/screen). *C-Spine,* Cervical spine; *IVP,* intravenous pyelography; *LGI,* lower gastrointestinal tract; *L-Spine,* lumbar spine; *T-Spine,* thoracic spine; *UGI,* upper gastrointestinal tract.

CR/DR Repeat Analysis Form

Room # _____ Date: _____ Technologist: _____

Patient ID	Exam	positioning	overexpose	underexpose	motion	wrong exam code	collimation	artifact	No exposure	Double expose	No marker	Marker over part	Wrong exam code	other

FIGURE 10-2 Repeat analysis worksheet (CR/DR).

Gelatin Buildup. Emulsion that has been removed from earlier images and either stuck on processor rollers or dissolved in the developer solution can be deposited on subsequent images. The primary cause is underreplenished developer solution or failure of the developer circulation system filter.

Curtain Effect. Solution dripping on, or "running down," a film can form patterns on the film that resemble a lace curtain (Fig. 10-3). This is more common in manually processed images but can occur in automatically processed images if the wash water is dirty or if a film has jammed and must be removed from the processor before passing through the dryer section.

Chemical Fog. Chemical fog is an overdevelopment of the film that results in excessive base + fog and minimum diameter (D_{min}) values with sensitometry images and excessive optical density with radiographic images (Fig. 10-4). The main cause is developer temperature, time, pH, or concentration above the manufacturer's specifications. It also may occur with overreplenishment of the developer solution.

Guide Shoe Marks. Guide shoe marks are scratches on images made by the jagged edges of the guide shoes because they may be bent, worn, damaged, incorrectly installed, or incorrectly adjusted. They also may occur with improperly seated transport racks or rollers (Fig. 10-5). Guide shoe marks caused by crossover assemblies usually occur at the top surface of the film. Guide shoe marks from turnaround assemblies tend to occur at the bottom surface of the film. These scratches

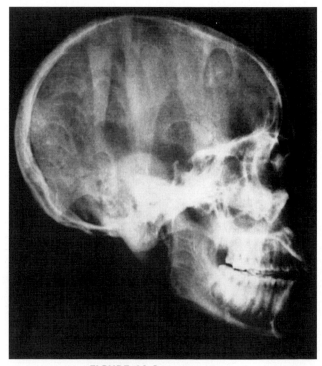

FIGURE 10-3 Curtain effect.

run parallel to (in the same direction as) the direction of film travel.

Pi Lines. Pi lines are artifacts that occur relative to the circumference of a roller and therefore occur at regular intervals (Fig. 10-6). These marks run perpendicular to

Normal fog

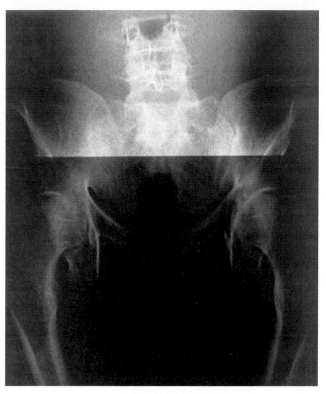

Severe fog

FIGURE 10-4 Chemical fog.

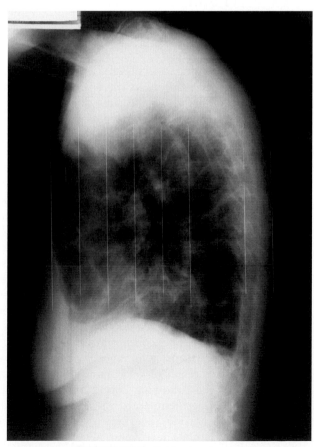

FIGURE 10-5 Guide shoe marks.

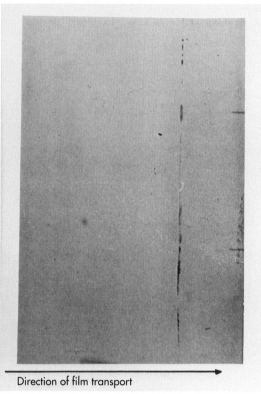

Direction of film transport

FIGURE 10-6 Pi lines.

the direction of film travel, and are usually caused by dirt or debris on the rollers.

Chatter. Chattering artifacts appear as bands of increased optical density that occur perpendicular to film direction. **Chatter** is caused by inconsistent motion of the transport system, usually because the drive gears or drive chain slips. Chemical buildup on gears or gears not seated properly can cause chatter marks that are approximately $^1/_8$ inch apart. A rusty or loose drive chain can cause chatter marks that are about $^3/_8$ inch apart.

Dichroic Stain. The term *dichroic* refers to "two colors," brown and greenish yellow. The presence of brown stains on a radiograph could indicate a film processed in oxidized developer or hyporetention that has been present during several years of storage. The greenish yellow type of stain indicates the presence of unexposed and undeveloped silver halide crystals remaining on the film after processing and is caused by incomplete fixation.

Reticulation Marks. When uneven solution temperatures cause excessive expansion and contraction of the film emulsion during processing, the result is a network of fine grooves in the film surface (**reticulation marks**).

Streaking. Streaking is uneven development of the image that can be caused by the failure of agitation in manual processing or the failure of the circulation system in automatic processing (Fig. 10-7).

Hesitation Marks. Hesitation marks (also known as *stub lines*) are stripes of decreased optical density where transport rollers are left in contact with the film and

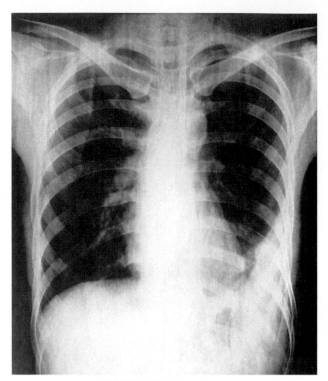

FIGURE 10-7 Streaking.

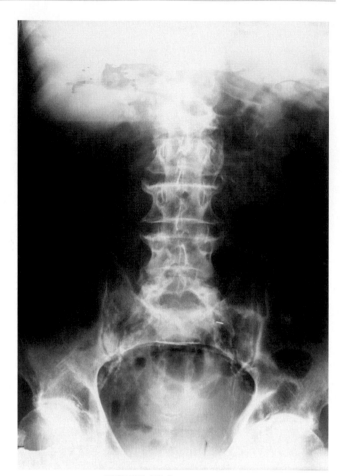

FIGURE 10-9 Water spots.

further development is prevented (Fig. 10-8). These artifacts occur when the processor is turned off or loses power while the film is in the developer section or if the film becomes jammed while in the developer section. They also can occur if the transport system speed decreases significantly.

Water Spots. Should water or other liquid come in contact with an unprocessed image, a pattern of increased optical density appears after processing (Fig. 10-9).

Wet-Pressure Sensitization. The entrance rollers on most processors are made of soft rubber rollers with grooves on the surface to grab the film from the feed tray. Should these rollers or the film become wet before the film is introduced, the combination of the pressure and the water marks forms a series of dark stripes that

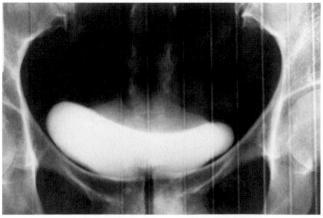

FIGURE 10-8 Hesitation marks.

match the grooves on the rollers (Fig. 10-10). The marks also may occur if the tension on the entrance rollers is too great. These marks run in the same direction as film travel. These artifacts also are known as *entrance roller marks.*

Hyporetention. Hyporetention is a white, powdery residue that remains on the film surface because of incomplete washing (Fig. 10-11). This residue forms when the fixer chemicals crystallize as the film dries. A lesser degree of hyporetention can result in brown dichroic stains, which were discussed previously.

Insufficient Optical Density. Images that lack sufficient optical density as a result of processing problems can occur because of the following conditions: developer temperature that is below accepted limits, insufficient developer time, underreplenished developer solution, a developer that is contaminated by the fixer, developer pH that is too low, or insufficient developer concentration.

Excessive Optical Density. Images with excessive optical density as a result of processing problems can occur because of the following conditions: the extension of the developer temperature's accepted limits, excessive developer time, overreplenishment, higher accepted limits of the developer pH, or excessive developer concentration.

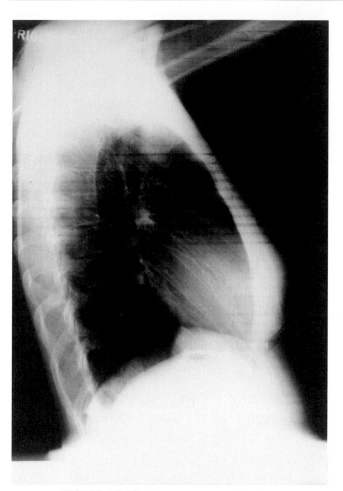

FIGURE 10-10 Wet-pressure sensitization.

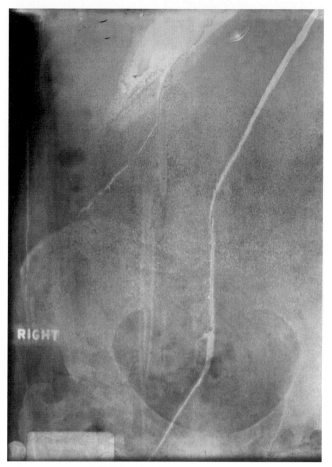

FIGURE 10-11 Hyporetention.

Exposure Artifacts

Exposure artifacts are caused by the patient, the technologist, or the equipment during a diagnostic procedure.

Motion. A motion artifact is a blurring of the image caused by the motion of the patient, x-ray source, or image receptor. This results in a significant loss of recorded detail. Patient motion can be reduced with short exposure time, immobilization, and proper instructions to the patient.

Patient Artifacts. Patient artifacts are caused by items that can be either on or within the patient when a diagnostic procedure is performed. Examples of patient artifacts include buttons, snaps, necklaces, earrings, hairpins, wet hair, and body piercing jewelry.

Improper Optical Density. Improper selection of technical factors by the technologist or improper cell selection with automatic exposure control results in improper optical density.

Improper Patient Position or Missing Anatomy of Interest. Improper patient position or missing anatomy of interest is the result of improper patient, x-ray, or image receptor position by the technologist or improper collimation, which can clip the anatomy of interest.

Quantum Mottle. Quantum mottle is a blotchy appearance in a radiograph that is caused by statistical variations in the number of x-ray photons covering a specific area. This is usually present when low milliampere-second (mAs) exposure factors (<2 mAs) are used. This can occur with film/screen radiography, computed radiography (CR), digital radiography (DR), fluoroscopy, computed tomography, and nuclear medicine imaging.

Poor Film-to-Screen Contact. Poor film-to-screen contact results in localized blurring of the radiographic image, which also may demonstrate slightly increased optical density in these regions.

Double Exposure. Double exposure occurs when an image receptor is exposed more than once before the image is processed.

Grid Artifacts. Improper use of a grid causes grid artifacts, which include grid lines, grid cutoff, and moiré effect.

Grid Lines. Grid lines are shadows of the lead strips that appear on the resulting image and are caused by failure of the grid to move during the exposure, improper grid-focusing distance, improper angulation of the central ray with respect to the grid lines, or improper centering (Fig. 10-12).

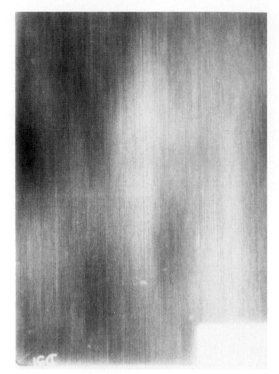

FIGURE 10-12 Grid lines.

Grid Cutoff. Grid cutoff is a decrease in optical density caused by primary radiation being absorbed by (or cut off by) the grid (Fig. 10-13). Any improper use of a grid can cause grid cutoff.

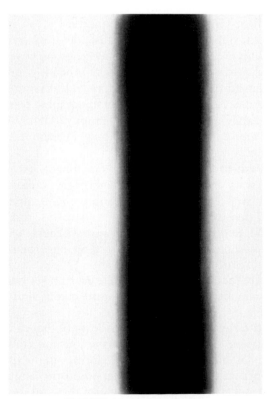

FIGURE 10-13 Grid cutoff.

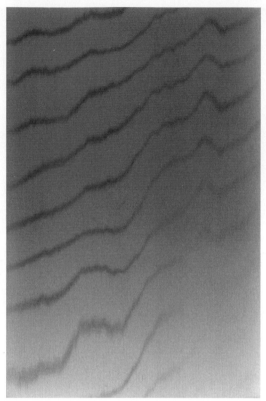

FIGURE 10-14 Moiré effect, or zebra pattern, artifact.

Moiré Effect. Moiré effect, or zebra pattern artifact, is a double set of grid lines caused by the placement of a grid cassette in a Bucky (Fig. 10-14). This artifact also can occur in CR systems when a stationary grid having a grid frequency in the range of 85 to 100 lines per inch is used, and the grid lines are parallel to the CR reader scan lines. This is due to the scan frequency of the laser in the image reader device (IRD) closely matching the grid frequency. To eliminate this particular cause of Moiré effect, the following steps can be taken:

1. Ensure grids are moving during the exposure.
2. Use a grid with a higher grid frequency.
3. Use a crosshatch grid or a multihole grid.
4. Change the orientation of the grid so that the grid lines are perpendicular to the CR reader scan lines

Handling and Storage Artifacts

Handling and storage artifacts occur during darkroom handling or during storage before use.

Light Fog. The light of any improper color that strikes the film before development fogs the film and therefore lowers the image contrast. Fog is any noninformational optical density present in a film image.

Age Fog. Age fog may occur in film that has been processed beyond the expiration date or has been stored in a warm, humid environment. It results in a lower image contrast.

Safelight Fog. Safelight fog is caused by an improper safelight filter, cracks or pinholes in the safelight filter, incorrect wattage of the safelight bulb, incorrect distance between the safelight and work surfaces, or widely open sodium vapor lamp shutters.

Radiation Fog. Radiation fog appears in film that has been exposed to ionizing radiation before development.

Pressure Marks. Excessive pressure, such as a heavy object placed on the film before development, causes pressure marks, which are areas of increased optical density. Pressure marks occur because the pressure splitting the bond between the silver and the halide ion in the film emulsion results in the presence of black metallic silver after processing. Film should be stored vertically to minimize the risk of pressure artifacts.

Static. The sparks from static electricity expose film and produce three types of static artifacts: tree static, crown static, and smudge static (Fig. 10-15).

Tree Static. Tree static resembles trees or bushes without leaves and is usually caused by low humidity conditions in the film processing area.

Crown Static. Crown static marks radiate in one direction so that they resemble a crown. Excessive friction from the pulling of the film (such as in a daylight system, in which the film is "squeezed" too tightly between the intensifying screens) can produce these marks.

Smudge Static. Smudge static consists of dark areas where excessive amounts of light have exposed the film and is usually caused by rough handling in the film processing area.

Crescent or Crinkle Marks. Crescent or crinkle marks are half-moon-shaped marks of increased optical density caused by bending of the film before processing (Fig. 10-16). The bending of a processed film image can result in crescent marks that are of decreased optical density because some of the silver can be moved from the area where the bending has occurred.

Scratches. Scratches are areas where the emulsion has been removed by sharp objects such as fingernails or sharp points on surfaces.

Cassette Marks. Cassette marks are white specks on the image caused by dirt or debris inside the cassette. This foreign matter blocks the light from the screen from reaching the film. Regular cleaning of the screens with an antistatic cleaner can minimize these artifacts (Fig. 10-17).

Computed Radiography and Digital Radiography Artifacts. Even though liquid processing and film/screen image receptors are not used with CR and DR systems, artifacts can still occur and therefore must have their sources recognized by radiographers in order to minimize their occurrence. This is in addition to the exposure artifacts listed earlier in the section on

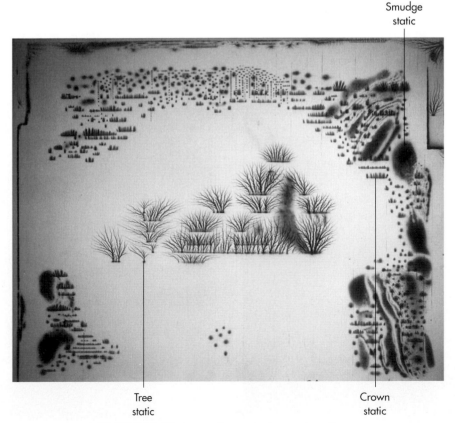

Smudge static

Tree static

Crown static

FIGURE 10-15 Image demonstrating static artifacts.

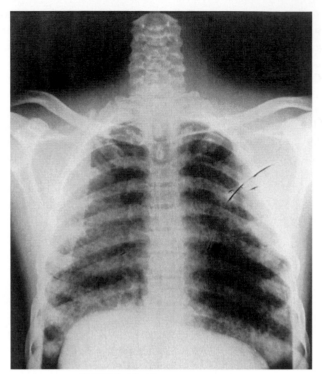

FIGURE 10-16 Crescent marks.

film/screen artifacts because these also will occur with CR and DR systems (except for poor film/screen contact). Artifacts occurring during preprocessing functions often cannot be corrected, while those occurring during postprocessing tend to be recoverable.

Heat Blur. This is a blurring of the image that can occur when a CR system imaging plate is exposed to intense heat before being processed within the CR reader system.

Improper Image Brightness. When CR systems are used, improper image brightness (optical density when placed onto a hard-copy image) can occur when an incorrect preprocessing histogram is selected (e.g., an adult histogram for the radiography of a pediatric chest). This is known as **histogram error.** Improper

optical density with CR systems also can occur because of nonparallel collimation. For the histograms used by CR systems to process the final image, the collimation edges of the radiation field should be parallel to the sides of the imaging plate. This way, the preprogrammed histogram in the CR system, the histogram created by the imaging plate match, and the computer can assign the correct optical density values to the appropriate region of the image. When collimation is not parallel, the histograms do not match correctly and the system then may be unable to determine the appropriate optical density value.

Quantum Mottle. Just as with film/screen systems (or any imaging system that relies on photons to cover an area of interest), quantum mottle can occur with digital imaging systems and create the same "blotchy" appearance. Oftentimes, it is even more common in digital systems as radiographers use low mAs values to decrease patient dose and use computer software to correct image brightness (Fig. 10-18).

Defects in the Imaging Plate. Scratches, scuff marks, or cracks in a CR image plate can mimic fractures and signs of pneumothorax (Fig. 10-19); therefore, image plates must be inspected periodically, and damaged plates must be removed from service.

Phantom Image Artifact. CR image plates must be properly erased before use, or data from previous images will interfere with current image data (Fig. 10-20).

Increased Sensitivity to Scatter. Both CR and DR systems have image receptors that are much more sensitive to scattered radiation due to lower K-edge values. This means the effects of scatter (and background

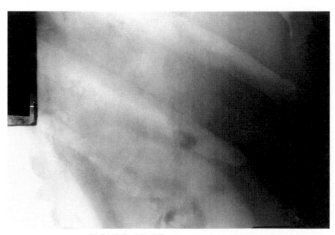

FIGURE 10-17 Cassette marks.

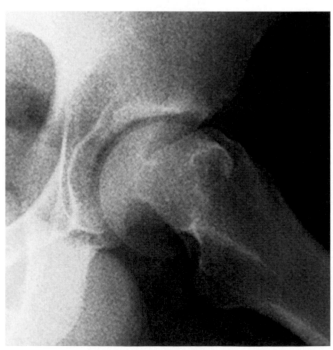

FIGURE 10-18 Quantum mottle occurring in a CR image.

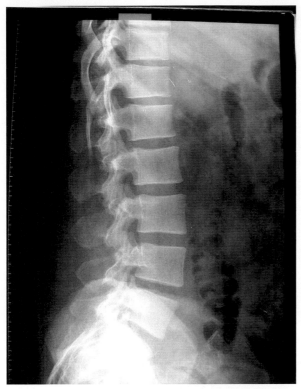

FIGURE 10-19 Artifact caused by scratches on a CR image plate. *(Courtesy of Janet Petersen, Elmhurst Memorial Hospital, Elmhurst, IL.)*

radiation) can cause a decrease in image contrast that postprocessing software may not be able to correct.

Double Exposure. As with film/screen image receptors, CR imaging plates can be double exposed, leading to both images being lost because data are entered during preprocessing functions (Fig. 10-21).

Computed Radiography Scanner Malfunction. CR scanner malfunction can cause skipped scan lines, missing pixels, and distorted images (Fig. 10-22). These also can be caused by memory problems, digitization problems, or communication errors. Dust and debris also can collect on the rotating polygonal mirror or light collection optics in the IRD. Lasers also have a limited life and must be replaced periodically.

Foreign Objects. Dirt and debris can find their way to CR image plates and DR flat panels, causing light-colored specks similar to those that occur with dirty intensifying screens in film/screen radiography (Fig. 10-23).

Halo Artifacts. Halo artifacts appear as dark bands at the interfaces of structures that differ widely in brightness level such as barium examinations or metal prosthesis.

Printer Errors. Both CR and DR systems rely on dry laser printers to produce hard copies of images. Even though these devices are generally more reliable than wet film processors, they are still subject to problems including incorrect density calibration, light leaks, transport problems, and laser misalignment. These can lead to artifacts such as shading, which results in dark areas

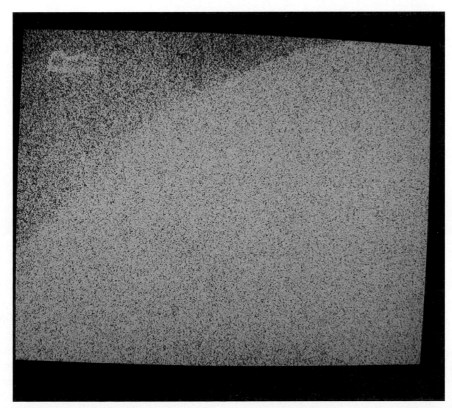

FIGURE 10-20 Phantom image caused by incomplete erasure of CR imaging plate. *(Courtesy of Janet Petersen, Elmhurst Memorial Hospital, Elmhurst, IL.)*

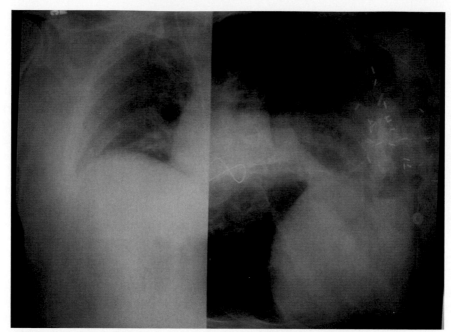

FIGURE 10-21 Double exposure. *(Courtesy of Pamela Verkuilen, Saint Alexius Medical Center, Hoffman Estates, IL.)*

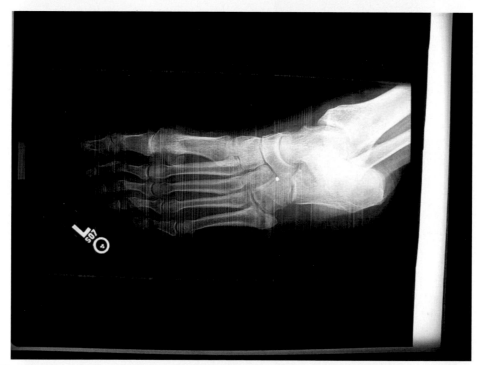

FIGURE 10-22 Scan lines appearing on digital image. *(Courtesy of Janet Petersen, Elmhurst Memorial Hospital, Elmhurst, IL.)*

in the image (Fig. 10-24) and the "corduroy effect" (Fig. 10-25), where scan lines caused by transport problems appear in the image.

DIAGNOSTIC PERFORMANCE MEASUREMENT

The main outcome of a diagnostic imaging examination is an accurate diagnosis of a patient's condition so that proper treatment can be administered. This is affected by factors such as image quality (for which the technical staff is responsible) and the competency of the radiologist to interpret the image (determining if the anatomy demonstrated in the image is healthy). In images of certain anatomic structures, the distribution of healthy patients follows a bell-shaped normal distribution. The distribution of patients with diseases also follows a normal distribution but with a different mean value (which can be larger or smaller depending on the patient population studied). Figure 10-26 shows the

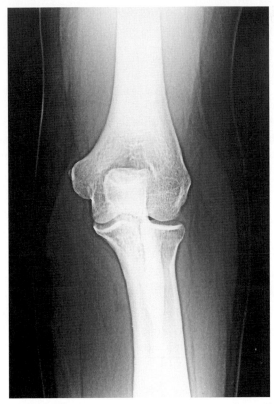

FIGURE 10-23 Artifact caused by dirt on CR imaging plate.

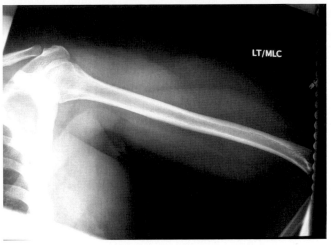

FIGURE 10-25 Corduroy effect. *(Courtesy of Pamela Verkuilen, Saint Alexius Medical Center, Hoffman Estates, IL.)*

distribution of these two groups. The two means are relatively far apart, so it should be easy to distinguish between the two.

The region where the two groups overlap indicates less of a distinction between them, and accurate diagnosis is more difficult. A diagnostic cutoff or threshold level is placed to distinguish a healthy diagnosis from a diagnosis of disease. Patients in whom the disease has been diagnosed are considered positive. If a test result (such as a biopsy) reveals that the diagnosis is correct, a designation of *true positive* (TP) is given. Patients are designated as *false positive* (FP) if further study indicates that they do not have the disease despite the positive finding from the image. Healthy patients with no disease present are considered negative. If a diagnosis of negative is determined from an image and supported by follow-up studies, it is designated as *true negative* (TN). If a negative diagnosis is given to a patient who later has the disease, then a designation of *false negative* (FN) is assigned. This information can be obtained from patient medical records and should be determined for high-risk studies such as angiographic procedures. The

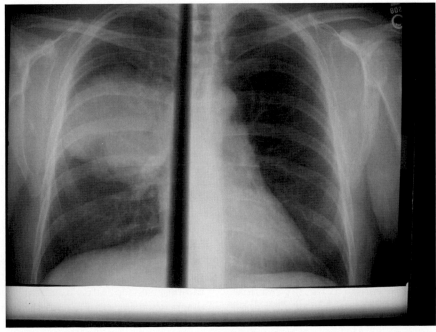

FIGURE 10-24 Shading occurring during hard copy printing. *(Courtesy of Pamela Verkuilen, Saint Alexius Medical Center, Hoffman Estates, IL.)*

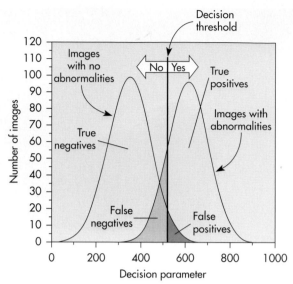

FIGURE 10-26 Graph showing patients with disease versus healthy patients.

FDA mandates that this information be derived for mammographic procedures. From this information, the values of accuracy, sensitivity, and specificity; **prevalence; positive predictive value;** and **negative predictive value** can be obtained.

Accuracy

Accuracy is the percentage or fraction of cases that are diagnosed correctly; it can be determined by the following equation:

$$Accuracy = \frac{(N_{TP} + N_{TN})}{N_{Total}} \times 100$$

N designates the number of cases. For example, if 210 mammograms are performed in 1 month and the number of TNs is 167 and the number of TPs is 36, then the accuracy rate of the image diagnosis is 0.967, or 96.7%.

Sensitivity

Sensitivity also is referred to as the *TP fraction* and indicates the likelihood of obtaining a positive diagnosis in a patient with the disease (or the ability to detect disease). A sensitive test has a low false-negative rate. Sensitivity is determined by the following equation:

$$Sensitivity = \frac{N_{TP}}{(N_{TP} + N_{FN})}$$

If a department demonstrates 36 TPs and 3 FNs, then the sensitivity is 0.92, or 92%.

Specificity. Specificity is also known as the *TN fraction* and indicates the likelihood of a patient obtaining a negative diagnosis when no disease is present. A specific test

has a low false-positive rate. Specificity is determined by the following equation:

$$Specificity = \frac{N_T}{(N_{TN} + N_{FP})}$$

A department receiving 167 TNs and 4 FPs has a specificity of 0.97, or 97%.

Positive Predictive Value. The positive predictive value is the probability of having the disease given a positive test and is determined by the following equation:

$$\frac{N_{TP}}{(N_{TP} + N_{FP})}$$

A department having 36 TPs and 4 FPs will have a positive predictive value of 0.9 or 90%.

Negative Predictive Value

The negative predictive value is the probability of not having the disease given a negative test and is determined by the following equation:

$$\frac{N_{TN}}{(N_{TN} + N_{FN})}$$

A department having 167 TNs and 3 FNs will have a negative predictive value of 0.98 or 98%.

The ideal for all of the previous values is 100%. In general, the diagnostic performance will depend on the disease prevalence, which is determined by the following equation:

$$\frac{[N_{TP} + N_{FN}]}{[N_{TP} + N_{FP} + N_{TN} + N_{FN}]}$$

A diagnostic imaging department is responsible for establishing its own threshold of acceptability for each value, with both internal and external factors being considered (see Chapter 1). Departments that want to improve accuracy, sensitivity, and specificity can use special statistical phantoms for radiographic, mammographic, and fluoroscopic analysis (Fig. 10-27). These specialized phantoms allow for the position of the phantom components (e.g., test wires, simulated bone fragments, and low-contrast objects) to be moved to different parts of the phantom each time it is used. This can eliminate the problem of "familiarity," whereby the observer is familiar with the phantom test pattern and begins to expect or predict that the objects are appearing at the appropriate location. By varying the location each time, the observer has to actually "see" the object at its location for the phantom testing to be valid. Many diagnostic imaging departments also use "double read" as a method to improve accuracy. With this method, two radiologists separately read the same case, and if their diagnoses differ from each other, they confer and decide conclusively.

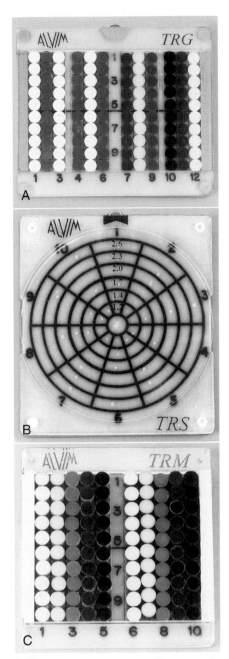

FIGURE 10-27 Statistical phantoms for **A**, radiographic; **B**, mammographic; and **C**, fluoroscopic images. *(Courtesy Nuclear Associates, Carle Place, N.Y.)*

Receiver Operator Characteristic Curve

A **receiver operator characteristic curve** (ROC, also known as a *relative operator characteristic curve*) is a plot of the true-positive probability (pTP) or sensitivity versus the false-positive probability (pFP), which also can be described as (1− specificity) (Fig. 10-28). An ideal image would yield a true-positive probability of 1 (100%) and a false-positive probability of 0. Data points that would fall toward the upper left-hand corner of an ROC curve would indicate an accurate diagnosis. If data points fall on a line that is at a 45-degree angle within the graph, it would indicate random guessing by the observer.

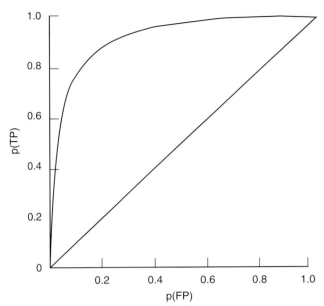

FIGURE 10-28 ROC Curve. The 45 degree diagonal line in the graph indicates pure guesswork by the observer. The curve on the left hand side of the graph depicts an accurate imaging procedure.

The area under the ROC curve is a measure of overall imaging performance and has a maximum value of 1 (100%). As image quality and performance improve, the curve will move toward the upper left hand corner, which increases the area under the curve. The area under the random guessing line is 0.5 (50%).

SUMMARY

Implementing a quality management program requires more than just equipment monitoring and maintenance. The outcomes assessment of diagnostic images also must be performed to evaluate the success of the procedure. In this way, future problems may be avoided by analyzing current causes of repeat images and artifacts. Continuous improvement of image quality and customer satisfaction can occur when diagnostic image quality and diagnostic accuracy are monitored on a routine basis.

Refer to the Evolve website at https://evolve.elsevier. com for Student Experiment 10.1: Reject-Repeat Analysis.

REVIEW QUESTIONS

1. In departments with a quality management program in place, the greatest number of repeat images is due to which of the following?
   a. Mechanical problems
   b. Image fog
   c. Patient motion
   d. Positioning error

2. If a department performs 1160 views during a 1-month period and 132 are repeated, the department repeat rate is which of the following?
   a. 9.5%
   b. 10.7%
   c. 11.4%
   d. 14.8%

3. Any repeat rate exceeding _____ should be seriously examined.
   a. 2% to 4%
   b. 4% to 6%
   c. 6% to 8%
   d. 10% to 12%

4. Which of the following processing artifacts run in the same direction as film travel?
   a. Pi lines
   b. Guide shoe marks
   c. Hesitation marks
   d. Chemical fog

5. Which of the following artifacts can occur in both CR and film/screen radiography?
   a. Static electricity
   b. Wet-pressure sensitization
   c. Moiré pattern
   d. Water spots

6. The types of static artifacts include (1) tree, (2) crown, and (3) smudge:
   a. 1 and 2
   b. 2 and 3
   c. 1 and 3
   d. 1, 2, and 3

7. Which of the following terms best describes the likelihood of obtaining a positive diagnosis in a patient with the disease actually present?
   a. Sensitivity
   b. Specificity
   c. Variance
   d. Frequency

8. Data for determining repeat rates should include at least _____ patients to obtain a statistical sample large enough for valid results.
   a. 100
   b. 150
   c. 250
   d. 500

9. Which of the following terms also is referred to as the TP fraction?
   a. Accuracy
   b. Sensitivity
   c. Specificity
   d. None of the above

10. Which of the following artifacts occurs as a result of patient motion during exposure?
   a. A processing artifact
   b. An exposure artifact
   c. A handling artifact
   d. No artifact

Mammographic Quality Standards

KEY TERMS

adverse event
annotations and measurements
beryllium window
compression
consumer
emission spectrum
extended processing

gray scale processing
image inversion
magnification
Mammography Quality
 Standards Act
postprocessing
serious adverse event

serious complaint
target composition
tomosynthesis
tissue equalization
workflow

OBJECTIVES

At the completion of this chapter the reader should be able to do the following:

- Explain the difference between dedicated mammography equipment and conventional equipment
- Describe the composition of the x-ray tube target in mammographic equipment
- Discuss the advantages of compression during mammographic procedures
- Describe the image receptor systems currently used in mammography
- Describe the basic differences between film/screen mammography and full-field digital mammography

- Indicate the quality control tasks relating to the radiologist and the medical physicist
- Describe the quality control duties of the mammographer on a daily, weekly, quarterly, and semiannual basis
- Describe the various components of a Food and Drug Administration/Mammography Quality Standards Act inspection

OUTLINE

Mammography is soft tissue radiography of the breast. It requires different equipment and techniques from conventional radiography because of the close similarities among anatomic structures (low subject contrast). Low kilovolt (peak) (kVp) in the 20- to 30-kVp range must be deployed to maximize the amount of photoelectric effect and enhance differential absorption. The side effect of using lower kilovolt (peak) exposure factors is correspondingly higher milliampere-second (mAs) values, which increase the total radiation dose to the patient. The American College of Radiology recommends that the average glandular dose for a 4.2-cm thick breast should be less than 300 millirad (3 milligray [mGy]) per view for film/screen image receptors used with a grid. If no grid is used, the average glandular dose should be less than 100 millirad (1 mGy) per view. Because the glandular tissue of the breast is inherently radiosensitive, care must be taken to minimize radiation exposure through dedicated equipment and quality control procedures.

DEDICATED MAMMOGRAPHIC EQUIPMENT

X-Ray Generator

The x-ray generators used in mammographic studies should be dedicated solely to mammographic imaging (Fig. 11-1). All current mammographic imagers are

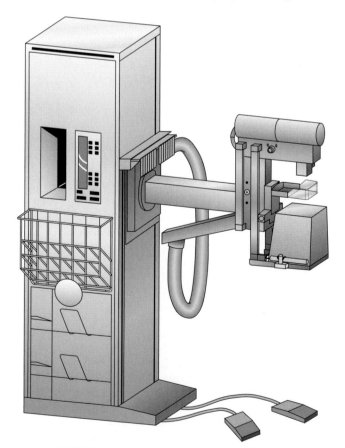

FIGURE 11-1 Dedicated mammographic unit.

high-frequency x-ray generators (see Chapter 7) that are smaller in size and less expensive than earlier single and three-phase mammographic units. High-frequency x-ray generators also provide exceptional exposure reproducibility, which is essential for consistent image quality. The kilovolt (peak) range available on most units is between 20 and 35 kVp, and typical x-ray tube currents are about 80 to 200 mA. Exposure times are usually about 1 second but can be as long as 4 seconds for dense or thick breasts or for those with implants. For a normal compressed breast (4.5 cm), a typical x-ray tube voltage is 25 kVp with an mA/exposure time combination of about 120 mAs. All systems with film/screen image receptors must be equipped with an automatic exposure control (AEC) system that consists of two to three sensors to regulate the optical density (OD) of the resulting image. Each film/screen system should provide an AEC mode that is operable in all combinations of equipment configuration provided (e.g., grid, nongrid, magnification, nonmagnification, and various target-filter combinations). The positioning or selection of the detector should permit flexibility in the placement of the detector under the target tissue. The size and available positions of the detector must be clearly indicated at the x-ray input surface of the breast compression paddle. The system also must provide a means for the operator to vary the selected OD from the normal (zero) setting. The x-ray tube/image receptor assembly must be capable of being fixed in any position and not undergo any unintended motion or fail in the event of power interruption.

X-Ray Tube

Modern mammographic x-ray units use rotating anode x-ray tubes just as conventional radiographic units do. However, some significant differences are present including the x-ray tube window, target composition, focal spot size, and source-to-image distance (SID).

X-Ray Tube Window. X-ray tubes used in conventional radiographic, fluoroscopic, and computed tomography units incorporate a window made primarily of glass (which is essentially silicon with an atomic number of 14). Because relatively high kilovolt (peak) exposure factors are used in these studies, absorption of lower-energy x-rays in the window material is acceptable and actually desired. Mammographic x-ray tubes use a thinner glass window or a **beryllium window** (atomic number of 4), which is less likely to absorb the low kilovolt (peak) x-rays used in mammographic procedures. The inherent filtration of the beryllium is about 0.1-mm aluminum (Al) equivalent compared with 0.5-mm Al equivalent for standard radiographic tubes.

Target Composition. Conventional radiographic x-ray tubes use a **target composition** of a tungsten-rhenium alloy. A mixture of x-rays produced by both bremsstrahlung (the slowing down of the projectile electron,

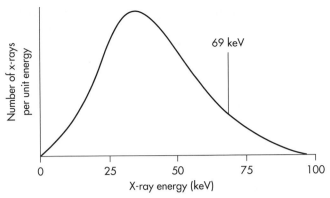

FIGURE 11-2 Emission spectrum for tungsten-rhenium target. *keV,* Kiloelectron volt.

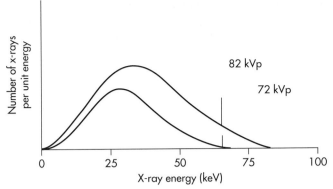

FIGURE 11-4 Effect of kVp on emission spectrum. *keV,* Kiloelectron; *kVp,* kilovolt (peak).

causing a wide range of x-ray energies) and characteristic radiation (x-rays created by electron transitions between orbits resulting in specific or discrete energies) exists in the x-ray beam created with these x-ray tubes. This effect can be demonstrated with an x-ray **emission spectrum** graph (Fig. 11-2). This wide band of energies may be desirable in conventional radiography but is not desirable in mammography because of the low subject contrast. Factors affecting the x-ray emission spectrum graph include milliampere, kilovolt (peak), added filtration, target material, and voltage waveform/ripple.

Milliampere. The factor of milliampere changes the amplitude of the curve (height of the y-axis) but not the shape of the curve (Fig. 11-3).

Kilovolt (Peak). The factor of kilovolt (peak) changes both the amplitude and the position of the spectrum curve. An increase in kilovolt (peak) shifts the spectrum to the right, indicating higher energy values (Fig. 11-4).

Added Filtration. Because filtration affects x-ray quality, the effect on the x-ray emission spectrum is similar to that of kilovolt (peak). If filtration is increased, the amplitude decreases and the spectrum shifts slightly to the right (Fig. 11-5).

Target Material. The amplitude and shape of the emission spectrum graph vary with any changes in the

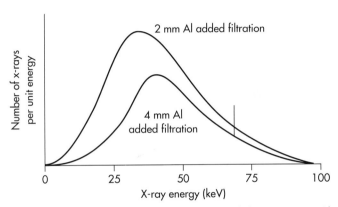

FIGURE 11-5 Effect of added filtration on emission spectrum. *Al,* Aluminum; *keV,* kiloelectron volt.

atomic number of the target material. If the atomic number increases, the continuous portion of the spectrum (bremsstrahlung) increases slightly in amplitude, especially to the high-energy side, whereas the discrete portion of the spectrum (characteristic x-rays) shifts to the right (Fig. 11-6). The target materials used in mammographic x-ray tubes can include tungsten, molybdenum, rhodium, or a combination of these.

Tungsten (Atomic Number, 74). Tungsten produces a wide band of x-ray energies including some that

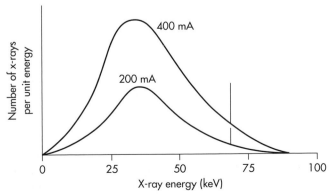

FIGURE 11-3 Effect of mA on emission spectrum. *keV,* Kiloelectron volt; *mA,* milliampere.

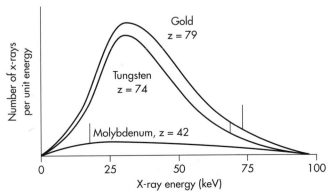

FIGURE 11-6 Effect of target material on emission spectrum. *keV,* Kiloelectron volt; *z,* atomic number.

are not useful in mammographic imaging. The emission spectrum is then shaped with filters that are made of aluminum, molybdenum, or rhodium.

Molybdenum (Atomic Number, 42). The lower atomic number significantly reduces the number of bremsstrahlung x-rays so that virtually all of the x-rays exiting the x-ray tube housing are characteristic x-rays of 17.9 and 19.5 kiloelectron volts (keV) (well within the K-edge of the image receptor being used). A 30- to 50-µm molybdenum filter is added to further eliminate any bremsstrahlung x-rays (which improves subject contrast). This target material is commonly used for normal or fatty breast composition.

Rhodium (Atomic Number, 45). Rhodium creates an emission spectrum similar to that of molybdenum. The characteristic x-rays have an energy of 20.2 and 22.7 keV (slightly higher than molybdenum, making it better for more dense breast tissue), and more bremsstrahlung x-rays are created. A 50-µm rhodium filter is used.

Molybdenum-Rhodium-Tungsten Alloy. Molybdenum-rhodium-tungsten alloy target material exhibits a mixed emission spectrum with characteristics of each element. With the selection of either an aluminum, rhodium, or molybdenum filter, the emission spectrum can be shaped to fit the image receptor that is used. When more than one target material is available with the mammographic unit, the system must indicate, before exposure, the preselected target material.

Voltage Waveform/Ripple. Three-phase and high-frequency x-ray generators create x-rays with a higher average energy (quality) and in greater number (quantity) than single-phase x-ray generators; therefore, the amplitude and relative position of the spectrum are different. With the three-phase and high-frequency generators, the increasing amplitude and the right-shifting spectrum indicate higher average energy (Fig. 11-7).

Focal Spot Size. The spatial resolution required in mammographic images is greater than that of conventional radiography because of the need to demonstrate microcalcifications. This must be accomplished with a small focal spot that ranges in size from 0.1 to 0.3 mm. When more than one focal spot is available on the unit, the system must indicate, before exposure, which focal spot is selected. Some manufacturers tilt the x-ray tube toward the cathode side (about 25 degrees), which reduces the effective focal spot size even further. Most mammographic x-ray tubes use a circular-shaped focal spot, rather than the rectangular-shaped focal spots found with conventional radiographic x-ray tubes. Circular focal spots provide better geometric sharpness but have a lower heat capacity because of less surface area of the anode under bombardment by the projectile electrons. The heel effect can be used by placing the cathode side of the tube toward the chest wall (not all units allow for rotation of the x-ray tube). However, since geometric unsharpness is also greater toward the cathode side of the x-ray field, any suspicious areas near the chest wall are often reimaged with the anode side closer to the chest wall.

Source-to-Image Distance and Target Angle. The source-to-image distance (SID) used in dedicated mammographic units ranges from 50 to 80 cm, with 65 cm being typical. Because of this relatively short SID, a larger target angle is necessary for mammographic x-ray tubes (22 to 24 degrees as compared to 7 to 13 degree angles for standard radiographic x-ray tubes) in order to create an x-ray field size large enough to cover the image receptor.

Compression

All modern mammographic units must be equipped with a compression device, usually made of radiolucent plastic. The amount of x-ray transmission through these devices is about 80% at 30 kVp. The function of these devices is to gently compress the breast tissue with a force of between 25 and 45 lb (111 and 200 N). An automatic adjust-and-release mechanism is found on most systems. Effective October 28, 2002, each mammographic system must provide (1) an initial power-driven compression activated by hands-free controls operable from both sides of the patient and (2) fine adjustment compression controls operable from both sides of the patient. The chest wall edge of the compression paddle shall be straight and parallel to the edge of the image receptor. The advantages of breast compression are shown in Box 11-1. The principal disadvantage of compression is patient discomfort.

Mammographic systems also must be equipped with various-sized compression paddles that match the sizes of all full-field image receptors provided for the system. The compression paddle should be flat and parallel to the breast support table and should not deflect from parallel by more than 1 cm at any point on the surface of the compression paddle when compression is applied.

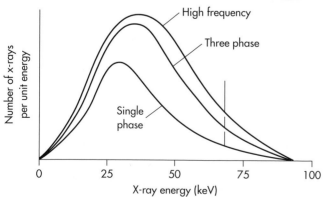

FIGURE 11-7 Effect of voltage waveform on emission spectrum. *keV*, Kiloelectron volt.

Grids

The presence of scattered radiation in a diagnostic image always reduces or lowers image contrast. Because mammographic images have an inherently low subject contrast, it is imperative that scattered radiation is reduced as much as possible. Carbon fiber-interspaced grids are often used to reduce scattered radiation (and therefore help increase image contrast). The grid ratios range from 3:1 to 5:1, and the grid frequency can range from 30 to 50 lines per centimeter. The mammographic grids also are focused to the x-ray source and move during the exposure to eliminate grid lines. Uniformity of construction and motion is paramount for proper image quality. A new type of crosshatch grid, called the *high transmission cellular* (HTC) *grid*, has been developed for mammographic systems. Crosshatch grids are superior at removing scattered radiation (compared with focused or parallel linear grids) but require significantly higher milliampere-second exposure because of increased absorption of primary radiation. For alleviation of this problem, the HTC mammographic grid uses copper as the grid strip material (as compared with lead in conventional grids) and air as the interspace material. The grid ratio of the HTC mammographic grid is 3.8:1. Systems with film/screen image receptors should be equipped with moving grids matched to all image receptor sizes provided. Systems used for magnification procedures should be capable of operation with the grid removed from between the x-ray source and the image receptor. Some studies have suggested that a grid can be omitted from mammographic exams performed with full-field digital mammography (FFDM) for breasts less than 5 cm thick when compressed, in order to decrease patient dose. This is because postprocessing of the digital images can maintain contrast despite the lack of a grid.

Image Receptors

Traditionally, most mammographic examinations that have been performed have utilized film/screen combinations as the primary image receptor. The film is most often single emulsion (to eliminate any parallax and crossover effects) and spectrally matched to the screen. Mammography films generally have a high average gradient (above 3) in order to deliver high inherent contrast but consequentially have a low or narrow exposure latitude (meaning that technique selection must be precise). The use of an AEC system and having a working technique chart available (Fig. 11-8) will help obtain precise techniques. The single-emulsion film is used with a single-screen image receptor. The mammographer must take special care to be sure that the emulsion side of the film faces the intensifying screen. Double-screen image receptors used with duplitized film also are available. Rare earth phosphors (often containing yttrium or gadolinium) are used in the intensifying screens to help reduce patient dose and increase image contrast. The absorption efficiency of these screens can be as high as 70% because low-energy x-ray photons are used. The main sources of image noise in film/screen mammography are quantum mottle and film granularity. It is also critical for film/screen image receptors to be kept clean to minimize artifacts. Systems with screen-film image receptors should provide, at a minimum, for operation with image receptors of 18 × 24 cm and 24 × 30 cm. Full-field digital mammographic systems are rapidly replacing film/screen image receptors and are discussed later in this chapter.

Film Processors

Mammographic images should have a dedicated film processor for conversion of the latent image into a manifest image. Mammography films tend to have a relatively thick single emulsion, making them much more sensitive to processor artifacts. Mammographic images require optical densities of between 1.5 and 2, which is a narrower range than that of conventional radiography (0.5 to 2.5). A common option for processing mammographic images is **extended processing**, which extends the standard cycle of a 20-second developing time to a cycle of 40 seconds and longer. The developer temperature, concentration, and composition remain unchanged. The main advantages of extended processing are greater image contrast (approximately 15%), increased image receptor sensitivity (about 30%), and reduced patient dose (about 30%). These improvements are seen only when single-emulsion films are used.

Magnification Mammography

Magnification studies are common during mammographic procedures to investigate small microcalcifications or lesions that may appear ambiguous at normal size. According to the Food and Drug Administration (FDA), mammographic systems that are used to perform noninterventional problem-solving procedures should have radiographic magnification capability available for use by the operator. These systems should provide, at minimum, at least one magnification value within the range of 1.4 to 2. This magnification factor is determined by the ratio of the image size as compared with

Mammography Phototimer Technique Chart
Room No._____ Unit _____

Compressed Breast Thickness	Fatty Breast				50% Fatty- 50% Dense				Dense breast			
	Target	Filter	kVp	Density	Target	Filter	kVp	Density	Target	Filter	kVp	Density
<3 cm												
3 to 5 cm												
5 to 7 cm												
>7 cm												

Techniques based upon proper photocell placement under the densest portion of the breast, screen-film combinations, and processing. Taut compression should be used for all patients except where noted.

Focal Spot size for:
    Nonmagnification Technique:_____mm
    Magnification Technique:_____mm

Special Techniques

Implant Displaced Views
    Phototiming same as above chart

Manual Techniques for Implant Views

Breast size	Target	Filter	kVp	mAs
Small				
Medium				
Large				

Apply minimal compression – enough to prevent motion.

Specimens: (Manual Technique Only)

Breast size	Target	Filter	kVp	mAs
Small				
Medium				
Large				

Specimens must be compressed.

FIGURE 11-8 Technique chart for mammographic imaging with AEC.

the object size or by the ratio of SID to source-to-object distance (SOD). Magnification of the image is achieved by increasing the object-to-image distance (OID), which reduces the SOD (typically 35 cm in magnification studies). Because this increase also reduces image sharpness, it is essential that the effective focal spot size for magnification studies not exceed 0.1 mm. However, the small focal spot can only tolerate low tube currents (25 mA), which can result in long exposure times of several seconds. The air gap created by the increased OID normally eliminates the need for a grid, thereby reducing the required mAs.

Digital Mammography Systems

Computed (CR) and digital radiographic (DR) systems have become relatively common imaging systems for conventional radiography. However, these systems tend to have lower spatial resolution than film/screen imaging systems and a high capital cost, which have slowed their application into mammographic imaging. On January 28, 2000, the FDA approved the Senographe 2000D Full-Field Digital Mammography (FFDM) system for marketing and immediate use in facilities that are already certified for film/screen imaging systems according to the

Mammography Quality Standards Act (MQSA). As of the writing of this edition, seven additional digital mammographic systems have been approved by the FDA (with other systems pending). They include the following:

- Fuji Computed Radiography Mammography Suite on 7/10/2006
- GE Senographe Essential FFDM system on 4/11/2006
- Siemens Mammomat Novation DR FFDM system on 8/20/2004
- GE Senographe DS FFDM System on 2/19/2004
- Lorad/Hologic Senia FFDM System on 10/2/2002
- Lorad Digital Breast Imager FFDM System on 2/15/2002
- Fischer Imaging SenoScan FFDM System on 9/25/2001

The GE and Fischer systems are indirect conversion systems with cesium iodide coupled to either a TFT assembly (GE) or a CCD assembly (Fischer). The Siemens and Lorad/Hologic systems use a direct conversion system with amorphous selenium coupled to a TFT assembly. The Fuji system is based on the computed radiography (CR) technology used in radiography. The typical matrix size in digital mammographic systems is

4096×6144 pixels, with pixel sizes ranging from about 24 to 100 μm.

The spatial resolution for these systems is on the order of 5 to 7 line pairs per millimeter (lp/mm), as compared with 11 lp/mm or more for film/screen mammography systems. This means that film/screen mammography is better at detecting subtle tissue changes, such as microcalcifications, that could indicate early cancer. However, a dual-energy subtraction technique that subtracts background objects from the image in digital systems could enable these systems to detect lesions that previously were masked by overlying structures. The limiting spatial resolution for digital mammography is about 10 lp/mm, which is inferior to film/screen systems that can reach 20 lp/mm. However, digital images produce better contrast resolution (especially in dense breast tissues), greater dynamic range (3200 gray shades are available for imaging breast structures versus less than 100 for film/screen systems) and have a higher detective quantum efficiency (DQE) than film/screen image receptor systems, which can be even more important in mammographic images. In digital mammography, the x-ray generator/x-ray tube combination is the limiting factor in determining the dynamic range. These images may be read directly from the monitor (soft-copy review) or from hard-copy images created by a laser camera or dry laser printer. These hard-copy images provide better contrast resolution and better visibility of detail than images from traditional film/screen mammography. The dry laser printer, with a D_{max} of 3.5 or greater, a base-plus-fog level of less than 0.25, and 16 bit images with at least 12-bit gray levels is recommended for printing hard copy digital mammographic images. They should support true-size printing, and images should be justified so that the chest wall is printed as close to the edge of the film as the printer server is capable. In addition, film artifacts are virtually completely eliminated. The Digital Mammographic Imaging Screening Trial (DMIST) which was sponsored by the National Cancer Institute and coordinated by the American College of Radiology Imaging Network (ACRIN), demonstrated that digital mammography systems are as effective as analog systems as a screening tool. For some women (such as those with dense breasts) digital mammography is more effective than film/screen in finding cancer.

A major advantage of digital imaging is postprocessing of the image, which can improve lesion visibility in underexposed or overexposed regions. **Postprocessing** is a manipulation of the image data in the memory of the computer, before display on a monitor. Postprocessing functions available with the FFDM and CR systems may include the following:

1. **Tissue Equalization**—image processing that compensates for varying breast tissue densities so that the entire breast (from the chest wall to the skin line) can be visualized in a single image.

2. **Magnification**—electronic digital zoom with software manipulation that can reduce the need to take additional magnification views, as with film/screen mammography.

3. **Image Inversion**—allows the converting of a negative image (standard radiographic image) into a positive image (meaning a reverse of the negative image where white areas on the negative image are black on the positive image and vice versa).

4. **Gray Scale Processing**—a manipulation of the gray scale values that are displayed in the image. This includes windowing (or window width), which controls image contrast and leveling (or window level), which controls image brightness (comparable to OD in film/screen imaging).

5. **Annotations and Measurements**—software manipulation allowing electronic annotation on the image and electronic measurement tools for calculating sizes and volumes.

Improved **workflow** (the number of patients imaged per hour) can be another advantage of FFDM and CR mammography. A report published by the London-based Centre for Evidence-based Purchasing (CEP) looked at an average of 16,000 screening mammograms per year between 2002 and 2006 and found the following times to produce four mammographic images:

Film/screen	3.5 to 6.5 minutes
CR	2.5 to 4 minutes
FFDM	1.3 to 4.7 minutes

Another advantage of digital systems is the use of scanning software (known as *computer-aided detection*, or CAD) to help radiologists locate suspicious areas of the images. Initial studies have shown that this type of software can have sensitivities as high as 90%, so they can help increase the accuracy of mammographic diagnosis. Film/screen mammographic images also can utilize CAD software, but the image must first be digitized with a scanner that was discussed in Chapter 9.

Patient dose in digital mammography is the same or less (up to 50% less in some studies) than that obtained with film/screen systems. Also contributing to lower patient dose is fewer recalls for additional imaging with digital mammography.

Patient Convenience/Satisfaction also is considered an advantage for digital mammography because less time is required to perform mammographic procedures, especially with FFDM. This is because the image is available in less than a minute with digital systems compared with 3.5 to 6.5 minutes with film/screen mammography.

A new application of digital mammography is tomosynthesis, which requires multiple images from many angles to generate tomographic slices that can eliminate overlapping structures. Playback of the sequence of slices is via a cine loop, similar to that used in CT imaging. These images can ultimately be used with 3-D visualization software to create 3-D images of breast structure. An emerging application of digital mammography is dual-energy subtraction imaging (similar to the type being used in chest imaging), which can enhance certain structures by subtracting background structures from the region of interest.

The main disadvantages of digital systems are lower spatial resolution (mentioned previously), higher capital cost for the equipment (currently about three to five times the cost of a film/screen system), higher maintenance costs, and higher adjunct costs (such as 5 megapixel viewing monitors that can cost up to $40,000 and last about 2 years). Because reimbursement of mammography services by private insurance companies and the federal government (e.g., Medicare, Medicaid) is relatively low, it has been difficult for healthcare organizations to recover their investment in these systems. Technological issues also can pose problems such as file storage issues (digital mammograms can have up to 200 MB of file size) and remote viewing (person accessing the image also must have a 5 megapixel high resolution monitor to be able to diagnose the image). Therefore PACS systems must be able to store up to 40 gigabytes of image data per month just for mammographic images and have a 5 megapixel monitor available to view the images for diagnosis, increasing both the cost and operational difficulties of these systems. For PACS systems to transmit digital mammographic images, lossless compression capability is essential. Magnification studies also can be of concern in digital mammography. Film/screen mammography utilizes geometric magnification (e.g., increased OID and/or decreased SID) to obtain magnification studies. Digital systems can utilize electronic magnification, which usually increases pixel size to magnify the image. This results in less exposure to the patient and shorter examination time, but greatly decreases the spatial resolution compared to those studies utilizing geometric magnification.

Stereotactic Localization

Stereotactic localization is a method that has been developed to perform core needle biopsies using mammographic imaging. As with the old process of stereoradiography, two views of the breast are acquired with the central ray at a different angle for each view (usually within 15 degrees of normal). Images of the lesion will shift by an amount depending on lesion depth, which permits a three-dimensional localization of the lesion. A biopsy needle gun is positioned at the correct location and then fired to obtain a core sample of the tissue. This type of biopsy is quick, accurate, and less invasive than other methods, with less scarring of the breast tissue. Full-field digital systems are better suited than film/screen systems for this technique because image acquisition is faster (no film processing is required), and the computer

software can align the two images for optimum visualization.

MAMMOGRAPHIC QUALITY ASSURANCE

The importance of mammography in the early diagnosis of breast cancer has been well demonstrated. Breast cancer can be detected by means of mammograms as early as 2 years before a lump can be felt during a manual examination. For breast cancer detection to be accomplished successfully, the images must be of the highest quality and the interpreting physician must be highly trained. This means that a detailed quality management program must be in place to minimize any variations, which are even more detrimental to image quality in mammography because of the low subject contrast.

MQSA and Mammography Quality Standards Reauthorization Act

Before 1992, quality standards for mammography were the responsibility of individual state agencies. The American College of Radiology (ACR) began a voluntary Mammography Accreditation Program (MAP) in 1987, which required specific quality control and quality assurance procedures for equipment and personnel. Approximately 30% of facilities that initially applied for ACR accreditation failed on their first attempt. Because so few facilities voluntarily sought and obtained ACR accreditation, concern of mammographic image quality prompted the U.S. Senate Committee on Labor and Human Resources to hold hearings on breast cancer in 1992. This committee discovered many problems with mammographic procedures in the United States including poor-quality equipment, a lack of quality assurance procedures, poorly trained interpreting physicians, and no consistent oversight or facility inspections. This led to the enactment of Public Law 102-539 (the MQSA), which passed on October 27, 1992. This law requires that all facilities (except for those of the Department of Veterans Affairs) be accredited by an approved accreditation body and certified by the Secretary of Health and Human Services to legally provide mammography services after October 1, 1994. The Secretary of Health and Human Services delegated the authority to approve accreditation bodies and to certify facilities to the FDA. Certification of facilities can be through the FDA, or by the states of Illinois, Iowa, or South Carolina. These state agencies use the same certification requirements as the FDA. The MQSA has been superseded by the Mammography Quality Standards Reauthorization Act (MQSRA) of 1998. As part of the new law, final FDA regulations regarding mammographic procedures became effective on April 28, 1999, replacing interim regulations that were used during the original law. In 2002 the amended final regulations were published with new subparts that included addressing alternatives such as digital mammographic systems. The final regulations emphasize performance objectives rather than specify the behavior and manner of compliance.

The main provisions of MQSA and MQSRA include the following:

- Accreditation of mammography facilities by private, nonprofit organizations (such as the ACR) or state agencies that have met the standards established by the FDA (including Iowa, Arkansas, and Texas) and have been approved by the FDA.
- An annual mammography facility physics survey, consultation, and evaluation performed by a qualified medical physicist are required.
- Annual inspection of mammography facilities performed by FDA-certified federal and state inspectors must occur.
- The establishment of initial and continuing qualification standards for interpreting physicians, radiologic technologists, medical physicists, and mammography facility inspectors.
- The specification of boards or organizations eligible to certify the adequacy of training and experience of mammography personnel.
- The establishment of quality standards for mammography equipment and practices including quality assurance and quality control programs.
- Establishment of infection control policy and procedures for cleaning and disinfecting mammographic equipment after contact with blood or other potentially infectious materials.
- Standards governing final assessment of findings in the evaluation of mammographic images. The final report should contain overall final assessment findings, classified in one of the following categories:
  1. Negative—nothing to comment on (if the interpreting physician is aware of clinical findings or symptoms, despite the negative assessment, these should be explained)
  2. Benign—also a negative assessment
  3. Probably benign—finding(s) have a high probability of being benign
  4. Suspicious—finding(s) without all of the characteristic morphology of breast cancer but indicating a definite probability of being malignant.
  5. Highly suggestive of malignancy—finding(s) have a high probability of being malignant.
  6. Incomplete: need additional imaging evaluation—should be assigned in cases where no final assessment category can be assigned because of incomplete workup. Reasons why no assessment can be made should be stated by the interpreting physician.
- Communication of mammography results to the patient. Each facility should send each patient a summary of the mammography report written in lay terms within 30 days of the mammographic examination. If assessments are "suspicious" or "highly suggestive of malignancy," the facility should make reasonable attempts to ensure that the results are communicated to the patient as soon as possible.
- Record keeping. Each facility that performs mammograms should maintain mammography images and reports in a permanent medical record of the patient for a period of not less than 5 years or not less than 10 years if no additional mammograms of the patient are performed at the facility, or a longer period of time if mandated by state or local law. This storage may be in either digital data or hard-copy films. Each facility should, on request or on behalf of the patient, permanently or temporarily transfer the original mammograms (hard-copy films) and copies of the patient's reports to a medical institution or to a physician or healthcare provider of the patient, or to the patient directly.
- Specific regulations for accrediting bodies.
- General facility provisions such as requirements for the content and terminology in the mammography report, specific guidelines for mammography reports, definition of the responsibilities of facility personnel, review of mammography medical outcomes data every 12 months, standards for examinees with breast implants, and the requirement of facilities to develop a system for collecting and resolving serious complaints.
- Personnel regulations for interpreting physicians, medical physicists, and mammographers. Facilities should maintain records to document the qualifications of all personnel who worked at the facility as interpreting physicians, radiologic technologists, or medical physicists. These records must be available for review for MQSA inspectors. Records of personnel no longer employed by the facility should not be discarded until the next annual inspection has been completed and the FDA has determined that the facility is in compliance with the MQSA personnel requirements.

Quality Control Responsibilities

The MQSA designates specific responsibilities for various members of the diagnostic imaging department.

Radiologist (Interpreting Physician). The primary responsibility for mammography quality control is the lead interpreting physician or radiologist. Minimum qualifications include a license to practice medicine and certification by the American Board of Radiology (ABR), the American Osteopathic Board of Radiology (AOBR), or the Royal College of Physicians and Surgeons of Canada (RCPSC) and at least 3 months of documented full-time training in the interpretation of mammograms. The physician or radiologist also must continue to read and interpret at least 40 patients per month over 24 months and obtain at least 15 category I continuing education units (CEUs) in mammography over a 36-month period. These individuals also have the responsibility of following up any patient with a positive diagnosis.

Medical Physicist. Medical physicists are responsible for the quality control evaluation of the mammographic equipment. They must have a license or state approval or be certified by an FDA-approved accrediting body. Their continuing experience must be maintained by surveying at least two mammography facilities and at least six mammography units in a 24-month period.

The FDA mandates that at least once a year, each facility must undergo a mammography equipment evaluation (MEE) that must be performed by a medical physicist and that the following quality control tests must be performed: AEC, kilovolt (peak) accuracy and reproducibility, focal spot condition, beam quality and half-value layer (HVL), breast entrance air kerma and AEC reproducibility, dosimetry, x-ray field/light field/image receptor/compression paddle alignment, uniformity of screen speed, system artifacts, radiation output, decompression, quality control tests—other modalities, viewbox illuminators and viewing conditions, comparison of test results with action limits, and additional evaluations.

Film/Screen Systems

Automatic Exposure Control. The AEC shall be capable of maintaining film OD within ± 0.15 of the mean OD when thickness of a homogenous material is varied over a range of 2 to 6 cm and the kilovolt (peak) is varied appropriately for such thickness over the kilovolt (peak) range used clinically in the facility. If this requirement cannot be met, a technique chart should be developed showing appropriate techniques (kilovolt [peak] and OD control settings) for different breast thicknesses and compositions that must be used so that ODs within ± 0.15 of the average under AEC-obtained conditions can be produced. Compliance with this requirement may be demonstrated by any of the following three methods:

1. Confirming AEC performance in the contact configuration. In the contact configuration, the AEC must maintain the film OD over the 2- to 6-cm-thick range within the action limit of ± 0.15 OD of the mean.

   AND

   Confirming AEC performance in all other clinically used configurations. This can be done by demonstrating that the AEC meets the OD and reproducibility limits established by the manufacturer for those other configurations.

   Note: Method #1 can be used *only* in those cases where the manufacturer has established AEC performance standards for the noncontact configurations provided.

2. Confirming AEC performance in the contact configuration. In the contact configuration, the AEC must maintain the film OD over the 2- to 6-cm-thick range within the action limit of ±0.15 of the mean.

   AND

   Confirming AEC performance in all other clinically used configurations. This can be done by comparing the mean film OD obtained from the data for the 2- to 6-cm thicknesses measured in the contact configuration with measurements obtained with the 4-cm-thick phantom in the other configurations used clinically at the facility. When results across *different configurations* are compared, the facility may use the action limit of ± 0.30 OD.

3. Confirming AEC performance by demonstrating that the AEC maintains the mean film OD within ± 0.15 OD in *all* configurations used clinically by the facility. The action limit applies only within each specific configuration tested and does not apply to data collected across the different configurations.

Kilovolt (Peak) Accuracy and Reproducibility. The kilovolt (peak) shall be accurate within ± 5% of the indicated or selected kilovolt (peak) at the lowest clinical kilovolt (peak) that can be measured by a kilovolt (peak) test device; the most commonly used clinical kilovolt (peak); or the highest available clinical kilovolt (peak). The coefficient of variation of reproducibility of the kilovolt (peak) shall be equal to or less than 0.02.

Focal Spot Condition. According to MQSA regulations, facilities shall evaluate focal spot condition only by determining the system resolution. The system resolution requirement is that the film/screen combination used in the facility should provide a minimum resolution of 11 lp/mm when a high-contrast resolution bar test pattern is oriented with the bars perpendicular to the anode-cathode axis and a minimum of 13 lp/mm when the bars are parallel to the axis. The bar pattern should be placed 4.5 cm above the breast support surface, centered with respect to the chest wall edge of the image receptor, and positioned with its edge within 1 cm of the chest wall edge of the image receptor. When focal spot dimensions are measured, standards of the National Electrical Manufacturers Association (NEMA) apply (Table 11-1).

Beam Quality and Half-Value Layer. The values for minimum acceptable HVL are listed in Table 11-2.

Breast Entrance Air Kerma and Automatic Exposure Control Reproducibility. The coefficient of variation for both air kerma and milliampere shall not exceed 0.05.

Dosimetry. The average glandular dose delivered during a single craniocaudal view of an FDA-accepted phantom (Fig. 11-9, *A*) simulating a standard breast shall not exceed 3 mGy (0.3 rad) per exposure. The dose shall be determined with technique factors and conditions used clinically for a standard breast.

TABLE 11-1 Standards of the National Electrical Manufacturers Association

Focal Spot Tolerance Limit

Nominal Focal Spot Size (mm)	Maximum Measured Dimensions	
	Width (mm)	Length (mm)
0.1	0.15	0.15
0.15	0.23	0.23
0.2	0.3	0.3
0.3	0.45	0.65
0.4	0.6	0.85
0.6	0.9	1.3

TABLE 11-2 Values for Minimum Acceptable Half-Value Layer X-Ray Tube Voltage (kVp) and Minimum HVL

Designed Operating Range (kVp)	Measured Operating Voltage (kVp)	Minimum HVL (mm of Aluminum)
Below 50	20	0.2
	25	0.25
	30	0.3

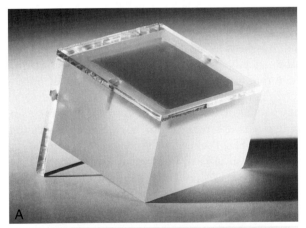

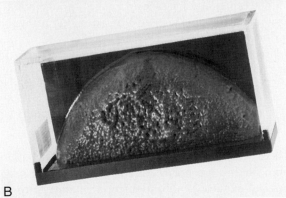

FIGURE 11-9 Conventional mammographic phantom **(A)** and anthropomorphic (lifelike) phantom **(B)**. *(Courtesy Nuclear Associates, Carle Place, N.Y.)*

X-Ray Field/Light Field/Image Receptor/Compression Paddle Alignment. All systems shall have beam-limiting devices that allow the entire chest wall edge of the x-ray field to extend to the chest wall edge of the image receptor and provide a means to ensure that the x-ray field does not extend beyond any edge of the image receptor by more than 2% of the SID. If a light field that passes through the x-ray beam limitation device is provided, it shall be aligned with the x-ray field so that the total of any misalignment of the edges of the light field and the x-ray field along either the length or the width of the visually defined field at the plane of the breast support surface does not exceed 2% of the SID. The chest wall edge of the compression paddle shall not extend beyond the chest wall edge of the image receptor by more than 1% of the SID when tested with the compression paddle placed above the breast support surface at a distance equivalent to standard breast thickness. The shadow of the vertical edge of the compression paddle should not be visible on the image.

Uniformity of Screen Speed. The uniformity of screen speed of all the cassettes in the facility shall be tested, and the difference between the minimum and maximum optical densities shall not exceed 0.30. Screen artifacts also should be evaluated during this test.

System Artifacts. System artifacts shall be evaluated with a high-grade, defect-free sheet of homogenous material large enough to cover the mammography image receptor and should be performed for all cassette sizes used in the facility with a grid appropriate for the cassette being tested. System artifacts also shall be evaluated for all available focal spot sizes and target filter combinations used clinically.

Radiation Output. The system shall be capable of producing a minimum output of 7 mGy air kerma per second (800 milliroentgen [mR]/sec) when operating at 28 kVp in the standard mammography (molybdenum per molybdenum) mode at any SID where the system is designed to operate and when measured by a detector with its center located 4.5 cm above the breast support surface with the compression paddle in place between the source and the detector. The system shall be capable of maintaining the required minimum radiation output averaged over a 3-second period. Instruments used by medical physicists in their annual survey to measure the air kerma or air kerma rate from a mammography unit should be calibrated at least once every 2 years and each time the instrument is repaired. The instrument calibration must be traceable to a national standard (either by the National Institute of Standards and Technology [NIST] or by a laboratory that participates in and has met the NIST's proficiency test requirements) and calibrated with an accuracy of ± 6% (95% confidence level) in the mammography energy range.

Decompression. If the system is equipped with a provision for automatic decompression after completion of an exposure or interruption of power to the system, the system shall be tested to confirm that it provides (1) an override capability to allow maintenance of compression, (2) a continuous display of the override status, and (3) a manual emergency compression release that can be activated in the event of power or automatic release failure.

Quality Control Tests-Other Modalities. For systems with image receptor modalities other than film/screen (e.g., full-field digital mammographic systems), the quality assurance program shall be substantially the same as the quality assurance program recommended by the image receptor manufacturer, except that the maximum allowable dose should not exceed the maximum allowable dose for film/screen systems (3 mGy or 0.3 rad per exposure).

Viewbox Illuminators and Viewing Conditions. These are not listed by the FDA in 21 Code of Federal Regulations (CFR) Part 900 as an annual duty but are recommended by the ACR in its 1999 edition of the *Mammography Quality Control Manual*. The acrylic plastic (Plexiglas) illuminator fronts should be clean and free of any loose dirt, marks from grease pens, or scratches. The viewbox luminance, color temperature, and ambient light conditions (room illuminance) should be measured with the equipment and procedures outlined in Chapter 3. The luminance from the center of the illuminator should be at least 3000 nit, and the room illuminance (ambient light) should be 50 lux or less. Fluorescent bulbs should be replaced at least every 2 years. MQSA specifies that facilities shall make special lights for film illumination (i.e., hot-lights) capable of producing light levels greater than that provided by the viewbox, available to the interpreting physicians. Facilities also must ensure that film masking devices that can limit the illuminated area to a region equal to or smaller than the exposed portion of the film are available to all interpreting physicians interpreting for the facility.

Comparison of Test Results with Action Limits. After completion of the annual quality control tests, the facility should compare the test results with the corresponding specified action limits or, for digital modalities, with the manufacturer's recommended action limits. If the test results fall outside of the action limits, the source of the problem should be identified and corrective actions taken:

1. Before any further examinations are performed or any films processed with a component of the mammography system that failed any tests of dosimetry or quality control tests for other modalities
2. Within 30 days for all other tests

Additional Evaluations. Additional evaluations of mammography units or image processors shall be conducted whenever a new unit or processor is installed, a unit or processor is disassembled and reassembled at the same time or a new location, or major components of a mammography unit or processor equipment are

changed or repaired. All problems shall be corrected before new or changed equipment is put into service for examinations or film processing. The mammography equipment evaluation should be performed by a medical physicist or by an individual who is directly supervised by a medical physicist. Major repairs would include the following:

- *AEC*—AEC replacement, thickness compensation internal* adjustment, AEC sensor replacement, AEC circuit board replacement
- *Bucky replacement*—If AEC systems also is replaced
- *Collimation system*—Collimator replacement, collimator reassembly with blade replacement
- Filter replacement
- Processor—installation, reassembly
- X-ray unit-kilovolt (peak), milliampere, or time internal* adjustments, high voltage generator replacement, x-ray tube replacement, installation, reassembly
- Software changes and upgrades for digital mammographic systems

The medical physicist's MQSA checklist form is found in Figure 11-10 and the QC test summary form for film/screen image receptors is found in Figure 11-11.

Digital Mammography Systems

Quality Control Tests—Other Modalities. For systems with image receptor modalities other than film/screen (e.g., full-field digital and CR mammographic systems), the quality assurance program shall be substantially the same as the quality assurance program recommended by the image receptor manufacturer, except that the maximum allowable dose should not exceed the maximum allowable dose for film/screen systems (3 mGy or 0.3 rad per exposure). However, medical physicists are required to have 8 hours' training in surveying FFDM and CR systems before conducting independent surveys or equipment evaluations, or both. Submission of images for accreditation consideration that are slightly different from film/screen images are:

- For FFDM and CR, the American College of Radiology accepts only hard-copy images for accreditation
- For phantom images, do not zoom or rotate, and print as close to true size as possible
- Clinical images must be of final interpretation quality, entire breast must fit on the image, no tiling, print as close to the true size as possible, and they must contain patient ID information
- Lead interpreting physician must review and approve all hard-copy images

There are also additional QC tests for FFDM and CR equipment that are not required for film/screen systems including monitor calibration/check, contrast-to-noise ratio (CNR), signal-to-noise ratio (SNR), and modulation

---

*Internal adjustments refer to equipment adjustments that typically cannot be made by the operator.

MAP ID#: _____

MEDICAL PHYSICIST'S CHECKLIST
MQSA REQUIREMENTS FOR MAMMOGRAPHY EQUIPMENT

Facility Name: _____

Unit Manufacturer: _____ **Model:** _____

Serial number: _____ **Year Mfr:** _____

Medical Physicist: _____ **Room ID:** _____

Signature: _____ **Survey Date:** _____

Feature	FDA Rule Section	Requirement	Applies to	Meets FDA Requirements? *(if NA, please explain)*
Motion of tube-image receptor assembly	3(i)	The assembly shall be capable of being fixed in any position where it is designed to operate. Once fixed in any such position, it shall not undergo unintended motion.	S-F & FFDM	☐ Yes ☐ No ☐ NA
	3(ii)	This mechanism shall not fail in the event of power interruption.	S-F & FFDM	☐ Yes ☐ No ☐ NA
Image receptor sizes	4(i)	Systems using screen-film image receptors shall provide, at a minimum, for operation with image receptors of 18 x 24 cm and 24 x 30 cm.	S-F	☐ Yes ☐ No ☐ NA
	4(ii)	Systems using screen-film image receptors shall be equipped with moving grids matched to all image receptor sizes provided.	S-F	☐ Yes ☐ No ☐ NA
	4(iii)	Systems used for magnification procedures shall be capable of operation with the grid removed from between the source and image receptor.	S-F & FFDM	☐ Yes ☐ No ☐ NA
Beam limitation and light fields	5(i)	All systems shall have beam limiting devices that allow the useful beam to extend to or beyond the chest wall edge of the image receptor.	S-F & FFDM	☐ Yes ☐ No ☐ NA
	5(ii)	For any mammography system with a light beam that passes through the x-ray beam-limiting device, the light shall provide an average illumination of not less than 160 lux (15 ft-candles) at 100 cm or the maximum source-image receptor distance (SID), whichever is less.	S-F & FFDM (except Fischer)	☐ Yes ☐ No ☐ NA
Magnification	6(i)	Systems used to perform noninterventional problem-solving procedures shall have radiographic magnification capability available for use by the operator.	S-F & FFDM	☐ Yes ☐ No ☐ NA
	6(ii)	Systems used for magnification procedures shall provide, at a minimum, at least one magnification value within the range of 1.4 to 2.0.	S-F & FFDM	☐ Yes ☐ No ☐ NA
Focal spot selection	7(i)	When more than one focal spot is provided, the system shall indicate, prior to exposure, which focal spot is selected.	S-F & FFDM	☐ Yes ☐ No ☐ NA
	7(ii)	When more than one target material is provided, the system shall indicate, prior to exposure, the preselected target material.	S-F & FFDM	☐ Yes ☐ No ☐ NA
	7(iii)	When the target material and/or focal spot is selected by a system algorithm that is based on the exposure or on a test exposure, the system shall display, after the exposure, the target material and/or focal spot actually used during the exposure.	S-F & FFDM	☐ Yes ☐ No ☐ NA
Application of compression	8(i)(A)	Each system shall provide an initial power-driven compression activated by hands-free controls operable from both sides of the patient.	S-F & FFDM	☐ Yes ☐ No ☐ NA
	8(i)(B)	Each system shall provide fine adjustment compression controls operable from both sides of the patient.	S-F & FFDM	☐ Yes ☐ No ☐ NA

FIGURE 11-10 American College of Radiology (ACR) Medical Physicist MQSA Checklist.

(Continued)

Feature	FDA Rule Section	Requirement	Applies to	Meets FDA Requirements? *(if NA, please explain)*
Compression paddle	8(ii)(A)	Systems shall be equipped with different sized compression paddles that match the sizes of all full-field image receptors provided for the system.	S-F & FFDM	☐ Yes ☐ No ☐ NA
	8(ii)(B)	The compression paddle shall be flat and parallel to the breast support table and shall not deflect from parallel by more than 1.0 cm at any point on the surface of the compression paddle when compression is applied.	S-F & FFDM (except Fischer)	☐ Yes ☐ No ☐ NA
	8(ii)(C)	Equipment intended by the manufacturer's design to not be flat and parallel to the breast support table during compression shall meet the manufacturer's design specifications and maintenance requirements.	S-F & FFDM	☐ Yes ☐ No ☐ NA
	8(ii)(D)	The chest wall edge of the compression paddle shall be straight and parallel to the edge of the image receptor.	S-F & FFDM	☐ Yes ☐ No ☐ NA
	8(ii)(E)	The chest wall edge may be bent upward to allow for patient comfort but shall not appear on the image.	S-F & FFDM	☐ Yes ☐ No ☐ NA
Technique factor selection and display	9(i)	Manual selection of mAs or at least one of its component parts (mA and/or time) shall be available.	S-F & FFDM	☐ Yes ☐ No ☐ NA
	9(ii)	The technique factors (kVp and either mA and seconds or mAs) to be used during an exposure shall be indicated before the exposure begins, except when AEC is used, in which case the technique factors that are set prior to the exposure shall be indicated.	S-F & FFDM	☐ Yes ☐ No ☐ NA
	9(iii)	Following AEC mode use, the system shall indicate the actual kVp and mAs (or mA and time) used during the exposure.	S-F & FFDM	☐ Yes ☐ No ☐ NA
Automatic exposure control	10(i)	Each screen-film system shall provide an AEC mode that is operable in all combinations of equipment configuration provided, e.g., grid, non-grid; magnification, nonmagnification; and various target-filter combinations.	S-F	☐ Yes ☐ No ☐ NA
	10(ii)	The positioning or selection of the detector shall permit flexibility in the placement of the detector under the target tissue. The size and the available positions of the detector shall be clearly indicated at the x-ray input surface of the breast compression paddle. The selected position of the detector shall be clearly indicated.	S-F	☐ Yes ☐ No ☐ NA
	10(iii)	The system shall provide means for the operator to vary the selected optical density from the normal (zero) setting.	S-F	☐ Yes ☐ No ☐ NA
X-ray film*	11	The facility shall use x-ray film for mammography that has been designated by the film manufacturer as appropriate for mammography.	S-F	☐ Yes ☐ No ☐ NA
Intensifying screens*	12	The facility shall use intensifying screens for mammography that have been designated by the screen manufacturer as appropriate for mammography and shall use film that is matched to the screen's spectral output as specified by the manufacturer.	S-F	☐ Yes ☐ No ☐ NA
Film processing solutions*	13	For processing mammography films, the facility shall use chemical solutions that are capable of developing the films used by the facility in a manner equivalent to the minimum requirements specified by the film manufacturer.	S-F	☐ Yes ☐ No ☐ NA
Lighting*	14	The facility shall make special lights for film illumination, i.e., hot-lights, capable of producing light levels greater than that provided by the view box, available to the interpreting physicians.	S-F & FFDM (for hardcopy comparison)	☐ Yes ☐ No ☐ NA
Film masking devices*	15	Facilities shall ensure that film masking devices that can limit the illuminated area to a region equal to or smaller than the exposed portion of the film are available to all interpreting physicians interpreting for the facility.	S-F & FFDM (for hardcopy comparison)	☐ Yes ☐ No ☐ NA

* NA is acceptable for new units at existing facilities if these were previously evaluated and have not changed

FIGURE 11-10—cont'd.

MEDICAL PHYSICIST'S MAMMOGRAPHY QC TEST SUMMARY
Screen-Film Systems

Site Name	
Address	
Medical Physicist's Name	
X-Ray Unit Manufacturer	
Date of Installation	
Film (mfr & type)	

Report Date	
Survey Date	
Signature	
Model	
Room ID	
Screen (mfr & type)	

Survey Type: ☐ Mammo Eqpt Evaluation of new unit (include MQSA Rqmts for Mammo Eqpt checklist)   ☐ Annual Survey

Medical Physicist's QC Tests

	PASS/FAIL	
	ACR Guides	**MQSA Regs**

1. Mammographic Unit Assembly Evaluation

2. Collimation Assessment
   Deviation between x-ray field and light field ≤2% of SID
   X-ray field does not extend beyond any side of the IR by more than 2% of SID
   Chest wall edge of compression paddle doesn't extend beyond IR by more than 1% of SID

3. Evaluation of Focal Spot Performance
   Measured performance within acceptable limits for large focal spot
   Measured performance within acceptable limits for small focal spot

4. Automatic Exposure Control (AEC) System Performance
   Exposure reproducibility is within acceptable limits
   AEC compensation for kVp, breast thickness and image mode is adequate
   AEC density control function is adequate

5. Uniformity of Screen Speed
   Optical density range is ≤0.30

6. Artifact Evaluation
   Artifacts were not apparent or not significant

7. Phantom Image Quality Evaluation
   4 largest fibers, 3 largest speck groups and 3 largest masses are visible
   Phantom image quality scores: Fibers
                                         Specks
                                         Masses

8. kVp Accuracy and Reproducibility
   Measured average kVp within ± 5% of indicated kVp
   kVp coefficient of variation ≤0.02

9. Beam Quality (Half-Value Layer) Assessment
   Half-value layer is within acceptable lower and upper limits at all kVp values tested

10. Breast Entrance Exposure, Average Glandular Dose and Radiation Output Rate
   Average glandular dose for average breast is below 3 mGy (300 mrad)
   Average glandular dose to a 4.2-cm-thick breast on your unit is ____ mrad
   Radiation output rate is ≥800 mR/sec (7.0 mGy/sec) at 28 kVp with Mo/Mo ____ mR/sec

11. Viewbox Luminance and Room Illuminance
   Mammographic viewbox is capable of a luminance of at least 3000 nit
   Room illuminance (viewbox surface & seen by observer) is 50 lux or less

> **Important: If either test #7 (Phantom Image Quality Evaluation) or the Average Glandular Dose component of test #10 fail FDA's MQSA regulations, corrective action must be taken before any further examinations are performed. Corrective action must be taken within 30 days of the test date for all other MQSA failures.**

*****PLEASE HAVE YOUR MEDICAL PHYSICIST COMPLETE THIS SUMMARY FORM*****

FIGURE 11-11 American College of Radiology (ACR) Physicist's Mammography QC Test Summary for Film/Screen Systems.
(Continued)

MEDICAL PHYSICIST'S MAMMOGRAPHY QC TEST SUMMARY
(screen-film systems, continued)

Evaluation of Site's Technologist QC Program

New units: Medical physicists **must** review the site's technologist QC program within 45 days of installation and complete this section so that the facility may submit this form along with the entire Mammography Equipment Evaluation report to the ACR with their phantom and clinical images.

Renewing units: Medical physicists **must** complete this section as part of the unit's annual survey.

	FREQUENCY	PASS/FAIL ACR Guides	MQSA Regs
1. Darkroom cleanliness (daily)	Daily		
2. Processor QC *(performed, records maintained, action taken when needed)*	Daily		
3. Screen cleaning	Weekly		
4. Mammo phantom imaging *(performed, records maintained, action taken as need)*	Weekly		
5. Darkroom fog	Semi-annually		
6. Film-screen contact test	Semi-annually		
7. Compression pressure monitored	Semi-annually		
8. Repeat analysis *(performed, records maintained, reviewed by radiologist)*	Quarterly		
9. Viewboxes and viewing conditions	Weekly		
10. Analysis of fixer retention	Quarterly		
11. Visual checklist	Monthly		

Medical Physicist's Recommendations for Quality Improvement

FIGURE 11-11—cont'd.

transfer function (MTF) tests. Procedures for performing these tests vary by manufacturer and are located in the manufacturers' QC manuals. The name of each quality control test can vary from vendor to vendor. For example, for the flat field test, GE Healthcare and Fischer Medical Technologies refer to it as "flat field," while Lorad calls it "artifact evaluation" and Siemens Medical Solutions calls it "detector calibration." The medical physicists QC test summary forms for various FFDM and CR systems are found in Figures 11-12 through 11-16.

Radiologic Technologist (Mammographer). Technologists who perform mammograms must have at least 40 hours of training in mammography while they are under the supervision of a qualified instructor and must be licensed by the individual state or certified by an approved agency (e.g., the American Registry of Radiologic Technologists) to verify competency in radiography. The hours of documented training should include, but not necessarily be limited to, the following:

MEDICAL PHYSICIST'S MAMMOGRAPHY QC TEST SUMMARY
Full-Field Digital – General Electric

Site Name		Report Date	
Address		Survey Date	
Medical Physicist's Name		Signature	
X-Ray Unit Manufacturer	*General Electric*	Model	
Date of Installation		Room ID	

QC Manual Version: *(check one;* **must** *use version applicable to unit tested; contact mfr if questions)* ☐ 2000D 2371472-100 Rev 0, 2003

☐ DS 5133453-4-1EN, Rev 1, 2007   ☐ ESSENTIAL 5141465-5-1EN Rev 1, 2007   ☐ OTHER (write in):

Accessory Equipment:	Manufacturer	Model	Location	QC Manual Version
Review Workstation*			☐ On-site ☐ Off-site	
Laser Film Printer*			☐ On-site ☐ Off-site	

FDA recommends that only monitors and printers specifically cleared for FFDM use by FDA's Office of Device Evaluation (ODE) be used. See FDA's Policy Guidance Help System www.fda.gov/CDRH/MAMMOGRAPHY/robohelp/START.HTM

Survey Type: ☐ Mammo Eqpt Evaluation of new unit (include MQSA Rqmts for Mammo Eqpt checklist)   ☐ Annual Survey

Medical Physicist's QC Tests
("Pass" means all components of the test passes; indicate "Fail" if any component fails)

PASS/FAIL

1. **Flat Field**
2. **Phantom Image Quality**

	Fibers	Specks	Masses
Phantom IQ Test on AWS			
Phantom IQ Test on Printer			

3. **CNR Measurement** *(NA for **DS or Essential** if Sub-System MTF test done)*

   CNR [ ] *(Required for both new unit Mammography Equipment Evaluations and Annual Surveys)*

   Change in CNR ≤0.2 *(NA for Mammography Equipment Evaluations)*

4. **MTF Measurement** *(NA for **2000D, DS or Essential** if Sub-System MTF test done)*
5. **AOP Mode and SNR**
6. **Collimation Assessment**

	Mammo Equipment Evaluation			Annual Survey		
	Essential	DS	2000D	Essential	DS	2000D
24 cm x 30.7 cm	x	NA	NA	x	NA	NA
19 cm x 23 cm tests	x	x	x	NA	x	x

7. **Evaluation of Focal Spot Performance** *(NA for **2000D, DS or Essential** if Sub-System MTF test done)*
8. **Sub-System MTF** *(NA for **2000D** if MTF and Focal Spot Performance tests done; NA for **DS or Essential** if CNR, MTF and Focal Spot Performance tests done)*
9. **Breast Entrance Exposure, Average Glandular Dose and Reproducibility**

   Average glandular dose for average breast is ≤3 mGy (300 mrad)   [ ] mrad

   Exposure reproducibility (CV) for air kerma (R) and mAs is ≤0.05
10. **Artifact Evaluation and Flat Field Uniformity**
11. **kVp Accuracy and Reproducibility**
12. **Beam Quality Assessment (Half-Value Layer Measurement)**
13. **Radiation Output**

    Radiation output is ≥800 mR/s   [ ] mR/s
14. **Mammographic Unit Assembly Evaluation**

    Meets requirements for motion of tube-image receptor assembly

    Meets requirements for compression paddle decompression
15. **Review Workstation (RWS) Tests** *(for all RWS, even if located offsite)*

    Overall Results *("Pass" means all tests pass; indicate "Fail" if any test fails)*

*** *YOUR MEDICAL PHYSICIST MUST SUMMARIZE HIS/HER RESULTS ON* __THIS__ *FORM* ***

FIGURE 11-12 American College of Radiology (ACR) Physicist's Mammography QC Test Summary for GE FFDM Systems.

(Continued)

- Training in breast anatomy, physiology, positioning, compression, quality assurance/quality control techniques, and imaging of patients with breast implants
- The performance of a minimum of 25 examinations while under the direct supervision of a qualified individual
- At least 8 hours of training in each mammography modality to be used by the technologist in performing mammography examinations

A continuing experience requirement for technologists dictates that they must perform a minimum of 200 mammography examinations during a 24-month period. Technologists also should obtain 15 CEUs in mammography every 36 months or as individual state guidelines dictate. Quality control duties are specified for technologists for film/screen, CR, and FFDM systems at daily, weekly, monthly, quarterly, and semiannual intervals.

MEDICAL PHYSICIST'S MAMMOGRAPHY QC TEST SUMMARY
(General Electric, continued)

Evaluation of Site's Technologist QC Program

New units: Medical physicists must review the site's technologist QC program within 45 days of installation and complete this section so that the facility may submit this form along with the entire Mammography Equipment Evaluation report to the ACR with their phantom and clinical images

Renewing units: Medical physicists must complete this section as part of the unit's annual survey.

		FREQUENCY	PASS/FAIL
1.	Monitor Cleaning	Daily	
2.	Darkroom Cleanliness *(if applicable)*	Daily	
3.	Processor QC *(if applicable)*	Daily	
4.	Flat Field	Weekly	
5.	Phantom Image Quality	Weekly	
6.	CNR	Weekly	
7.	Viewbox and Viewing Conditions *(NA if no hardcopy interpreted or compared)*	Weekly	
8.	MTF Measurement	DS/Essential-Weekly; 2000D-Monthly	
9.	AOP Mode and SNR	Monthly	
10.	Visual Checklist	Monthly	
11.	Repeat Analysis	Quarterly	
12.	Analysis of Fixer Retention *(if applicable)*	Quarterly	
13.	Compression Force	Semi-annually	
14.	Darkroom Fog *(if applicable)*	Semi-annually	
15.	Review Workstation QC-Overall	See FDA guidance	
16.	Laser Film Printer QC *(GE requires laser printer mfr's manual)*	Printer mfr recommendations	
17.	Mobile Unit Quality Control *(if applicable)*	After every move	

Medical Physicist's Recommendations for Quality Improvement

Important:
1. The facility's "quality assurance program shall be **substantially the same** as the quality assurance program recommended by the ***image receptor [digital detector] manufacturer***." This is required by the FDA.
2. Use the QC manual version provided by the manufacturer ***for the digital system surveyed***.
3. If the RWS or printer is FDA-cleared for FFDM, their ***QC manual*** is considered to be ***"substantially the same"*** and may be followed. (Check with the RWS or printer manufacturers for their clearance status and QC manual.)
4. If the RWS or printer is not cleared by the FDA for FFDM, ***follow the QC manual provided by the image receptor manufacturer***. (Check with the image receptor manufacturer for their required tests.)
5. See the attached FDA-approved alternative standard for GE FFDM regarding corrective action periods when components fail QC. However, if these tests are performed as part of a Mammography Equipment Evaluation (e.g., for a new system), corrective action must be taken before mammographic images are acquired.

FIGURE 11-12—cont'd.

MEDICAL PHYSICIST'S MAMMOGRAPHY QC TEST SUMMARY
Full-Field Digital – Fischer

Site Name		**Report Date**	
Address		**Survey Date**	
Medical Physicist's Name		**Signature**	
X-Ray Unit Manufacturer	*Fischer*	**Model**	*Senoscan*
Date of Installation		**Room ID**	

QC Manual Version: *(check one;* **must** *use version applicable to unit tested; contact mfr if questions)*

☐ P-55943-OM Issue 1 Rev. 9 (July 2004)   ☐ OTHER (write in):

Accessory Equipment:

	Manufacturer	Model	Location	QC Manual Version
Review Workstation*			☐ On-site ☐ Off-site	
Laser Film Printer*			☐ On-site ☐ Off-site	

*FDA **recommends** *that only monitors and printers specifically cleared for FFDM use by FDA's Office of Device Evaluation (ODE) be used. See FDA's Policy Guidance Help System www.fda.gov/CDRH/MAMMOGRAPHY/robohelp/START.HTM*

Survey Type: ☐ Mammo Eqpt Evaluation of new unit (include MQSA Rqmts for Mammo Eqpt checklist)   ☐ Annual Survey

Medical Physicist's QC Tests
("Pass" means all components of the test passes; indicate "Fail" if any component fails)

PASS/FAIL

1. **X-Ray Field Size Alignment and Chest Wall Missed Tissue Checks**
   X-ray field size aligns with field area indicated on breast support within ≤2% SID
   Chest wall edge of the digital image to the ruler reference mark of breast support is ≤8.5 mm

2. **Compression Paddle Alignment**
   Compression paddle edges not visible within field of view
   Chest wall edge of compression paddle extends beyond image by ≤1% SID

3. **kVp Accuracy Test**
   Measured average kVp within ±5% of indicated kVp
   kVp coefficient of variation ≤0.02

4. **Linearity, Reproducibility and Accuracy**
   Linearity <0.08
   Reproducibility <0.035 for each technique

5. **Half-Value Layer and Output** *(HVL ≤0.33 mm Al at 30 kVp, 100 mA)*

6. **Dosimetry – Average Glandular Dose and Output**
   Average glandular dose for average breast is ≤3 mGy (300 mrad)   mrad

7. **Phantom Image Acquisition Test** *(values required for all tests)*
   No obvious artifacts
   Background StDev   within +50/-0 ADU counts of baseline *(NA for Equipment Evaluations)*
   Background mean   within ±100 ADU counts of baseline *(NA for Equipment Evaluations)*
   ADU level difference   within ±300 ADU counts of baseline *(NA for Equipment Evaluations)*

8. **Image Quality**
   Largest 4 fibers, 3 speck groups and 3 masses

Fibers	Specks	Masses

   Phantom IQ Test on Review Work Station

9. **System Resolution/Scan Speed Uniformity**
   Standard imaging mode @ 7 lp/mm: ≥5 transitions, ≥10% modulation
   High resolution imaging mode @ 11.1 lp/mm: ≥5 transitions, ≥5% modulation

10. **Flat Field Test**
    Flat field test
    Deviations between corner ROIs and center within ±20%

11. **Geometric Distortion and Resolution Uniformity**

12. **Automatic Decompression Control**

13. **System Artifacts**

14. **Image Viewing Room Illuminance Test** *(≤50 lux)*

15. **Review Workstation (RWS) Tests** *(for all RWS, even if located offsite)*
    Overall Results *("Pass" means all tests pass; indicate "Fail" if any test fails)*

**** **YOUR MEDICAL PHYSICIST MUST SUMMARIZE HIS/HER RESULTS ON** THIS **FORM** ****

FIGURE 11-13 American College of Radiology (ACR) Physicist's Mammography QC Test Summary for Fischer FFDM System.

(Continued)

MEDICAL PHYSICIST'S MAMMOGRAPHY QC TEST SUMMARY
(Fischer, continued)

Evaluation of Site's Technologist QC Program

New units: Medical physicists *must* review the site's technologist QC program within 45 days of installation and complete this section so that the facility may submit this form along with the entire Mammography Equipment Evaluation report to the ACR with their phantom and clinical images.

Renewing units: Medical physicists *must* complete this section as part of the unit's annual survey.

	FREQUENCY	PASS/FAIL
1. Laser Image Quality Test	Daily	
2. Phantom Image Acquisition Test	Weekly	
3. Phantom Image Quality Test	Weekly	
4. Detector Calibration and Flat-Field Test	Weekly	
5. System Resolution (Detector Alignment/Scan Speed Uniformity)	Monthly	
6. System Operation	Monthly	
7. Reject/Repeat Analysis	Quarterly	
8. Compression Force Test	Semi-annually	
9. Review Workstation QC-Overall	See FDA guidance	

Medical Physicist's Recommendations for Quality Improvement

Important:

1. The facility's "quality assurance program shall be *substantially the same* as the quality assurance program recommended by the *image receptor [digital detector] manufacturer*." This is required by the FDA.

2. Use the QC manual version provided by the manufacturer *for the digital system surveyed*.

3. If the RWS or printer is FDA-cleared for FFDM, their *QC manual* is considered to be *"substantially the same"* and may be followed. (Check with the RWS or printer manufacturers for their clearance status and QC manual.)

4. If the RWS or printer is not cleared by the FDA for FFDM, *follow the QC manual provided by the image receptor manufacturer*. (Check with the image receptor manufacturer for their required tests.)

FIGURE 11-13—cont'd.

Film/Screen Systems

Daily Duties

Darkroom Cleanliness. The floor, countertops, processor feed tray, and passboxes should be cleaned with a damp cloth to remove any loose dirt that could get into the cassette and cause artifacts. Safelights and overhead air vents should be cleaned weekly.

Processor Quality Control. The processor must be cleaned daily and must operate according to the manufacturer's specifications. Variations in developer temperature cannot exceed ± 0.5° F (0.3° C) and must be checked with a digital thermometer only. Film immersion time should not vary by more than ± 2% from the manufacturer's specifications. After it has been determined that the processor is operating within accepted parameters, a sensitometric

MEDICAL PHYSICIST'S MAMMOGRAPHY QC TEST SUMMARY
Full-Field Digital – Lorad

Site Name		**Report Date**	
Address		**Survey Date**	
Medical Physicist's Name		**Signature**	
X-Ray Unit Manufacturer	*Lorad*	**Model**	*Selenia*
Date of Installation		**Room ID**	

QC Manual Version: *(check one;* **must** *use version applicable to unit tested; contact mfr if questions)*

☐ MAN-00093, Rev. 008 (2007)   ☐ MAN-00523, Rev. 003 (2007)   ☐ OTHER (write in):

Accessory Equipment:	Manufacturer	Model	Location	QC Manual Version
Review Workstation*			☐ On-site ☐ Off-site	
Laser Film Printer*			☐ On-site ☐ Off-site	

FDA recommends that only monitors and printers specifically cleared for FFDM use by FDA's Office of Device Evaluation (ODE) be used. See FDA's Policy Guidance Help System www.fda.gov/CDRH/MAMMOGRAPHY/robohelp/START.HTM.

Survey Type: ☐ Mammo Eqpt Evaluation of new unit (include MQSA Rqmts for Mammo Eqpt checklist)   ☐ Annual Survey

Medical Physicist's QC Tests
("Pass" means all components of the test passes; indicate "Fail" if any component fails)

PASS/FAIL

1. **Mammographic Unit Assembly Evaluation**
2. **Collimation Assessment**
3. **Artifact Evaluation**
4. **kVp Accuracy and Reproducibility**
5. **Beam Quality Assessment - HVL Measurement**
6. **Evaluation of System Resolution**
7. **Automatic Exposure Control (AEC) Function Performance** *(NA for systems without AEC)*
8. **Breast Entrance Exposure, AEC Reproducibility and Average Glandular Dose**

    Average glandular dose for average breast is ≤3 mGy (300 mrad) ⬜ mrad
9. **Radiation Output Rate**
10. **Phantom Image Quality Evaluation**

    Phantom image scores: Fibers ⬜   Specks ⬜   Masses ⬜
11. **Signal-To-Noise Ratio and Contrast-To-Noise Ratio Measurements** *(values required for all tests)*

    SNR *(value)* ⬜

    CNR *(value)* ⬜ *(Required for both new unit Mammography Equipment Evaluations and Annual Surveys)*

    CNR should not vary by more than ±15% *(NA for Equipment Evaluation)*
12. **Viewbox Luminance and Room Illuminance**
13. **Review Workstation (RWS) Tests** *(for all RWS, even if located offsite)*

    Overall Results *("Pass" means all tests pass; indicate "Fail" if any test fails)*

*** YOUR MEDICAL PHYSICIST MUST SUMMARIZE HIS/HER RESULTS ON __THIS__ FORM ***

FIGURE 11-14 American College of Radiology (ACR) Physicist's Mammography QC Test Summary for Lorad FFDM Systems.
(Continued)

strip should be created and analyzed. The sensitometer should be spectrally matched with the type of film used (usually orthochromatic). If a single-sided film is used, then the sensitometer should be a single-sided device. For dual-emulsion film, a dual-sided device should be used. The exposed sensitometric film always should be processed in the same manner each day, usually first thing in the morning before any mammograms. The least exposed end should be fed into the processor first, and the same side of the feed tray should be used, with the emulsion side down to avoid bromide drag and location effect

(see Chapter 5). The ODs of the processed strip should be measured immediately, and the following indicators of processor performance determined:

- Base + fog (B + F). This refers to the OD of the clear portion of the film and must not vary by more than ± 0.03 from the initial control value.
- Minimum density (D_{min}), or low density (LD). This is the OD of the step closest to 0.25 above the B + F and should not vary by more than ± 0.05 from the accepted value.

MEDICAL PHYSICIST'S MAMMOGRAPHY QC TEST SUMMARY
(Lorad, continued)

Evaluation of Site's Technologist QC Program

New units: Medical physicists **must** review the site's technologist QC program within 45 days of installation and complete this section so that the facility may submit this form along with the entire Mammography Equipment Evaluation report to the ACR with their phantom and clinical images.

Renewing units: Medical physicists **must** complete this section as part of the unit's annual survey.

	FREQUENCY	PASS/FAIL
1. DICOM Printer Quality Control	Weekly	
2. Viewboxes and Viewing Conditions	Weekly	
3. Artifact Evaluation	Weekly	
4. Signal-To-Noise and Contrast-To-Noise Measurements	Weekly	
5. Phantom Image	Weekly	
6. Detector Flat-Field Calibration	Weekly	
7. Compression Thickness Indicator	Bi-weekly	
8. Visual Checklist	Monthly	
9. Reject Analysis	Quarterly	
10. Compression	Semi-annually	
11. Review Workstation QC-Overall	See FDA guidance	

Medical Physicist's Recommendations for Quality Improvement

Important:

1. The facility's "quality assurance program shall be **substantially the same** as the quality assurance program recommended by the **image receptor [digital detector] manufacturer**." This is required by the FDA.

2. Use the QC manual version provided by the manufacturer **for the digital system surveyed**.

3. If the RWS or printer is FDA-cleared for FFDM, their **QC manual** is considered to be **"substantially the same"** and may be followed. (Check with the RWS or printer manufacturers for their clearance status and QC manual.)

4. If the RWS or printer is not cleared by the FDA for FFDM, **follow the QC manual provided by the image receptor manufacturer**. (Check with the image receptor manufacturer for their required tests.)

5. See the attached FDA-approved alternative standard for Lorad FFDM regarding corrective action periods when components fail QC. However, if these tests are performed as part of a Mammography Equipment Evaluation (e.g., for a new system), corrective action must be taken before mammographic images are acquired.

Phantom image scores: Fibers [   ]   Specks [   ]   Masses [   ]

FIGURE 11-14—cont'd.

MEDICAL PHYSICIST'S MAMMOGRAPHY QC TEST SUMMARY
Full-Field Digital – Siemens

Site Name		Report Date	
Address		Survey Date	
Medical Physicist's Name		Signature	
X-Ray Unit Manufacturer	*Siemens*	Model	
Date of Installation		Room ID	

QC Manual Version: *(check one; **must** use version applicable to unit tested; contact mfr if questions)*

☐ Novation DR Order No: SPB7-250.623.50.05.24. Ver05/AG 04/07   ☐ OTHER (write in): _____

☐ Novation S Order No: SPB7-250.621.60.01.24. Ver01/AG 12/07

Accessory Equipment:	Manufacturer	Model	Location	QC Manual Version
Review Workstation*			☐ On-site ☐ Off-site	
Laser Film Printer*			☐ On-site ☐ Off-site	

FDA recommends that only monitors and printers specifically cleared for FFDM use by FDA's Office of Device Evaluation (ODE) be used. See FDA's Policy Guidance Help System www.fda.gov/CDRH/MAMMOGRAPHY/robohelp/START.HTM.

Survey Type: ☐ Mammo Eqpt Evaluation of new unit (include MQSA Rqmts for Mammo Eqpt checklist)   ☐ Annual Survey

Medical Physicist's QC Tests
("Pass" means all components of the test passes; indicate "Fail" if any component fails)

PASS/FAIL

1. **Site Audit/Evaluation of Technologist QC Program**
2. **Mechanical Inspection**
3. **Acquisition Workstation Monitor Check**
4. **Detector Uniformity and Artifact Detection**
5. **Collimation, Dead Space and Compression Paddle Position**
6. **AEC Thickness Tracking Test**
7. **Spatial Resolution**
8. **SNR, CNR and AEC Repeatability**

   Measured values: SNR ☐   CNR ☐   *(values required for all tests)*

   SNR and CNR within ± 15% baseline values *(NA for Equipment Evaluations)*

9. **Image Quality** *(5 largest fibers, 4 largest speck groups and 4 largest masses are visible)*

   Phantom image scores: Fibers ☐   Specks ☐   Masses ☐

10. **Radiation Dose**

    Average glandular dose for average breast is ≤3 mGy (300 mrad) ☐ mrad

11. **HVL and Radiation Output**
12. **Tube Voltage Measurement & Reproducibility**
13. **Printer Check**
14. **Review Workstation (RWS) Tests** *(for all RWS, even if located offsite)*

    Overall Results *("Pass" means all tests pass; indicate "Fail" if any test fails)*

*** *YOUR MEDICAL PHYSICIST MUST SUMMARIZE HIS/HER RESULTS ON* <u>THIS</u> *FORM* ***

FIGURE 11-15 American College of Radiology (ACR) Physicist's Mammography QC Test Summary for Siemens FFDM.

(Continued)

- Speed indicator, or medium density. This is the OD of the step closest to 1.0 above the B + F and cannot vary by more than ± 0.15 from the accepted value. If this variance occurs, all mammogram procedures must be halted and the cause of the variation must be found and corrected.
- Maximum density (D_{max}), or high density (HD). This is the OD of the step closest to 2 above the B + F, and it cannot vary by more than ± 0.15 from the accepted value.
- Contrast indicator, or density difference (DD). This value is obtained by subtracting the D_{min} from the

D_{max}. The result should not vary by more than ± 0.15 from the accepted value.

The B + F, speed indicator, and contrast indicator are plotted daily on a control chart (Fig. 11-17) for documentation purposes.

During the MQSA inspections, the inspector performs the Sensitometric Technique for the Evaluation of Processing (STEP) test on the processor. This involves comparing the ODs of FDA control film processed in the facility processor with the same film developed in an FDA processor. If the ODs of the two films are the

MEDICAL PHYSICIST'S MAMMOGRAPHY QC TEST SUMMARY
(Siemens, continued)

Evaluation of Site's Technologist QC Program

New units: Medical physicists must review the site's technologist QC program within 45 days of installation and complete this section so that the facility may submit this form along with the entire Mammography Equipment Evaluation report to the ACR with their phantom and clinical images

Renewing units: Medical physicists must complete this section as part of the unit's annual survey.

		FREQUENCY	PASS/FAIL
1.	Phantom image quality	Daily	
2.	Detector calibration	Weekly	
3.	Artifact detection	Weekly	
4.	SNR and CNR measurements	Weekly	
5.	Repeat analysis	Quarterly	
6.	Compression force	Semi-annually	
7.	Printer check	Daily, when images printed	
8.	Review workstation QC-overall	See FDA guidance	

Medical Physicist's Recommendations for Quality Improvement

Important:
1. The facility's "quality assurance program shall be ***substantially the same*** as the quality assurance program recommended by the ***image receptor [digital detector] manufacturer***." This is required by the FDA.
2. Use the QC manual version provided by the manufacturer ***for the digital system surveyed***.
3. If the RWS or printer is FDA-cleared for FFDM, their ***QC manual*** is considered to be ***"substantially the same"*** and may be followed. (Check with the RWS or printer manufacturers for their clearance status and QC manual.)
4. If the RWS or printer is not cleared by the FDA for FFDM, ***follow the QC manual provided by the image receptor manufacturer***. (Check with the image receptor manufacturer for their required tests.)

FIGURE 11-15—cont'd.

same, a relative processing speed of 100 is given for standard cycle and between 130 and 140 for extended cycles. Standard cycles with a speed of less than 80 or an extended cycle with a speed of less than 100 are cited as a Level 2 noncompliance.

Weekly Duties

Screen Cleanliness. Intensifying screens should be cleaned at least weekly or as needed. This can be accomplished with a screen cleaner recommended by the screen manufacturer and a lint-free gauze pad. Screens should be allowed to air dry while standing vertically before use. Alternative cleaning methods include the use of compressed air (available in cans from a photographic supply store) or dusting with a camel's hair brush. The detailed procedure for cleaning intensifying screens is presented in Chapter 3.

MEDICAL PHYSICIST'S MAMMOGRAPHY QC TEST SUMMARY
Full-Field Digital – Fuji

Site Name		Report Date	
Address		Survey Date	
Medical Physicist's Name		Signature	
X-Ray Unit Manufacturer		Model	
Date of Unit Installation		Room ID	
FFDM Image Receptor Mfr	*Fuji*	FFDM Model	*FCRm*

FFDM QC Manual Version: *(check one; **must** use version applicable to system tested; contact mfr if questions)*

☐ 3rd edition, 02.2007 897N0602B, 2007   ☐ OTHER (write in):

Accessory Equipment:

	Manufacturer	Model	Location	QC Manual Version
Review Workstation*			☐ On-site ☐ Off-site	
Laser Film Printer*			☐ On-site ☐ Off-site	

*FDA **recommends** that only monitors and printers specifically cleared for FFDM use by FDA's Office of Device Evaluation (ODE) be used. See FDA's Policy Guidance Help System www.fda.gov/CDRH/MAMMOGRAPHY/robohelp/START.HTM

Survey Type: ☐ Mammo Eqpt Evaluation of new unit (include MQSA Rqmts for Mammo Eqpt checklist)   ☐ Annual Survey

Medical Physicist's QC Tests
("Pass" means all components of the test passes; indicate "Fail" if any component fails)

PASS/FAIL

1. **S Value Confirmation** *(≤120 ± 20% [96 ≤ corrected S value <144])*
2. **System Resolution** *(8 lp/mm ± 2 lp/mm in both directions)*
3. **CR Reader Scanner Performance**
4. **Mammography Unit Assembly Evaluation**
5. **Collimation Assessment**   *Test date if different from above:*
   - Chest wall edge of X-ray field extends to edge of IR
   - Deviation between X-ray field and light field ≤2% of SID
   - X-ray field does not extend beyond any side of the IR by more than 2% of SID
   - Paddle chest wall edge not beyond IR by more than 1% of SID or appear on the image
6. **Automatic Exposure Control (AEC) System Performance Assessment**
   - AEC density control function meets Fuji performance criteria
   - Reproducibility (CV) for either exposure or mAs is ≤0.05
   - Image mode tracking meets Fuji performance criteria
   - CNR per object thickness meets Fuji performance criteria
7. **System Artifact Evaluation**
8. **Phantom Image Quality Evaluation**

	Fibers	Specks	Masses	*(at least 4 fibers, 3 speck groups & 3 masses)*
Phantom IQ (printed images)				
Phantom IQ (softcopy)				

   - Other tests meet Fuji performance criteria *(mAs, OD & DD for hardcopy, S value for soft copy)*
9. **Dynamic Range**
10. **Primary Erasure (Additive and Multiplicative Lag Effects)**
11. **Inter-Plate Consistency** *(variation of mAs within ± 10%; SNR within ± 15%)*
12. **kVp Accuracy and Reproducibility**   *Test date if different from above:*
    - Measured average kVp within ±5% of indicated kVp
    - kVp coefficient of variation ≤0.02
13. **Dose** *(average glandular dose for average breast is ≤ 3 mGy [300 mrad])*   mrad
14. **Beam Quality Assessment & HVL Measurement**   *Test date if different from above:*
    - HVL ≥kVp/100 mm Al
15. **Radiation Output**   *Test date if different from above:*
    - Radiation output rate is ≥800 mR/sec (7.0 mGy/sec) at 28 kVp with Mo/Mo
16. **Viewing and Viewing Conditions**   *Test date if different from above:*
    - Mammographic viewbox luminance ≥3000 cd/m² (nit)
    - Room illuminance ≤20 lux or as recommended by the monitor manufacturer
17. **Review Workstation (RWS) Tests** *(for all RWS, even if located offsite)*
    - Overall Results *("Pass" means all tests pass; indicate "Fail" if any test fails; NA if only hardcopy read)*
18. **Printer Tests** *(for all printers used for mammography, even if located offsite)*
    - Overall Results *("Pass" means all tests pass; indicate "Fail" if any test fails)*

*** YOUR MEDICAL PHYSICIST MUST SUMMARIZE HIS/HER RESULTS ON <u>THIS</u> FORM ***

FIGURE 11-16 American College of Radiology (ACR) Physicist's Mammography QC Test Summary for Fuji FCRm.

(Continued)

MEDICAL PHYSICIST'S MAMMOGRAPHY QC TEST SUMMARY
(Fuji, continued)

Evaluation of Site's Technologist QC Program

New units: Medical physicists **must** review the site's technologist QC program within 45 days of installation and complete this section so that the facility may submit this form along with the entire Mammography Equipment Evaluation report to the ACR with their phantom and clinical images.

Renewing units: Medical physicists **must** complete this section as part of the unit's annual survey.

		FREQUENCY	PASS/FAIL
1.	CNR Weekly Check	Weekly	
2.	Phantom Image	Weekly	
3.	Visual Checklist	Monthly	
4.	Repeat Analysis	Quarterly	
5.	Compression	Semi-annually	
6.	Imaging Plate (IP) Fog	Semi-annually	
7.	Printer QC	See FDA guidance	
8.	Review Workstation QC-Overall	See FDA guidance	

Medical Physicist's Recommendations for Quality Improvement

Important:
1. The facility's "quality assurance program shall be **substantially the same** as the quality assurance program recommended by the **image receptor [digital detector] manufacturer**." This is required by the FDA.
2. Use the QC manual version provided by the manufacturer **for the digital system surveyed**.
3. Fuji specifies that the **printer and monitor manufacturers' QC program must be followed**; if no manufacturer-provided QC is available, the Fuji manual includes testing information.
4. See the attached FDA-approved alternative standard for Fuji FFDM regarding corrective action periods when components fail QC. However, if these tests are performed as part of a Mammography Equipment Evaluation (e.g., for a new system), corrective action must be taken before mammographic images are acquired.

FIGURE 11-16—cont'd.

Phantom Images. Phantom images are taken to assess OD, contrast, uniformity, and image quality. An ACR accreditation or equivalent phantom is required, along with an acrylic disk that is 4-mm thick and 1 cm in diameter (Fig. 11-18). The phantom is approximately equivalent to a 4.2-cm thick compressed breast consisting of 50% glandular and 50% adipose tissue. The phantom includes appropriate details that range from visible to invisible on a standard mammographic image. The phantom has fibers with diameters of 1.56, 1.12, 0.89, 0.75, 0.54, and 0.4 mm; specks with diameters of 0.54, 0.4, 0.32, 0.24, and 0.16 mm; and masses with decreasing diameters of 2, 1, 0.75, 0.5, and 0.25 mm. A magnifying glass, densitometer, and specialized control chart (Fig. 11-19) also are required.

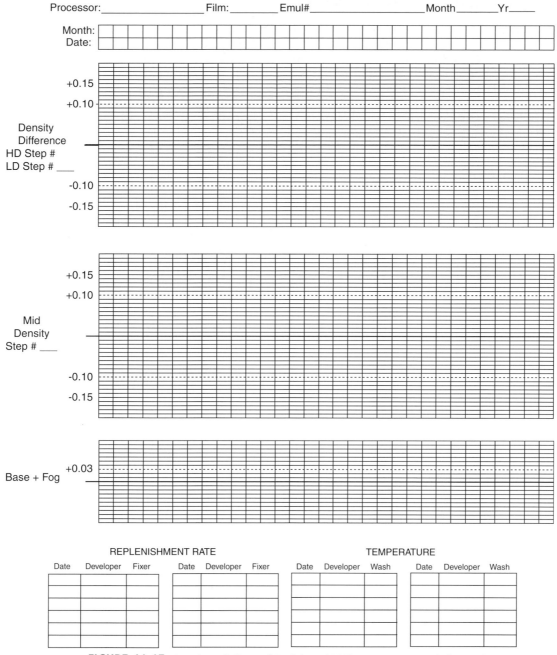

FIGURE 11-17 American College of Radiology (ACR) processor control chart.

A checklist for documentation of daily and weekly duties is found in Figure 11-20.

Monthly Duties. The FDA does not specify monthly duties for mammographers in 21 CFR Part 900. However, the ACR recommends a monthly visual checklist of mammographic equipment by mammographers to obtain their accreditation. This visual inspection evaluates certain equipment characteristics on a pass/fail basis. An example of the Mammography Quality Control Visual Checklist is found in Figure 11-21.

Quarterly Duties

Repeat Analysis. All rejected films should be collected, examined for the specific cause, and recorded on a repeat analysis form (Fig. 11-22). At least 250 patients are necessary for valid results. The total repeat rate and causal repeat rate should be calculated with the equations

PROCEDURE

1. Place the phantom on the cassette holder, and position it so that the edge of the phantom is aligned with the chest wall side of the image receptor. Place the acrylic disk on top of the phantom, but position it so that it does not obscure details of the phantom. The disk must be placed in the same location each time this test is performed. (*Note:* For GE Senographe 2000D, the contrast disk must not be used with the phantom.)
2. Next, bring the compression device into contact with the phantom. If the AEC system is used, the same sensor should be used for each phantom image and the phantom must completely cover the sensor. If manual technique is used, select the appropriate milliampere and exposure time.
3. Make the exposure at 28 kVp (or the most common clinically used kilovolt [peak]) and record the milliampere-second from the display on the control panel onto the control chart. This value should stay within a range of ± 15%.
4. After the image is processed, measure the OD at the center of the image of the phantom with a densitometer (for FFDM and CR units, print a hard copy with a dry laser printer). This OD value is referred to as the *background density*. This background density should be at least 1.2 when exposed under a typical clinical condition. For all future phantom image tests, the background density should not change by more than ± 0.2 from the established operating level. Plot this value on the control chart.
5. Using the densitometer, take the OD reading of the area of the image from under the acrylic disk. Subtract this value from the background density to determine the DD. This value should be approximately 0.4, with an allowed range of ± 0.05 on subsequent phantom images. The DD value is also plotted on the control chart.
6. Next, determine the total number of simulated masses, speck groups, and fibers visible in the image. A mass is counted as 1 point if a DD is seen at the correct location, with a circular border and a DD noted. A score of 0.5 points is awarded if it is visible but the shape is not circular. A fiber is counted as 1 if its entire length is visible at the correct location and with correct orientation. If one half or more of its length is visible, a value of 0.5 is assigned. Less than one half is assigned a value of zero. The speck groups consist of six individual specks and should be viewed with a magnifying glass. If four or more of the six groups are visible, a value of 1 is assigned. If at least two of the six groups are visible, a value of 0.5 is given. Each score should be plotted on the control chart. The minimum scores required to pass ACR accreditation are 4 fibers, 3 speck groups, and 3 masses, for a total of 10 objects. The score of phantom objects on subsequent images should not decrease by more than 0.5. (*Note:* For the Lorad Selenia FFDM system, the minimum phantom scores must be 4 for fibers, 4 for speck groups, and 3 for masses).

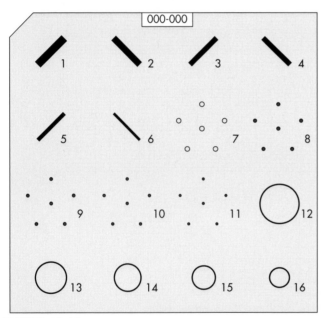

FIGURE 11-18 American College of Radiology (ACR) accreditation phantom.

listed in Chapter 10. If the total repeat rate or reject rate changes from the previously determined rate by more than 2% of the total films included in the analysis, any reasons for the change should be determined. Any corrective actions should be recorded, and the results of these corrective actions assessed.

Archival Quality. The amount of hyporetention in mammographic films should be evaluated with a test kit such as the one described in Chapter 4. The residual fixer shall be no more than 5 μg/cm² (Fig. 11-23).

PROCEDURE

1. Place a drop of solution on a sheet of unexposed but processed film, and allow it to stand for 2 minutes.
2. Remove the excess solution, and compare the stain on the film with the test strip supplied by the manufacturer (see Fig. 11-23). If the amount of hyporetention exceeds 5 μg/cm², the processor should be inspected and the reason for the discrepancy investigated.

Semiannual Duties

Darkroom Fog. Inspection should be performed semi-annually to ensure that darkroom safelights and other light sources do not fog mammographic films (because contrast is reduced). Safelight filters and bulb wattage should be inspected, and proper distance from work surfaces verified. Personnel performing the inspection should turn off all lights in the darkroom and remain in the dark for 5 minutes to allow the eyes to become adjusted to minimal light conditions. Personnel should observe and correct any obvious light leaks, especially around doors, passboxes, processors, or ceiling. They should turn on all fluorescent lights in the darkroom for 2 minutes, turn them off, and observe for any obvious afterglow (more than 1 minute). A darkroom fog test should be performed using the procedure discussed in Chapter 3 of this text, whereby a pre-exposed film is placed on the counter in the darkroom with half of it covered by a sheet of cardboard (or other opaque material) for 2 minutes. After processing, OD readings of the covered and uncovered halves are taken and compared. Any differences between the two sides should be ≤0.05.

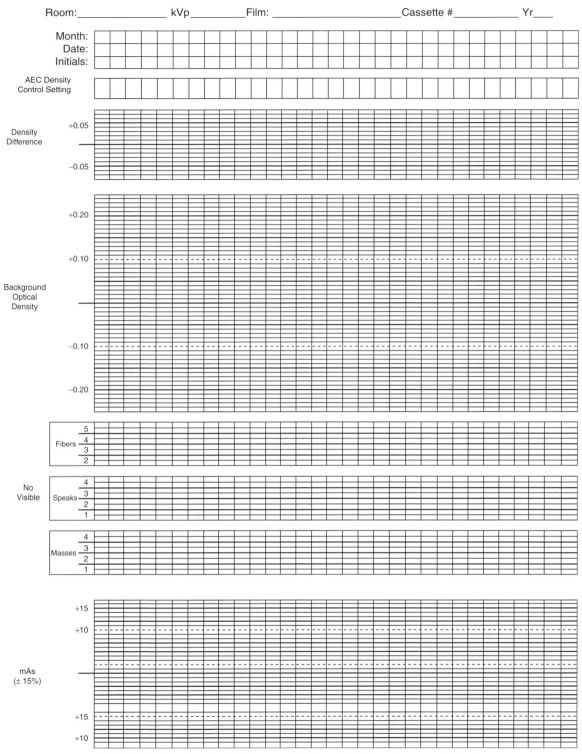

FIGURE 11-19 American College of Radiology (ACR) phantom control chart.

Mammography Quality Control Checklist

Department of Diagnostic Radiology

Daily and Weekly Tests

Year																																	
Month																																	
Date																																	
Initials																																	
Darkroom Cleanliness (daily)																																	
Processor QC (daily)																																	
Phantom Images (weekly)																																	
Screen Cleanliness (weekly)																																	
Viewing Conditions (weekly)																																	

Year																																	
Month																																	
Date																																	
Initials																																	
Darkroom Cleanliness (daily)																																	
Processor QC (daily)																																	
Phantom Images (weekly)																																	
Screen Cleanliness (weekly)																																	
Viewing Conditions (weekly)																																	

Year																																	
Month																																	
Date																																	
Initials																																	
Darkroom Cleanliness (daily)																																	
Processor QC (daily)																																	
Phantom Images (weekly)																																	
Screen Cleanliness (weekly)																																	
Viewing Conditions (weekly)																																	

FIGURE 11-20 American College of Radiology (ACR) Mammographer QC checklist for daily/weekly duties.

PROCEDURE

1. Take a mammographic phantom and film/screen image receptor into the mammographic examination room.
2. Place the image receptor into the image receptor holder of the mammographic unit.
3. Place the mammographic phantom on top of the image receptor holder, and position the edge of the phantom with the chest wall side of the image receptor. Place the compression device in contact with the phantom.
4. Make an exposure that would be appropriate for a 4- to 4.5-cm compressed breast using either manual technique or AEC device. If using AEC, be sure to use the same sensor as all previous phantom images. The exposure should produce an OD of between 1.2 and 1.5.
5. Bring the image receptor into the darkroom and place the film on the loading bench with the emulsion side up under the safelight. All lights (including the safelight) should be off at this time. Cover half the phantom image with cardboard or opaque paper. The cardboard or opaque paper should be perpendicular to the chest wall edge of the film.
6. Turn on all safelights, let the film lie on the countertop for 2 minutes, and then process the film.
7. Using a densitometer, measure the OD of both the covered and uncovered sides of the film. Do not obtain any readings where there are test objects. The difference between the two values should not exceed an OD value of 0.05. If the difference does exceed this value, corrective action must be taken.

| | Mammography Quality Control Visual Checklist | | Visual Quality Control Checks |

Building: _____ Room No. _____ Tube: _____

C-Arm	SID indicator or marks													
	Angulation indicator													
	Locks (all)													
	Field light													
	High tension cable/other cables													
	Smoothness of motion													
	_____													
Cassette holder	Cassette lock													
	Compression device													
	Compression scale													
	Amount of compression: Automatic													
	Manual													
	Grid													
	_____													
Control booth	Hand switch placement													
	Window													
	Panel switches/lights/meters													
	Technique charts													
	_____													
Other	Gonad shield/aprons/gloves													
	Cones													
	Cleaning solution													
	_____													
	_____													
	_____													
Pass = ✝	Month:													
Fail = F	Date:													
Does not apply = NA	Initials:													

Visual checklist (may be reproduced for use).

FIGURE 11-21 American College of Radiology (ACR) visual checklist.

Mammography Repeat-Reject Analysis

From _____   To _____

Reason for Reject	Projection Repeated (mark one for each repeated film)						Number of Films	% of Repeats
	Left CC	Right CC	Left MLO	Right MLO	Left Other	Right Other		
1. Positioning								
2. Patient Motion								
3. Light Films								
4. Dark Films								
5. Black Films								
6. Static, Artifacts								
7. Fog								
8. Incorrect ID or Double Exposure								
9. Mechanical								
10. Miscellaneous								
11. Good Films (No apparent reason)								
12. Clear Film								
13. Wire Localization								
14. Q.C.								

	Number	%
Repeats (1-11)		
Rejects (All; 1-14)		

Total Films Used [   ]

Remarks: _____
_____
_____

Corrective Action: _____
_____

FIGURE 11-22 American College of Radiology (ACR) Repeat-Reject Analysis Chart.

Film/Screen Contact. Mammographic image receptors must provide spatial resolution of at least 11 lp/mm, which is significantly greater than that of conventional image receptors (2 to 5 lp/mm). For this level of spatial resolution to be maintained, the contact between the film and screen must be as close as possible. A mammography film/screen contact test tool consisting of a copper screen with 40 wires per inch is required (Fig. 11-24). This is usually laminated in plastic with the equivalent density of 4 cm of acrylic.

PROCEDURE

1. Place the contact tool over the cassette, move the compression device as close as possible to the x-ray tube, and expose at 28 kVp and enough milliampere-second to produce an OD between 0.7 and 0.8 when measured over the mesh area near the chest wall side of the film.
2. After processing, place the film on a viewbox and look for clarity and nonuniformity in OD. Dark or "fuzzy" areas indicate poor film/screen contact. Areas that are larger than 1 cm or more than two areas of less than 1 cm should not be tolerated.

Hypoestimator

1   2

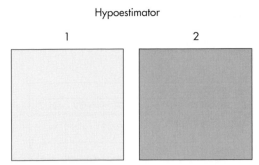

FIGURE 11-23 Hyporetention estimator test strip.

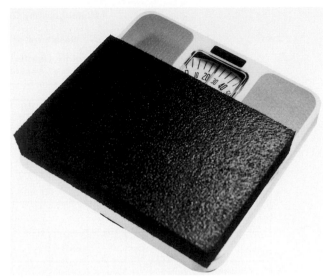

FIGURE 11-25 Mammographic compression scale. *(Courtesy Nuclear Associates, Carle Place, N.Y.)*

Compression. For adequate compression of the breast, the compression force should range from at least 111 newton (N) (25 lb) to a maximum of 200 N (45 lb) in both manual and power-drive modes. This compression should be held for at least 15 seconds. This can be evaluated with a scale placed directly under the compression device. A bathroom scale is acceptable; however, commercially available mammography compression scales are available and are more accurate (Fig. 11-25). Any compression more than 45 lb is dangerous to the patient. If the power drive fails to cease compression when more than 45 lb is measured, then a service engineer is required.

A checklist for documentation of monthly, quarterly, and semiannual testing is found in Figure 11-26.

Full-Field Digital Mammography Systems

Daily Duties. As with film/screen systems, mammographers have daily responsibilities for FFDM systems as well. However, each system manufacturer lists slightly different duties. They generally include monitor cleaning and testing, darkroom cleanliness and processor QC (if applicable), and laser imager quality test. The manufacturer's QC manual and your medical physicist should be consulted for the exact procedure to perform these duties.

Weekly Duties. The weekly duties performed by mammographers for FFDM systems again vary by manufacturer but generally include phantom image testing, detector flat-field calibration, viewbox and viewing conditions, signal-to-noise ratio (SNR) and contrast-to-noise ratio (CNR) measurements, and modulation transfer function (MTF) measurements. The

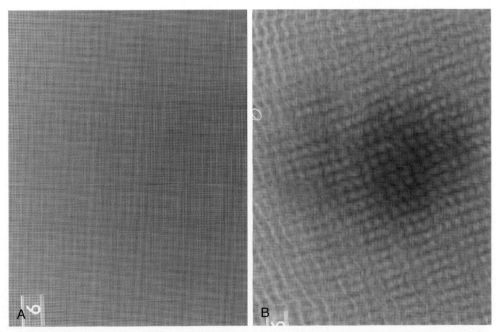

FIGURE 11-24 Wire mesh test images showing **(A)** good and **(B)** poor film screen contrast. *(Courtesy Sharon Glaze; from Bushong SC: Radiologic science for technologists, ed 6, St Louis, 1997, Mosby.)*

Mammography Quality Control Checklist

Department of Diagnostic Radiology

Monthly, Quarterly, and Semiannual Tests

(date, initial, and enter number where appropriate)

Year / Month	JAN	FEB	MAR	APR	MAY	JUN	JUL	AUG	SEP	OCT	NOV	DEC
Visual checklist (Monthly)												
Repeat Analysis (≤2% change) (quarterly)												
Fixer (≤0.05 gm/m²) (quarterly)												
Darkroom Fog (≤0.05) (semiannually)												
Screen-film contact (semiannually)												
Compression (25-45 lb) (semiannually)												

Date: **Test:**   **Comments:**

FIGURE 11-26 American College of Radiology (ACR) Mammographer QC checklist for monthly, quarterly, and semi-annual duties.

manufacturers' QC manuals and a medical physicist should be consulted for the exact procedure to perform these duties.

The quality control checklists for daily and weekly duties for GE, Lorad, Siemens, and Fischer FFDM systems, along with Fuji CR systems are found in Figures 11-27 through 11-31.

Monthly Duties. Again, these duties vary by manufacturer but generally include visual checklist, system resolution, detector alignment, scan speed uniformity, and monitor calibration check. The manufacturer's QC manual and your medical physicist should be consulted for the exact procedure to perform these duties.

Quarterly Duties. The quarterly duties are essentially the same of those for film/screen systems and include repeat analysis and hyporetention analysis (laser cameras only).

Semi-annual Duties. Semi-annual duties for FFDM systems also are essentially the same as those of film/

screen systems and include the compression force test and darkroom fog test (laser cameras only). Fuji CR systems require an imaging plate (IP) fog test be performed semi-annually.

The quality control checklists for monthly, quarterly, and semi-annual tests for GE, Lorad, Siemens, and Fischer FFDM systems, along with Fuji CR systems are found in Figures 11-32 through 11-36.

After completion of the required quality control tests, the facility should compare the test results with the corresponding specified action limits or, for nonscreen/film modalities, with the manufacturer's recommended action limits. If the test results fall outside of the action limits, the source of the problem should be identified and corrective actions should be taken:

1. Before any further examinations are performed or any films processed with a component of the mammography system that failed any tests of daily processor performance tests, phantom image tests,

FULL-FIELD DIGITAL MAMMOGRAPHY QUALITY CONTROL CHECKLIST – GENERAL ELECTRIC MODEL *(circle all that apply)* : 2000D DS Essential

Daily and Weekly Tests

Year																																
Month																																
Date																																
Initials																																
Monitor Cleaning *(daily)*																																
Darkroom Clean- liness *(daily, if app)*																																
Processor QC *(daily, if app)*																																
Flat Field *(weekly)*																																
Phantom Image Quality *(weekly)*																																
CNR *(weekly)*																																
Viewbox and Viewing Conditions *(weekly)*																																
MTF *(DS/Essential-weekly)*																																
Laser Film Printer QC *(printer mfr rec)*																																
Review Workstation QC *(See QC Manual)*																																

Year																																						
Month																																						
Date																																						
Initials																																						
Monitor Cleaning *(daily)*																																						
Darkroom Clean- liness *(daily, if app)*																																						
Processor QC *(daily, if app)*																																						
Flat Field *(weekly)*																																						
Phantom Image Quality *(weekly)*																																						
CNR *(weekly)*																																						
Viewbox and Viewing Conditions *(weekly)*																																						
MTF *(DS/Essential-weekly)*																																						
Laser Film Printer QC *(printer mfr rec)*																																						
Review Workstation QC *(See QC Manual)*																																						

FIGURE 11-27 American College of Radiology (ACR) Mammography QC checklist for daily and weekly tests for GE FFDM systems.

FULL-FIELD DIGITAL MAMMOGRAPHY QUALITY CONTROL CHECKLIST – LORAD MODEL: _____

Daily and Weekly Tests

Year																																
Month																																
Date																																
Initials																																
DICOM Printer QC (weekly)																																
Viewboxes and Viewing Conditions (weekly)																																
Artifact Evaluation (weekly)																																
SNR & CNR Measurements (weekly)																																
Phantom Image (weekly)																																
Detector Flat-Field Calibration (weekly)																																
Compression Thickness Indicator (biweekly)																																
Review Workstation QC (See QC Manual)																																

Year																																
Month																																
Date																																
Initials																																
DICOM Printer QC (weekly)																																
Viewboxes and Viewing Conditions (weekly)																																
Artifact Evaluation (weekly)																																
SNR & CNR Measurements (weekly)																																
Phantom Image (weekly)																																
Detector Flat-Field Calibration (weekly)																																
Compression Thickness Indicator (biweekly)																																
Review Workstation QC (See QC Manual)																																

FIGURE 11-28 American College of Radiology (ACR) Mammography QC checklist for daily and weekly tests for Lorad FFDM systems.

darkroom fog, film/screen contact, or compression device performance

2. Within 30 days for all other tests

Table 11-3 summarizes the responsibilities for the radiologist, radiographer, and medical physicist.

Inspection by the Food and Drug Administration. As a result of the MQSA, only FDA-certified (or those certified by the states of Illinois, Iowa, and South Carolina) facilities may lawfully conduct mammography. To maintain its certified status, each facility must do the following:

- Have an annual survey performed by a qualified medical physicist
- Undergo periodic audits or clinical image reviews by their accreditation body
- Undergo annual inspection by an FDA-certified inspector (or those certified by the states of Illinois, Iowa, and South Carolina)

FULL-FIELD DIGITAL MAMMOGRAPHY QUALITY CONTROL CHECKLIST – FISCHER MODEL: _____

Daily and Weekly Tests

Year																																			
Month																																			
Date																																			
Initials																																			
Laser Imager Quality Test (daily, if app)																																			
Phantom Image Acquisition Test (weekly)																																			
Phantom Image Quality Test (weekly)																																			
Detector Calibration and Flat Field Test (weekly)																																			
Review Workstation QC (See QC Manual)																																			

Year																																			
Month																																			
Date																																			
Initials																																			
Laser Imager Quality Test (daily, if app)																																			
Phantom Image Acquisition Test (weekly)																																			
Phantom Image Quality Test (weekly)																																			
Detector Calibration and Flat Field Test (weekly)																																			
Review Workstation QC (See QC Manual)																																			

FIGURE 11-29 American College of Radiology (ACR) Mammography QC checklist for daily and weekly tests for Fischer FFDM systems.

- Pay an inspection fee or re-inspection fee if necessary
- Correct any deficiencies found during the inspections

The FDA-MQSA inspection covers equipment performance, technologist and physicist quality control tests, medical audit and outcome analysis records, medical records (mammography reports and films), and personnel qualification records. Completing an inspection of a facility with a single mammographic unit takes approximately 6 hours.

Equipment Performance. For equipment performance, the inspector assesses the following:

- Collimation system (x-ray field/image receptor and image receptor/compression device alignments)
- Entrance skin exposure and exposure reproducibility
- Beam quality (HVL) measurement
- Phantom image quality evaluation (including phantom scoring)
- Processor evaluation and darkroom fog measurement

Records. The records that the inspector asks to review include the following:

- Records for the previous 12 months for the technologist quality control tests/tasks mentioned previously

FULL-FIELD DIGITAL MAMMOGRAPHY QUALITY CONTROL CHECKLIST – SIEMENS MODEL: _____

Daily and Weekly Tests

Year																																												
Month																																												
Date																																												
Initials																																												
Phantom Image Quality (daily)																																												
Detector Calibration (weekly)																																												
Artifact Detection (weekly)																																												
SNR and CNR Measurement (weekly)																																												
Printer Check (daily, when images printed)																																												
Review Workstation QC *(See QC Manual)*																																												

Year																																												
Month																																												
Date																																												
Initials																																												
Phantom Image Quality (daily)																																												
Detector Calibration (weekly)																																												
Artifact Detection (weekly)																																												
SNR and CNR Measurement (weekly)																																												
Printer Check (daily, when images printed)																																												
Review Workstation QC *(See QC Manual)*																																												

FIGURE 11-30 American College of Radiology (ACR) Mammography QC checklist for daily and weekly tests for Siemens FFDM systems.

- Actual sensitometric film strips for the previous 30 days of mammographic film processing and charting of the strips for the previous 12 months
- Images from film/screen contact and darkroom fog tests for the previous 12 months
- Phantom images and charting for the previous 12 months
- Annual medical physicist's report for each x-ray unit

- Quality assurance/quality control documentation forms
- The latest version of all QC manuals for digital equipment
- Whether all QC tests listed in the manuals have been conducted
- Whether all monitor and printer QC tests for digital equipment have been performed per manufacturer's manual

FULL-FIELD DIGITAL MAMMOGRAPHY QUALITY CONTROL CHECKLIST – FUJI FCRm

Daily and Weekly Tests

Year																																	
Month																																	
Date																																	
Initials																																	
CNR Weekly Check (weekly)																																	
Phantom Image (weekly)																																	
Printer QC (See FDA guidance)																																	
Review Workstation QC (See QC Manual)																																	

Year																																	
Month																																	
Date																																	
Initials																																	
CNR Weekly Check (weekly)																																	
Phantom Image (weekly)																																	
Printer QC (See FDA guidance)																																	
Review Workstation QC (See QC Manual)																																	

FIGURE 11-31 American College of Radiology (ACR) Mammography QC checklist for daily and weekly tests for Fuji FCRm systems.

- Whether timely corrective actions have been taken for any tests that have failed
- Personnel orientation program for technologists
- Procedures for equipment use and maintenance
- Mammographic technique charts including information pertinent to optimizing mammographic quality such as positioning and compression.
- Radiation safety policy and responsibilities.
- Medical audit and outcomes analysis. This is a system to track positive mammograms and a process to correlate the findings with the surgical biopsy results obtained. Analysis of these outcome data should be made individually and collectively for all interpreting physicians at the facility. In addition, any cases of breast cancer among women who underwent imaging at the facility that subsequently become known to the facility should prompt the facility to initiate follow-up on surgical or pathologic results and review of the mammograms taken before the diagnosis of a malignancy.

- Examine permanent records, which include the actual film images and the mammography report of the interpreting physician. In digital departments, facilities must keep, in retrievable form, the original raw mammographic image as well as the lossless compressed data, or hard-copy films that duplicate the soft copies interpretive quality.
- Infection control policy. Facilities that perform mammographic procedures must establish and comply with a system that specifies procedures to be followed by the facility for cleaning and disinfecting mammography equipment after contact with blood or other potentially infectious materials. This system must specify the methods for documenting facility

FULL-FIELD DIGITAL MAMMOGRAPHY QUALITY CONTROL CHECKLIST–
GENERAL ELECTRIC MODEL *(circle all that apply)* : 2000D DS Essential

Monthly, Quarterly, and Semi-Annual Tests
(date, initial and enter number where appropriate)

Year / Month	JAN	FEB	MAR	APR	MAY	JUN	JUL	AUG	SEP	OCT	NOV	DEC
MTF *(2000D-monthly)*												
AOP Mode and SNR *(monthly)*												
Visual Checklist *(monthly)*												
Repeat Analysis (≤2% change) *(quarterly)*												
Analysis of Fixer Retention (≤0.05 gm/m²) *(quarterly, if app)*												
Compression Force (25-45 lb) *(semi-annually)*												
Darkroom Fog (≤0.05) *(semi-annually, if app)*												
Review Workstation QC *(See QC Manual)*												

Date: **Test:**   **Comments:**

FIGURE 11-32 American College of Radiology (ACR) Mammography QC checklist for monthly, quarterly, and semi-annual duties for GE FFDM systems.

compliance with the infection control procedures. It should comply with all applicable federal, state, and local regulations that pertain to infection control; with the manufacturer's recommended procedures for the cleaning and disinfection of the mammography equipment used in the facility; or, if adequate manufacturer's recommendations are unavailable, with generally accepted guidance on infection control, until such recommendations become available.

- Consumer complaint mechanism. Each facility performing mammograms must establish a written and documented system for collecting and resolving consumer complaints. It also must maintain a record of each serious complaint received by the facility for at least 3 years from the date the complaint was received. The facility also must provide the consumer with adequate directions for filing serious complaints with the facility's accreditation body if the facility is unable to resolve a serious

FULL-FIELD DIGITAL MAMMOGRAPHY QUALITY CONTROL CHECKLIST–
LORAD MODEL: _____

Monthly, Quarterly, and Semi-Annual Tests
(date, initial and enter number where appropriate)

Year / Month	JAN	FEB	MAR	APR	MAY	JUN	JUL	AUG	SEP	OCT	NOV	DEC
Visual Checklist (monthly)												
Reject Analysis (≤2% change) (quarterly)												
Compression (25-45 lb) (semi-annually)												
Review Workstation QC (See QC Manual)												

Date: **Test:**   **Comments:**

FIGURE 11-33 American College of Radiology (ACR) mammography QC checklist for monthly, quarterly, and semi-annual duties for Lorad FFDM systems.

complaint to the consumer's satisfaction. Each facility also is required to report unresolved serious complaints to the accreditation body in a manner and time frame specified by the accreditation body. An example of an acceptable system for collecting and documenting the consumer complaint is described as follows:

Inspection Report. After the inspection, a report summarizing the inspection findings is sent to the institution. The findings belong to one of the following categories.

Level 1. A Level 1 finding is a deviation from the MQSA standards that may seriously compromise the quality of mammography services offered by a facility. For example, a Level 1 finding for the phantom image test exists when the score is less than 3 fibers, less than 2 speck groups, or less than 2 masses, or if the raw score is less than 6. A Level 1 finding also is issued if the interpreting physician is not certified by a board, has not had the initial (2 or 3 months) training in mammography, or has never had a valid license to practice medicine. A warning letter is sent if this type of finding exists, to allow the facility to

FULL-FIELD DIGITAL MAMMOGRAPHY QUALITY CONTROL CHECKLIST– FISCHER MODEL: _____

Monthly, Quarterly, and Semi-Annual Tests
(date, initial and enter number where appropriate)

Year / Month	JAN	FEB	MAR	APR	MAY	JUN	JUL	AUG	SEP	OCT	NOV	DEC
System Resolution (Detector Alignment/ Scan Speed Uniformity) (monthly)												
System Operation (monthly)												
Reject/Repeat Analysis ($\leq 2\%$ change) (quarterly)												
Compression Force Test (25-45 lb) (semi-annually)												
Review Workstation QC (See QC Manual)												

Date: **Test:**   **Comments:**

FIGURE 11-34 American College of Radiology (ACR) Mammography QC checklist for monthly, quarterly, and semi-annual duties for Fischer FFDM systems.

PROCEDURE

1. The facility designates a facility contact person with whom consumers, the accreditation body, and the FDA can interact regarding serious consumer complaints. The contact person and other health professionals at the facility develop a clear understanding of the definitions of "consumer," "adverse event," "serious adverse event," and "serious complaint" so that all parties are knowledgeable about the requirements of the consumer requirements of the consumer complaint mechanism (Box 11-2).

2. If the facility cannot resolve a complaint to the consumer's satisfaction, the facility provides the consumer with directions for filing serious complaints with the facility's accreditation body. These directions are to be provided in writing. The facility may want to post a sign to explain how to file complaints. In this case, the facility could use messages such as, "We care about our patients. If you have comments or concerns, please direct them to (the name of the person in the facility who is responsible for complaints)." This would be in addition to the name and address of the accreditation body, which is listed on the facility's certificate. The facility is required by law to post the certificate prominently in the facility.

PROCEDURE—CONT'D

3. The facility keeps documentation of the complaint on file for a period of 3 years from the date the complaint was received. The facility may develop a form to record, at a minimum, the following items concerning "serious complaints": the name, address, and telephone number of the person making the complaint; date of the complaint; date the serious adverse event occurred; precise description of the serious adverse event (including the name[s] of the individual[s] involved); the manner of the complaint's resolution; and the date of the complaint's resolution. This record can be either manually written or computerized, depending on the facility's preference.

4. The facility acknowledges the consumer's complaint, investigates the complaint, makes every effort to resolve the complaint, and responds to the individual filing the complaint within a reasonable time frame (these steps can usually be accomplished within 30 days).

5. The facility ensures that the complaint and any information about the complaint or its follow-up are shared only with those needed to resolve the complaint. In addition, facilities should design their complaint procedures to be responsive to the particular needs of the patients they serve. Patients or their representatives may complain in person or in writing.

6. The facility reports unresolved serious complaints to its accreditation body in a manner and time frame specified by the body. The facility may want to contact its accreditation body about this requirement. For easy reference, facilities may want to keep a separate listing of unresolved serious complaints, with the date of referral; summary; and date of response, if any, from the accreditation body. (This is in addition to the record described in number 3.)

FULL-FIELD DIGITAL MAMMOGRAPHY QUALITY CONTROL CHECKLIST–
SIEMENS MODEL : _____

Monthly, Quarterly, and Semi-Annual Tests
(date, initial and enter number where appropriate)

Year												
Month	JAN	FEB	MAR	APR	MAY	JUN	JUL	AUG	SEP	OCT	NOV	DEC
Repeat Analysis (quarterly)												
Compression Force (25-45 lb) (semi-annually)												
Review Workstation QC (See QC Manual)												

Date: _____

Test: _____

Comments: _____

FIGURE 11-35 American College of Radiology (ACR) Mammography QC checklist for monthly, quarterly, and semi-annual duties for Siemens FFDM systems.

FULL-FIELD DIGITAL MAMMOGRAPHY QUALITY CONTROL CHECKLIST–
FUJI FCRm

Monthly, Quarterly, and Semi-Annual Tests
(date, initial and enter number where appropriate)

Year / Month	JAN	FEB	MAR	APR	MAY	JUN	JUL	AUG	SEP	OCT	NOV	DEC
Visual Checklist *(monthly)*												
Repeat Analysis *(≤2% change)* *(quarterly)*												
Compression *(25-45 lb)* *(semi-annually)*												
Imaging Plate Fog *(semi-annually)*												
Review Workstation QC *(See QC Manual)*												

Date: **Test:**   **Comments:**

FIGURE 11-36 American College of Radiology (ACR) Mammography QC checklist for monthly, quarterly, and semi-annual duties for Fuji FCRm system.

TABLE 11-3	Summary of Responsibilities for Mammography	
Radiologist	**Medical Physicist**	**Radiographer**
Ensures that QC program is implemented	Ensures proper functioning of mammography equipment	Monitors darkroom and processor on a daily basis
Ensures that the technical staff has adequate mammography training and maintains continuing education	Performs yearly evaluation of mammographic systems	Maintains screen cleanliness and viewing conditions on a weekly basis
Identifies primary QC		Performs a visual inspection on a monthly basis
Technologist and medical physicist		Performs a repeat analysis and hyporetention test on a quarterly basis
Reviews technologist and medical physicist test results		Evaluates darkroom fog, film/screen contact and compression on a semiannual basis
Ensures that procedures on infection control, QC, radiation safety, and patient follow-up are maintained and updated		

QC, Quality control.

BOX 11-2	Definitions by the Food and Drug Administration

1. **Consumer**: An individual who chooses to comment or complain in reference to a mammography examination including the patient or representative of the patient (e.g., family member or referring physician).
2. **Adverse event**: An undesirable experience associated with mammography activities within the scope of the MQSRA. Adverse events include, but are not limited to, poor image quality, the failure to send mammography reports to the referring physician within 30 days or to the self-referred patient in a timely manner, or the use of unqualified personnel (i.e., they do not meet the applicable requirements of 21 CFR Part 900, Section 12[a]).
3. **Serious adverse event**: An adverse event that may significantly compromise clinical outcomes or an adverse event for which a facility fails to take appropriate corrective action in a timely manner.
4. **Serious complaint**: A report of a serious adverse event.

Courtesy Code of Federal Regulations.
CFR, Code of Federal Regulations; *MQRSA,* Mammography Quality Standards Reauthorization Act.

correct the problem before any enforcement action is implemented.

Level 2. A Level 2 finding is not as serious a deviation from the MQSA standards as a Level 1 finding, but it still may compromise the quality of a facility's mammography program and should be corrected as soon as possible. Facilities with these findings are rated "acceptable" but must submit an acceptable corrective action plan to the FDA.

Level 3. A Level 3 finding is a minor deviation from the MQSA standards. Facilities with only Level 3 findings are rated "satisfactory" but should institute policies and procedures to correct these conditions.

No Findings. A report of no findings shows that the facility has met all requirements of the MQSA.

SUMMARY

Quality control and quality assurance for mammographic equipment and procedures are mandatory for compliance with the MQSA. Proper documentation of these procedures is essential for a facility to remain accredited to perform mammographic procedures.

Refer to the Evolve website at https://evolve.elsevier. com for Student Experiment 11.1: Daily Mammographic Quality Control, and 11.2: Phantom Image and Visual Inspection.

REVIEW QUESTIONS

1. What kilovolt (peak) range should be used during film/screen mammography?
   a. 15 to 20 kVp
   b. 20 to 28 kVp
   c. 30 to 40 kVp
   d. 40 to 50 kVp
2. Which of the following value ranges is the correct focal spot size for most mammographic x-ray tubes?
   a. 0.1 to 0.6 mm
   b. 0.6 to 1 mm
   c. 1 to 1.5 mm
   d. 1.5 to 2.5 mm
3. Which type of filter material should be used with a molybdenum target x-ray tube?
   a. Aluminum
   b. Copper
   c. Rhodium
   d. Molybdenum

4. Which of the following does not change the shape of the x-ray emission spectrum?
   a. Milliampere
   b. Kilovolt (peak)
   c. Exposure time
   d. Target material
5. What is the usual range of force for mammographic system compression devices?
   a. 5 to 20 lb
   b. 15 to 30 lb
   c. 25 to 45 lb
   d. 45 to 60 lb
6. Which of the following is not an advantage of extended film processing in mammography?
   a. Greater image contrast
   b. Increased image receptor sensitivity
   c. Reduced patient dose
   d. Increased recorded detail
7. The light field/x-ray field alignment for mammographic units must be accurate to within ± _____ % of the SID.
   a. 2
   b. 3
   c. 4
   d. 5

8. The B + F value of a mammographic sensitometry film should not vary by more than ± _____ from the initial control value.
   a. 0.02
   b. 0.03
   c. 0.05
   d. 0.1
9. The contrast indicator, or DD, of mammographic sensitometry films should not vary by more than ± _____ from the initial control value.
   a. 0.03
   b. 0.05
   c. 0.1
   d. 0.15
10. At a minimum, how often should phantom images with an ACR accreditation phantom be obtained?
    a. Daily
    b. Weekly
    c. Monthly
    d. Yearly

Quality Control in Computed Tomography

Lorrie Kelley

OBJECTIVES

At the completion of this chapter the reader will be able to do the following:

- Differentiate between high- and low-contrast resolution
- Describe how basic quality control tests for computed tomography are conducted

- Describe the selection factors for quality control measurements
- Identify the parameters under the technologist's control that influence noise and spatial resolution

The goal of any quality control program is to ensure that the imaging equipment is producing the best possible image quality with a minimal radiation dose to the patient. The image quality in computed tomography (CT) can be difficult to maintain because of the complex nature of image acquisition and display. A contemporary CT system is composed of numerous electronic parts and computers that generate and process huge amounts of data. Because of the system's complexity, a quality assurance program is essential to ensure optimal system performance and image quality with the least amount of radiation dose to the patient. Quality assurance programs

in CT are designed to provide certain performance parameters that allow for comparisons between two scanners and help determine whether a newly installed unit meets the specifications set by the vendor. A CT quality assurance program is conducted by a qualified team of medical physicists and radiologic technologists.

ACCEPTANCE TESTING

Typically, the installation of most CT units is immediately followed by extensive acceptance testing by qualified medical physicists. The purpose of the acceptance tests is to ensure that the equipment is performing according to the manufacturer's specifications before it is released for clinical use. **Acceptance testing** consists of measuring radiologic and electromechanical performance, analyzing image performance, and evaluating the system components. The results of the acceptance tests are used to identify system components that may need only slight adjustments and defective parts that should be replaced. At the end of the acceptance testing, scans are taken of standard objects so that their images, CT numbers, and **standard deviations** can be recorded as a baseline for future measurements of the system's performance.

ROUTINE TESTING

In order to provide more consistency in the performance measurements of CT scanners, federal performance standards state that the vendors of CT systems manufactured after September 1985 are required to supply the following: instructions for performing quality control tests, a schedule for testing, allowable variations for the indicated parameters, a method to store and record the quality assurance data, and dose information in the form of a CT dose index. In addition, each vendor is required to supply **phantoms** capable of testing the following parameters: **contrast scale,** noise, slice thickness, spatial resolution capabilities for both high- and low-contrast objects, and the **mean CT number** for water or other reference material. Many routine quality control tests can be performed by a CT technologist. In most instances, vendors specify the test conditions for evaluating their system's performance; therefore, specific procedures for evaluating a system's performance may vary among manufacturers. Also, there is some disagreement among manufacturers about the proper monitoring frequency for high- and low-contrast resolution, alignment, contrast scale, and slice thickness. Until standards for monitoring frequency can be agreed on, it is best to follow those recommended by the manufacturer.

The performance of CT scanners is evaluated with a phantom as a test object. The phantoms that are supplied by the manufacturer can vary among vendors because of the differing requirements for performance evaluations and quality control testing. However, a typical phantom used to assess the performance of a CT system is a multisectioned phantom, which enables the separate evaluation of different parameters (Figs. 12-1 and 12-2). In general, a phantom is constructed from plastic cylinders, with each section filled with water or other test objects to measure specific parameter performance. Some phantoms are designed so that numerous parameters can be evaluated with a single scan.

CT has undergone significant technologic advancements in recent years, resulting in new clinical applications and changes in clinical protocols in numerous CT departments across the country. In 2002, in an effort to establish a reasonable standard of image quality, the

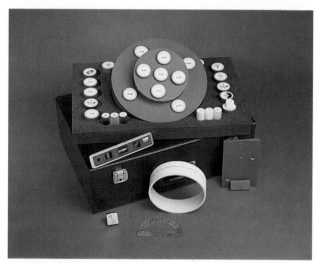

FIGURE 12-1 This computed tomography (CT) phantom is used to evaluate noise, spatial resolution, contrast resolution, slice thickness, linearity, and uniformity. *(Courtesy Gammex/RMI, Middleton, WI.)*

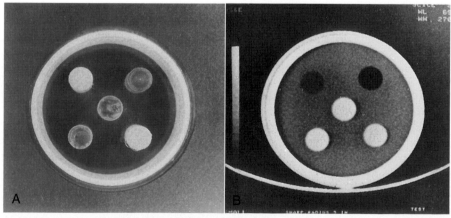

FIGURE 12-2 Photograph **(A)** and computed tomography (CT) image **(B)** of the five-pin test phantom designed by the American Association of Physicists in Medicine. The attenuation coefficient for each pin is known precisely and the CT number computed. *(From Bushong S: Radiologic science for technologists, ed 6, St Louis, 1997, Mosby.)*

American College of Radiology (ACR) approved the implementation of an Accreditation Program for CT. The CT Accreditation Program was designed to evaluate the primary determinants of clinical image quality including the qualifications of the radiologists, medical physicists and technologists; equipment performance; effectiveness of quality control tests and measures; and clinical image quality and examination protocols. The ACR CT Accreditation Committee developed a specially designed CT phantom, along with test protocols for use in the accreditation process and for establishing QA programs for clinical CT scanners. The multisectioned ACR CT accreditation phantom was designed to examine a wide variety of scanner parameters including: positioning accuracy, CT number accuracy, slice thickness, low-contrast resolution, high-contrast resolution, image uniformity and noise, distance measurement accuracy, section sensitivity profiles, and image artifacts. In the summer of 2008, Congress passed the Medicare Improvements for Patients and Providers Act of 2008 (MIPPA), which mandates that any nonhospital institution performing advanced diagnostic services (such as CT) must be accredited (by January 1, 2010) in order to receive federal funding (Medicare reimbursement). The CARE bill (discussed in Chapter 1) if passed, would make similar requirements for hospital-based facilities. Therefore, accreditation programs are becoming mandatory for CT departments to succeed.

All quality control tests described in this chapter should be performed according to the following three basic tenets of quality control:

- The quality control tests should be performed on a regular basis.
- All quality control test measurements should be documented with the data form provided by the manufacturer (Fig. 12-3).
- The quality control test should indicate whether the tested parameter is within specified guidelines.

In order to maintain ACR CT accreditation status, the ACR states that a QC program must be implemented under the direction of a qualified medical physicist. The medical physicist is responsible for the annual performance evaluations of each CT unit, as well as the establishment of a continuous quality control program for implementation by a qualified CT technologist. The medical physicist will determine the frequency that each test must be performed on the basis of the facility and CT usage. The ACR recommends that a continuous quality control program include, but not be limited to, evaluations of the following: alignment light accuracy, slice thickness, image quality, high-contrast resolution, low-contrast resolution, image uniformity, noise, artifact evaluation, CT number accuracy, and display devices.

The methodology of most of the following QC tests uses the ACR CT Accreditation Phantom and testing criteria, but the same tests can be performed with phantoms supplied by the CT system's vendor. When using a vendor-supplied phantom, test measures should be compared with the limits specified by the vendor or during acceptance testing.

The ACR CT Accreditation Phantom is a solid phantom constructed primarily from a water-equivalent material. It consists of four contiguous modules, each 4 cm in width and 20 cm in diameter. Various test objects are embedded within the phantom in order to measure the various image quality parameters of a QC program.

Before starting any QC tests, it is important to complete a tube warm-up and daily system calibrations recommended by the manufacturer in order optimize image quality.

Alignment Light Accuracy

Internal and external laser lights are used extensively for patient positioning and alignment. Accurate laser light performance is critical during stereotactic and interventional procedures.

Measurements to determine laser light accuracy can be made with the manufacturer's specific phantoms or a piece of covered, unexposed x-ray film.

After the x-ray film has been processed, the two sets of holes represent the internal and external light fields and the two dark bands from radiation exposure represent the radiation field. To measure the accuracy of the laser lights, one should check to see if the dark bands of exposure fall directly over the associated holes (Fig. 12-4). For optimal performance, the light field should coincide with the radiation field to within 2 mm.

An alternative method to measure laser light accuracy is to scan the phantom and place a grid over the resultant image. The grid should line up accurately with the lines on the phantom.

PROCEDURE

1. Tape the unexposed x-ray film securely to the CT table.
2. To measure the accuracy of the internal laser lights, turn on the internal laser lights and poke two or three small holes through the wrapper and x-ray film at the exact location of the light field. The holes should be located near the right and left edges and center of the film.
3. Perform a scan through the location specified by the internal laser lights.
4. To measure the accuracy of the external laser lights, turn on the external laser lights and poke two small holes through either edge of the film at the exact location of the external light field.
5. Advance the table so that it is in position to scan, and perform a scan at that location.

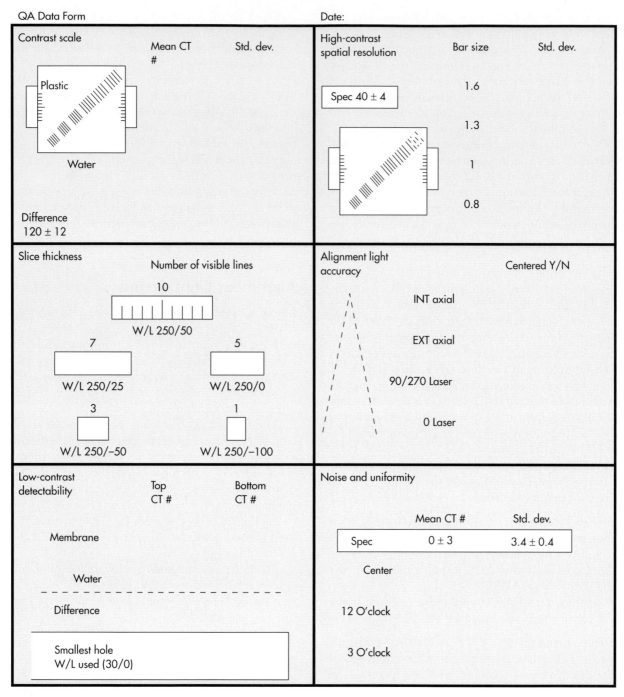

FIGURE 12-3 Sample quality assurance data form.

Image Quality

High-Contrast (Spatial) Resolution. High-contrast spatial resolution is described as the minimum distance between two objects that allows them to be seen as separate and distinct. The parameters that influence the high-contrast spatial resolution of a CT scanner include the following:

1. Scanner design (focal spot size, detector size and spacing, magnification)
2. Image reconstruction (pixel size, reconstruction algorithm, slice thickness)

3. Sampling (number of rays per projection and number of projections)
4. Image display capabilities (display matrix)

Two procedures can be used to evaluate the spatial resolution capabilities of a CT scanner. In the first method an edge is measured to determine the point spread function (PSF). The PSF is then mathematically transformed to obtain the modulation transfer function (MTF). This process takes considerable time and is

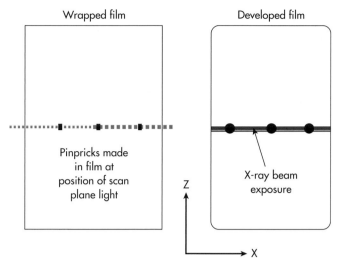

Wrapped film   Developed film

Pinpricks made
in film at
position of scan
plane light

X-ray beam
exposure

Z

X

FIGURE 12-4 Technique for assessing laser light accuracy. *(Courtesy ImPACT, a Medical Devices Agency Evaluation Group, London, UK.)*

usually completed by the medical physicist. In the second method a bar or hole pattern is used to determine the spatial resolution. This method is commonly performed by the CT technologist and is explained in the following procedure.

PROCEDURE

1. Take a single scan through the test object.
2. On the resultant image, determine which row has the smallest set of holes in which all of the holes can be clearly identified. This is known as the *limiting resolution* of the CT scanner.

The ACR CT Accreditation Phantom contains eight bar resolution patterns, which represent spatial frequencies corresponding to: 4, 5, 6, 7, 8, 9, 10, and 12 lp/cm, each fitting into a 15-mm × 15-mm square region on module 4.

Test—High-Contrast Resolution

1. Scan module 4 with adult abdomen and high-resolution chest protocols making sure to use the appropriate reconstruction algorithm.
2. Display the images with a window width of 100 and window level ≈1100.
3. Record the bar pattern for which the bars and spaces are distinctly visualized for both images.

American College of Radiology Acceptance Criteria

- The adult abdomen and high-resolution chest protocols must be used
- Window width = 100
- Window level ≈ 1100
- The 5 lp/cm bar pattern must be clearly resolved for adult abdomen protocol
- The 6 lp/cm bar pattern must be clearly resolved for adult high-resolution chest protocol

The limiting high-contrast spatial resolution of a CT scanner is measured in line pairs per centimeter (lp/cm). Even though many modern scanners have the ability to resolve holes as small as 0.3 mm, the spatial resolution of CT scanners is still lower than that of conventional radiography. The results of this test can be compared with the baseline measurement of the scanner collected during optimal system performance or compared with the manufacturer's specifications. Comparative measurements over time provide an index of the performance reproducibility of the CT system.

Low-Contrast Resolution. Low-contrast resolution refers to the capability of the CT system to demonstrate subtle differences in tissue densities from one region of anatomy to another. Compared with conventional radiography, CT provides superior low-contrast resolution. Typically, contrast resolution is expressed in one of two ways: the smallest diameter of an object with a specific contrast that can be detected or the smallest difference in x-ray attenuation that can be discriminated for an object of a specific diameter.

A phantom consisting of test objects such as holes drilled into plastic is used for this test. The rows of holes should be of varying sizes and filled with a liquid that has a CT number different from the CT number for the plastic by approximately 0.6%.

PROCEDURE

1. Scan the phantom, and determine the smallest row of holes that can be seen clearly.
2. Current CT scanners are capable of displaying 3-mm objects with density differences of 0.5% or less.

The ACR CT Accreditation Phantom uses module 2 to assess low-contrast resolution. It consists of a series of cylinders of varying diameters with a 0.6% Hounsfield unit (HU) difference from the background material, which has a CT number of approximately 90 HU. Four cylinders exist for each of the following diameters: 2 mm, 3 mm, 4 mm, 5 mm, and 6 mm. The space between each cylinder is equal to the diameter of the cylinder. An additional 25 mm cylinder is used to verify the contrast between the cylinders and the background material.

Test—Low-Contrast Resolution

1. Scan module 2 with the adult abdomen and adult head protocols.
2. Display images with window width of 100 and window level of 100.
3. Record the diameter of the smallest set of cylinders for which all four cylinders can be resolved.
4. Place a 100 mm ROI within the 25 mm diameter cylinder and outside the cylinder over the background material. Record the mean CT number of each ROI and calculate the difference. Low contrast = 6 HU ± 0.5 HU (Fig. 12-5).

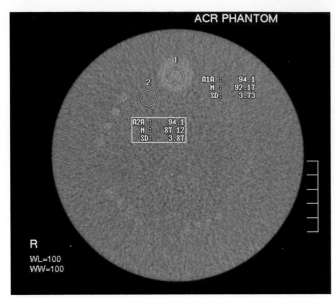

FIGURE 12-5 CT image from module 2 of the ACR, CT accreditation Phantom demonstrating placement of ROIs for assessing low-contrast resolution. *(Courtesy of Intermountain Medical Imaging.)*

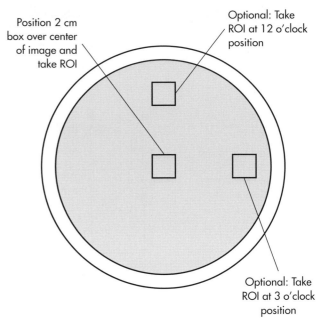

FIGURE 12-6 Test for noise and uniformity. *ROI,* Region of interest.

American College of Radiology Acceptance Criteria

- The adult abdomen and head protocols must be used.
- Window width = 100.
- Window level = 100.
- All four of the 6 mm cylinders must be clearly visible.

The primary factor limiting low-contrast resolution in CT is image noise caused by quantum mottle. As noise increases in an image, the edge definition of anatomic borders and subtle differences in attenuation between tissues decreases.

Image Uniformity. *Uniformity* refers to the ability of the CT scanner to yield the same CT number regardless of the location of the **region of interest** (ROI) within a homogenous object.

A simple 20-cm water phantom can be used to measure noise and uniformity in CT. Module 3 of the ACR CT Accreditation Phantom is used to assess image uniformity. Module 3 consists of a uniform, tissue-equivalent material with two small BBs placed at known distances within the material for optional measurements of in-plane distance measurements (Fig. 12-6).

PROCEDURE

1. Take a scan through the water phantom and position a cursor over the resultant image in three different locations.
2. The cursor should be positioned in the center, at the top, and at the side of the image (see Fig. 12-6).
3. At each cursor location, take an ROI measurement and record the standard deviation and mean CT number.

   For noise measurements, the noise in a CT system should not exceed ± 10 HU. However, if the scanner is used for quantitative CT, tighter specifications might be necessary.

Test—Image Uniformity

1. Scan module 3 with adult abdomen protocol.
2. Display the image with a window width of 100 and window level of 0.
3. Place an ROI, approximately 400 mm in diameter, at the center of the image and record the HU and standard deviation.
4. Place the same size ROI at peripheral edges of the phantom at positions 12, 3, 6, and 9 o'clock. Record the HU and standard deviation for each ROI.
5. Determine the difference between the mean CT number of the center ROI to the mean CT numbers for all four edge ROIs (mean CT number of center ROI − mean CT number of edge ROI).
6. Assess the image for streaking or artifacts.

American College of Radiology Acceptance Criteria

- Edge-to-center mean CT number difference must be less than 5 HU for all four edge positions
- Correct size and location of ROIs
- The center CT number must be between −7 and +7 HU (± 5 HU preferred)
- Adult abdomen protocol must be used
- Window width = 100
- Window width = 0
- No image artifacts

Noise. **Noise** represents the portion of the CT image that contains no useful information. It is defined as the random variation of CT numbers about a mean value when an image of a uniform object is obtained. The contrast resolution of a CT system is primarily determined by the amount of noise in the images. Noise produces a "salt-and-pepper" appearance or grainy quality in the image. The sources of noise in a CT image include quantum (statistical) noise, electronic noise, object size, reconstruction algorithms, detector efficiency, and artifacts. Of these, the predominant source of noise is quantum noise, which is defined as the statistical variation in the number of photons detected.

Factors under the influence of the technologist that affect the amount of noise in an image are pixel size, slice thickness, reconstruction algorithm, and technique factors. Simple methods to minimize noise and help provide uniform images include tube warm-ups and daily system calibrations. Because the amount of noise contained in an image is inversely proportional to the total amount of radiation absorbed, noise can be measured by obtaining the mean and standard deviation of the CT numbers within an ROI.

Test—Noise.
1. Scan module 3 with adult abdomen protocol.
2. Display the image with a window width of 100 and window level of 0.
3. Place an ROI, approximately 20 mm in diameter, at the center of the image and record the HU and standard deviation.

American College of Radiology Acceptance Criteria.
No value given, compare with manufacturer's specifications.

Computed Tomography Number Accuracy

CT numbers represent the attenuation values of different structures within the body according to their atomic number and physical density. The CT numbers are assigned a shade of gray corresponding with the attenuation value they represent. This constitutes the gray-scale or contrast scale of the displayed image. The contrast scale is determined by the CT numbers for air (-1000 HU) and water (0 HU). In CT the scanner assigns CT numbers according to the attenuation values of x-rays passing through tissue. Water is the reference material used to determine CT numbers because it constitutes up to 90% of soft tissue mass, is easy to obtain, and is completely reproducible. Because water has a CT number value of zero, tissues with densities greater than water have positive CT numbers and those with densities less than water have negative CT numbers (Fig. 12-7).

PROCEDURE

1. Using a specific technique, take a single scan through the phantom.
2. On the reconstructed image, select a 2- to 3-cm area in the center of the phantom and measure the ROI (see Fig. 12-7).
3. From the pixels located within the ROI, calculate the two parameters, the mean CT number, and the standard deviation of the CT numbers.
4. On a monthly basis, move the cursor outside of the phantom on the reconstructed image and perform the ROI function over air.

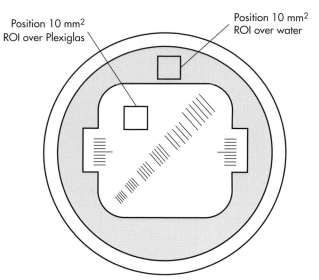

FIGURE 12-7 Test for contrast scale. *ROI,* Region of interest.

This test is performed to determine if the scanner is assigning CT numbers that accurately correspond to the appropriate tissue. Many radiologists use CT numbers as quantitative parameters to identify suspected pathologic conditions in the image. Calculating the CT number of known materials is necessary to measure the accuracy of the CT numbers.

Test–Computed Tomography Number Accuracy
1. Align module 1 to lasers. Module 1 consists of water embedded with four cylinders of known reference materials (air, polyethylene, bone, and acrylic).
2. Scan with adult abdomen protocol and at all kilovolt (peaks) (kVps) available.
3. Place an ROI approximately 200 mm over the center of each cylinder and the water. Record all HUs.
4. Scan varying slice thicknesses and repeat step 3.

The contrast scale can vary with different x-ray energies; therefore, for quality control testing, each test should be repeated at the same kVp setting and for each kVp setting that can be selected. For consistent results, the same cursor size and location should be used each time the test is performed.

American College of Radiology Acceptance Criteria
- ROIs must be placed within the cylinders
- Polyethylene mean CT number must be between -107 and -87 HU
- Water mean CT number must be between -7 and $+7$ HU (± 5 HU preferred)
- Acrylic mean CT number must be between $+110$ and $+130$ HU
- Bone mean CT number must be between $+850$ and $+970$ HU
- Air mean CT number must be between -1005 and -970 HU
- Image data are required for all selectable kVp settings

Slice Thickness. The slice thickness in single-slice CT is determined primarily by the collimators. The position of the collimators determines the width of the slice that falls within the view of each detector. In multidetector CT, the slice thickness is determined by the width of the active detector elements. Another factor affecting slice thickness is the focal spot size. The focal spot size can influence the penumbra, or sharpness of the edge of the x-ray beam, which can cause the edge of the slice to spread. Focal spot size in CT is determined by the technique factors or algorithm selected for the scan parameters. Slice thickness is a primary factor of image quality and spatial resolution.

Measurements of slice thickness are determined with a phantom that includes a ramp, spiral, or step wedge in the test objects. The test objects have known measurements and provide a standard to compare with the scanner. Typically, the test objects are aligned obliquely to the scan plane (Fig. 12-8).

If it is 5 mm or more, the slice thickness should not vary more than ± 1 mm from the intended slice thickness. If it is 5 mm or less, the slice thickness should not vary more than ± 0.5 mm.

Module 1 of the ACR CT Accreditation Phantom is used to assess slice thickness. Embedded within module 1 are a series of discrete wires that are positioned on a ramp inclined with respect to the axial plane such that the spacing between them equals 0.5 mm along the z-axis.

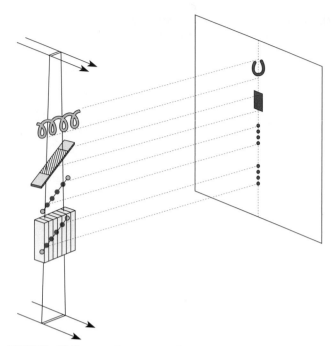

FIGURE 12-8 Test objects used for determining slice thickness. *(From Marshall C: The physical basis of computed tomography, St Louis, 1982, Warren H Green.)*

> **PROCEDURE**
>
> 1. Perform three separate scans through the test object, each with a specified thickness (10, 5, and 1 mm).
> 2. Display the images using the manufacturer's recommendations.
> 3. If a ramp is used, the length of the resultant image gives the slice width. For a spiral test object, the resultant image contains an arc, with the arc length giving the slice width. When a step wedge is used, the slice width can be determined according to the number of steps that are imaged.

Test—Slice Thickness

1. Scan module 1 with 3, 5, 7 mm and high resolution chest slice thicknesses.
2. Use a WW = 400 and a WL = 0 to view images.
3. Count the number of wires visualized in each of the two slice thickness ramps at each slice thickness (count the number of wires in the top and bottom ramps separately).
4. Estimate the slice thickness by counting the number of well-visualized wires at the top and bottom of each slice and divide by two. For example, if you can visualize 11 wires, 11 ÷ 2 is 5.5 mm.

American College of Radiology Acceptance Criteria

- Image data required for HRC, 3, 5, 7 mm slice thicknesses
- The slice width must be within 1.5 mm of the prescribed width

Linearity. Linearity refers to the relationship between CT numbers and the linear attenuation values of the scanned object with a particular kVp value. When linearity is present within an image, it is an indication that subject contrast is constant across the range of CT numbers within the image.

A standard phantom containing materials with known physical and x-ray absorption properties is used for this test (Fig. 12-9).

Over time, these values can vary because of changes in system components. Daily calibrations help maintain image quality by compensating for changes in detector channel variations and responses.

The plotted values should demonstrate a straight line between the average CT numbers and the linear attenuation coefficients (Fig. 12-10). Any deviation from the straight line can indicate that inaccurate CT numbers are being generated or the scanner is malfunctioning.

> **PROCEDURE**
>
> 1. Take a single scan through the appropriate phantom.
> 2. Plot the average CT numbers as a function of the attenuation values corresponding to the materials within the phantom.

Patient Dose. Personnel should monitor the amount of radiation to which patients and staff are exposed. It is equally important for a CT technologist to realize that the patient dose can increase with changes in slice thickness, kVp, and milliampere-seconds (mAs). In addition,

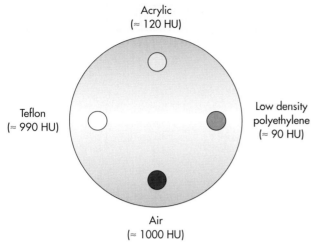

FIGURE 12-9 Phantom with known physical and x-ray absorption properties used for measuring linearity. *HU,* Hounsfield unit. *(Courtesy ImPACT, a Medical Devices Agency Evaluation Group, London, UK.)*

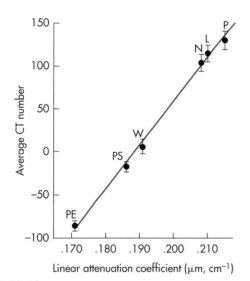

FIGURE 12-10 Graph showing computed tomography (CT) linearity. *L,* Lexan; *N,* nylon; *P,* Plexiglas; *PE,* polyethylene; *PS,* polystyrene; *W,* water. *(From Bushong S: Radiologic science for technologists, ed 6, St Louis, 1997, Mosby.)*

PROCEDURE

1. Along with a standard phantom, position the radiation-detecting device at the location and intervals of the desired radiation measurements.
2. Initiate the appropriate scans at the selected locations, and measure the resultant radiation dose. Some facilities prefer to take two scans at each location, but with a change in the technique factors to simulate the difference between head and body examinations. This gives a more reliable dose estimate for a particular CT examination.

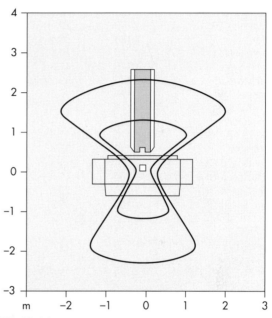

FIGURE 12-11 Isodose curves for a typical computed tomography (CT) scanner. *(From Wegener OH: Whole body computed tomography, Cambridge, Mass, 1992, Blackwell Scientific.)*

---

if it is necessary for ancillary personnel to remain within the scan room, all CT technologists should be able to direct them to the safest location within the room to avoid unnecessary radiation exposure. Figure 12-11 provides representative isodose curves for a typical CT scanner.

Specially designed ionization chambers or thermoluminescent dosimeters (TLDs) are used to measure the radiation dose. These specially designed radiation detectors are capable of providing measurements from which the dose can be calculated for the exposure factors used (slice thickness, mAs, and kVp).

No acceptable maximum levels of radiation are specified for the permissible dose to a patient during a CT procedure. In addition, the results can vary according to patient location and distance from the x-ray source. However, most experts agree that the values should remain within ± 10% of the manufacturer's specifications when a fixed technique is used (Table 12-1).

For ACR CT accreditation purposes, a medical physicist is required to perform CTDI testing on every CT unit at the clinical facility. In order for the CT unit to pass the phantom image quality tests, it has to be demonstrated that the scanner meets the ACR dose reference levels. The ACR has recently updated the ACR CT accreditation dose pass/fail criteria and reference levels (Table 12-2).

TABLE 12-1 Computed Tomography Dose Index

Scanner	kVp	CTDI (Head) (mGy/100 mAs)			CTDI (Body) (mGy/100 mAs)		
		Air	Center	Periphery	Air	Center	Periphery
CGR CE 10000, 12000	130	—	—	—	—	—	—
ElscintExel 2400 Elect	120	18.8	13.2	14.5	18.5	3.5	6.2
Elscint Exel 2400 Elect	140	—	—	—	25.8	5.2	6.6
Elscint CT Twin, Helicat	120	18.6	12.9	13.9	19	3.8	6.5
GE 8800/9000 Series	120	14.1	6.5	6.1	14.6	2.1	4.2
GE 9800 Series	120	26	14.1	14.9	26	3.9	7.4
GE 9800 Series	140	34.1	19.4	20	34.1	5.7	10
GE HiLight, HiSpeed,	80	8.5	4.2	4.5	8.5	1	1.9 CT/i (No SmB)
GE HiLight, HiSpeed,	100	14	8.2	8.3	14	2.2	4.3 CT/i (No SmB)
GE HiLight, HiSpeed,	120	19.3	11.4	11.9	18.8	3.2	6.1 CT/i (No SmB)
GE HiLight, HiSpeed,	140	27	16.8	17.2	25.8	4.8	9 CT/i (No SmB)
GE HiSpeed CT/i	80	8.5	4.2	4.5	8.5	1	2.7 with SmartBeam
GE HiSpeed CT/i	100	14	8.2	8.3	13.9	2.5	5.6 with SmartBeam
GE HiSpeed CT/i	120	19.3	11.4	11.9	20.4	3.8	7.3 with SmartBeam
GE HiSpeed CT/i	140	27	16.8	17.2	27.7	5.8	10.7 with SmartBeam
GE Max	120	38.4	18.8	17.7	38.4	5	8.8
GE Pace, Sytec	80	20.1	8	10	19.2	1.9	5.3
GE Pace, Sytec	120	41.6	22.1	23.8	41	6.3	13.2
GE Pace, Sytec	140	55.5	30.7	33.5	54.1	9.5	18.5
GE Prospeed	120	36.6	20.8	22.2	35	5.4	11
GE Prospeed	140	43.6	22.2	25.8			
GE FX/i, LX/i	80	16.3	6.7	8.2	16.3	1.5	4.3
GE FX/i, LX/i	120	33.4	18	19.4	33.4	5.1	10.2
GE FX/i, LX/i	140	33.4	18	19.4	43.2	7.3	13.9
GE LightSpeed QX/i	80	11.8	6.4	6.7	11.8	1.5	3.6
GE LightSpeed QX/i	100	19.8	12	12	19.8	3.2	6.8
GE LightSpeed QX/i	120	29	18.6	18.2	29	5.5	10.7
GE LightSpeed QX/i	140	39.3	26.2	25.2	39.3	8.2	15.1
Philips 310, 350 (GE2, no Cu)	120	32.8	18.7	21.2	—	—	—
Philips 310, 350 (GE2, w. Cu)	120	15.8	11.2	11.6	—	—	—
Philips 310, 350 (GE3, no Cu)	120	—	—	—	21.7	4.2	10.2
Philips 310, 350 (GE3, w. Cu)	120	—	—	—	—	—	—
Philips AV, LX, SR7000 PH.e	80	4.3	2.6	3	8.7	1.4	3.5
Philips AV, LX, SR7000	100	13.2	8.8	9.6	13.2	2.6	5.7
Philips AV, LX, SR7000	120	19.2	13.6	14.8	19.3	4.3	9
Philips AV, LX, SR7000	130	22.6	16	17.6	22.8	5.3	11.1
Philips AV, LX, SR7000	140	26	19	20.3	26	6.2	12.4
Philips CX, CX/S	120	20.5	14.2	15.4	19.2	4	7.4
Philips SR 4000	120	18.2	12.5	13.5	18.2	3.8	7.8
Philips SR 5000	120	18	11.8	13	18	3.6	7.7
Philips SR 5000	130	20.8	14.1	15.1	20.8	4.4	10.1
Philips M/ EG	120	58.4	34.8	45.2	58.4	11.3	39.1
Philips M/ EG	130	67.6	41.6	53.8	67.6	13.9	47.9
Philips TX	100	—	—	—	—	—	—
Philips TX	120	7.8	5.2	5.5			
Philips TX	130	—	—	—	—	—	—
Picker 1200SX	80	—	—	—	16.3	1.3	5.3
Picker 1200SX	120	30.3	12.1	11.2	30	4.3	11.2
Picker 1200SX	130	31.8	12.3	12.6	32.6	4.8	12.6
Picker 1200SX	140	38	16.9	14.3	38.8	6.4	15.5
Picker PQ Series	120	30.1	14	13.3	30	4.8	11.8
Picker PQ Series	130	36.8	17.5	16.2	36.8	6	15.5
Picker PQ Series	140	38.2	19.1	17.7	38	7	16.8
Picker UltraZ	80	16.5	5.6	6.2	17.7	1.2	5.2
Picker UltraZ	100	23.7	9.7	10.3	25.3	3	8.4
Picker UltraZ	120	31.4	14.3	13.8	33.6	4.9	11.9

TABLE 12-1	Computed Tomography Dose Index—cont'd						
	CTDI (Head) (mGy/100 mAs)			**CTDI (Body) (mGy/100 mAs)**			
Scanner	kVp	Air	Center	Periphery	Air	Center	Periphery
Picker UltraZ	130	35.6	16.9	16	38.1	6	14.2
Picker UltraZ	140	39.7	19.5	18.3	42.5	7.1	16.3
Shimadzu SCT	80	5.6	3.6	4.4	5.4	1	3.3
Shimadzu SCT	120	15.6	12	13.4	15.6	4	10.1
Shimadzu SCT	130	17.4	13.5	14.9	17.3	4.6	11.5
Siemens CR, CR512, DRH	125	12.4	9.3	10.9	13.2	3.5	9.6
Siemens Somatom 2, DR1/2/3	125	8.9	6.5	7.6	8.9	2.3	6.5
Siemens DRG, DRG1	125	—	—	—	—	—	—
Siemens Somatom	80	5.6	3.7	4.3	5.6	1.1	2.9 Plus 4 Series
Siemens Somatom	120	17.7	13.6	15.1	17.9	4.4	9.6 Plus 4 Series
Siemens Somatom	140	25.1	19.5	21.3	25.2	6.6	13.9 Plus 4 Series
Siemens Somatom	110	24.5	16.2	18.1	24.5	4.9	10.9 AR-C, AR.SP, AR-T
Siemens Somatom	130	35.7	25.2	27.7	35.7	7.8	16.4 AR-C, AR.SP, AR-T
Siemens AR.HP	130	33.5	26.2	27.6	33.5	8.9	16.4
Siemens Plus, DXP,	120	12.2	9.4	10.8	12.2	3.2	7.0 Plus-S
Siemens Plus, DXP,	137	15.6	12.2	13.5	16.2	4.3	9 Plus-S
Siemens HI Q	133	17.6	12.9	14.5	17.6	4	10.3
Toshiba TCT 800	120	22.3	16.1	15.8	18.3	3.9	7
Toshiba Xspeed II	120	30.7	21.4	21.2	11.8	2.9	5.5
Toshiba Xpress GX	120	33.6	17.8	18.7	—	—	— (Pre '98)
Toshiba Xvision/EX	120	25.6	17	15.8	22	4.8	7.4
Toshiba Xpress HS1	120	30.6	19.7	20.8	22	5.3	8.2
Toshiba Xpress HS	120	17.4	12.9	12.9	22	4.7	7.3
Toshiba Xpress GX	120	21.6	13	13.7	22.2	4.4	7.8 (Post '98), Asteion
Toshiba Xpress GX	130	24.9	15.3	15.6	23.1	4.7	8.1 (Post '98), Asteion

Courtesy ImPACT, a Medical Devices Agency Evaluation Group, London.

CTDI, Computed tomography dose index; *kVp,* kilovolt (peak); *mAs,* milliampere-second; *mGy,* milligray.

Note: These are average dose values from our dose survey. Great care has been taken to exclude potentially incorrect data, but there are variations from one scanner to another. Although the scanner groups have been carefully selected, there is always the possibility that design features will change, altering the CTDI characteristics.

TABLE 12-2	ACR CT Accreditation Dose Pass/Fail Criteria and Reference Levels	
Examination	Pass/Fail Criteria CTDI$_{vol}$ (mGy)	Reference Levels CTDI$_{vol}$ (mGy)
Adult head	80	75
Adult abdomen	30	25
Pediatric abdomen (5 yrs)	25	20

SUMMARY

An effective quality assurance program provides a method for systematic monitoring of the CT system's performance and image quality. The collected data are beneficial in identifying specific problems or malfunctions. Increasingly, it is becoming the responsibility of the CT technologist to perform and document the routine quality control tests. However, more extensive quality assurance procedures should be performed periodically by the department physicist or service engineer. Like all quality management and accreditation processes, documentation of all quality control testing and maintenance of all records is imperative for program success.

Refer to the Evolve website at https://evolve.elsevier. com for Student Experiment 12.1: Computerized Tomography (CT) Quality Control.

REVIEW QUESTIONS

1. What is used as the reference material for CT number calibrations?
   a. Bone
   b. Liver
   c. Water
   d. Lung
2. Which of the following is the expected result of a CT number calibration test?
   a. 0 ± 5
   b. 1000 ± 5
   c. 0 ± 3
   d. 1000 ± 3

3. Which of the following is the primary determination of slice thickness?
   a. Spacing between detectors
   b. Collimators
   c. Focal spot size
   d. Field of view (FOV)

4. Which term describes the ability of a CT scanner to differentiate objects with minimal differences in attenuation coefficients?
   a. Spatial resolution
   b. Contrast resolution
   c. Linearity
   d. Modulation

5. Which of the following factors can affect the accuracy of a density (HU) measurement in a CT image?
   a. System calibration
   b. Window width setting
   c. Window level setting
   d. Display FOV

6. Increasing which of the following factors can improve spatial resolution?
   a. FOV
   b. Matrix
   c. Pixel size
   d. Slice thickness

7. Which of the following is the main limiting factor for contrast resolution?
   a. Noise
   b. Pixel depth
   c. Voxel volume
   d. Focal spot size

8. Which of the following is measured using the MTF method?
   a. Low-contrast resolution
   b. High-contrast spatial resolution
   c. Attenuation
   d. Section thickness

9. A contemporary CT system should be able to detect 3-mm objects with which of the following density differences?
   a. 0.05%
   b. 0.5%
   c. 1%
   d. 1.5%

10. What is the tolerance limit for noise in a CT image?
    a. ± 3
    b. ± 5
    c. ± 10
    d. ± 15

Quality Control for Magnetic Resonance Imaging Equipment

Lorrie Kelley

KEY TERMS

center frequency
geometric accuracy
high-contrast resolution

image intensity uniformity
low-contrast resolution
signal-to-noise ratio

slice position accuracy
transmit gain

OBJECTIVES

At the completion of this chapter the reader will be able to do the following:
- Describe the various types of phantoms used in magnetic resonance (MR) scanners
- Understand the frequency of quality control testing of various MR parameters
- Describe the concept of signal-to-noise ratio (SNR)
- Understand the concept of center frequency
- Perform quality control testing for center frequency, transmit gain, geometric accuracy, and high-contrast and low-contrast resolution

OUTLINE

Quality assurance procedures for magnetic resonance imaging (MRI) equipment are designed to establish a standard of measurement for daily system performance and the documentation of any variance thereof. Although the definition of *standard* varies from scanner to scanner, the goal of quality control is the detection of any changes or potential changes in the system performance. Documentation of daily quality control measurements is considered an essential part of the MRI quality control program and must be done properly.

The ultimate goal is to maintain high image quality and patient safety.

MRI is a relatively new imaging modality that has seen tremendous growth and technologic advancements in recent years. The rapid proliferation of new and used MR units in conjunction with the older units still in place has contributed to increasing variation in MR image quality across the country. In an effort to address those concerns and to establish a reasonable standard of image quality, the American College of Radiology

(ACR) developed an MRI Accreditation Program. The MRI Accreditation Program was designed to review the qualifications of the radiologists, MR scientists/medical physicists and technologists, as well as the clinical image quality and effectiveness of QC testing procedures of each site applying for accreditation. In November 1996 the ACR approved the MRI Accreditation Program for implementation. More information about the MRI accreditation process can be obtained by contacting the ACR *(www.acr.org)*. In the summer of 2008, Congress passed the Medicare Improvements for Patients and Providers Act of 2008 (MIPPA), which mandates that any nonhospital institution performing advanced diagnostic services (such as MRI) must be accredited (by January 1, 2010) in order to receive federal funding (Medicare reimbursement). The CARE bill (discussed in Chapter 1) if passed, would make similar requirements for hospital-based facilities. Therefore, accreditation programs are becoming mandatory for MRI departments to succeed.

PHANTOMS

Typically, the phantoms for routine quality control tests are provided by the manufacturer of the MR system. A user's manual and charts for documenting standardized tests also are provided. Use of the equipment can be easily taught to the technologists during the site installation. Specific actions for obtaining and documenting quality control results vary among manufacturers.

Generally, quality control phantoms are paramagnetic materials in an oil or water solution. Ions such as copper, aluminum, manganese, and nickel often are used. The materials used are designed to mimic biologic tissues or to shorten T1 relaxation times for strong MR signals. The relaxation rates vary with each material, main magnetic field strength (B_0), and temperature. Other considerations for materials are minimal chemical shifts and thermal and chemical stability. For the sake of the scan time, when quality control tests are performed, the T1 repetition time (TR) of the phantom material should be compatible with a short TR, and the T2 repetition time should be long enough for any echo-time (TE) value that can be obtained. Figure 13-1 demonstrates a copper (II) sulfate ($CuSO_4$) phantom used daily at a clinical site.

Quality control phantoms are designed with various shapes, sizes, and geometric variables. The same type of phantom may be used for signal-to-noise ratio (SNR) and resonant frequency tests, whereas a different phantom is required for spatial resolution and linearity tests. Regardless of the type of test being performed, any quality control phantom must be placed in the magnet at the isocenter, unless specified otherwise. The scanning parameters used (e.g., TR, TE, flip angle, slice thickness, matrix, and coil) should be documented.

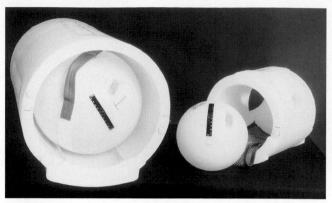

FIGURE 13-1 *Left,* Body coil phantom and holder. *Right,* Head coil phantom and holder.

The ACR MRI Accreditation Committee developed a specially designed MR phantom along with test protocols for use in establishing QA programs for clinical MR scanners. The ACR MRI accreditation phantom is designed to examine several important instrument parameters within a single phantom, which means that each test can be accomplished in a reasonable amount of time. The phantom is a short, hollow cylinder constructed of acrylic plastic and is filled with a solution of nickel chloride and sodium chloride to simulate biologic tissue relaxation properties. Structures located within the phantom provide the tools necessary for quantitative assessment of seven important equipment performance parameters affecting image quality.

QC TESTING FREQUENCY

Quality control tests should be performed regularly by an MR technologist and/or service engineer under the supervision of a qualified MR scientist/medical physicist. Planning and preparing for the quality control tests should be a part of the site installation process. The ACR states that a qualified medical physicist must have the responsibility of overseeing the equipment quality control program. The medical physicist, in conjunction with the service engineer, system manufacturer specialist, and site technologist, should discuss goals and potential outcomes for regular quality control tests. It can then be decided which tests should be performed at certain intervals and by which personnel. Although all of the tests are important, not all are required at the same frequency. Testing can be thought of as monitoring essential fluids in a car: The windshield washer fluid may be checked infrequently, the oil checked more regularly, and the gasoline monitored daily. The ACR requires that at a minimum, the clinical site perform the following tests on a weekly basis: center frequency, table positioning, set-up and scanning, geometric accuracy, high-contrast resolution, low-contrast resolution, artifact analysis, film quality control and visual checklist. In addition to the weekly test requirements, the

ACR requires the following tests be performed annually: magnetic field homogeneity, slice position accuracy, slice thickness accuracy, radiofrequency (RF) coil checks, and soft-copy display devices. The decision of how frequently to perform QC testing is commonly dictated by personnel convenience and time constraints. However, performing QC tests daily will provide a site with enough quantitative data to spot negative trends much faster than if QC testing is done weekly, which might take several months to acquire enough data to spot the trends. The factors listed here are unanimously believed to be essential indicators of MR system performance. For information on MRI safety, refer to the website *www.MRIsafety.com*.

Although the following tests can be performed with phantoms supplied by the MR system's vendor, where appropriate, the methodology of the following QC tests will include the ACR MR Accreditation phantom and testing criteria.

WEEKLY TESTS

Setup and Table Positioning Accuracy

This entails an overview of the general condition of the system's functions including: table movement, console function, prescan, and table positioning. The goal is to ensure the safe operation of the scanner during patient setup.

Any problems noted with the scanner interface, computer boot up, table movement (including docking), or table positioning should be noted.

PROCEDURE

1. Place the ACR phantom in the head coil, making sure that the crosshairs engraved on the phantom are moved into the center of the magnet.
2. Fine tune the position of the phantom along all three axes with the nonmetallic bubble level enclosed with the ACR phantom.
3. Verify the accuracy of the phantom positioning by performing sagittal and, if necessary, coronal localizer scans.
4. Once the phantom is correctly aligned, leave the phantom in place for the rest of the series of scans used for QC testing.

Center (Resonance) Frequency

Center frequency is defined as the radiofrequency that matches the static magnetic field (B_0) according to the Larmor equation. It is recommended that the resonance frequency be checked before quality assurance procedures are initiated and each time the phantom is changed. An example of the Larmor equation follows, where B_0 is the magnetic field strength, and the gyromagnetic ratio for hydrogen 5 42.57 MHz/T.

$$B_0 \times \text{gyromagnetic ratio} = \text{Resonance frequency}$$
$$\text{Examples}: 1.5 \text{ T} \times 42.57 \text{ MHz/T} = 63.86 \text{ MHz}$$
$$1 \text{ T} \times 42.57 \text{ MHz/T} = 42.57 \text{ MHz}$$
$$0.5 \text{ T} \times 42.57 \text{ MHz/T} = 21.29 \text{ MHz}$$
$$0.3 \text{ T} \times 42.57 \text{ MHz/T} = 12.77 \text{ MHz}$$

The term *center frequency* is used interchangeably with *resonance frequency* and *Larmor frequency*. Conveniently, the center frequency can be obtained during the prescan mode of the ACR phantom test. Most manufacturers provide an automated way to determine the resonance frequency.

PROCEDURE

1. Use the ACR phantom.
2. Place the phantom in the center of the magnet.
3. Use the ACR T1-weighted axial series protocol and perform a prescan. Record the center frequency on the required data form.
4. If the prescribed action limit is exceeded, repeat the prescan a second time.
5. If the action limit is still exceeded, report the change to the service engineer and medical physicist.

If a notable change in the resonance frequency occurs, the service engineer should be notified. As determined by the Larmor equation (mentioned previously), a change in the center frequency indicates that there is a change in the strength of the main magnetic field, B_0. This could be a result of cryogen boiloff, the presence of external ferromagnetic materials, shim coil failure, and/or changes in the current of the main coil windings.

Checking the center frequency is important in magnets that undergo frequent ramping of the magnetic field (e.g., mobile units and resistive magnets). In a superconducting magnet, the cryogen levels should be routinely monitored. Although most systems have a cryogen alarm, monitoring is the best way to avoid an urgent situation (similar to running out of gas in a car). If the superconductor uses liquid helium and liquid nitrogen, both should be monitored. The service organization should be notified if the cryogens seem to be decreasing more than usual between replenishments.

Significant changes in the center frequency indicate changes in the SNR.

The center frequency should not deviate by more than 1.5 parts per million (ppm) between successive measurements.

Transmit Gain (Attenuation)

Transmit gain is a measure of the RF power that is required to produce a 90-degree flip of the patient's magnetic vector during imaging. During the prescan process and after establishing the center frequency, the system acquires several signals with varying levels of transmit gain to determine the appropriate RF flip angles for a given pulse sequence. Fluctuations in the transmit gain could indicate problems in the RF transmitter or the receive coils anywhere along the RF chain or circuitry. Transmitter gain or attenuation values are usually recorded in units of decibel (dB). The decibel provides a logarithmic scale where a small change in dB represents a large change in the transmit gain.

The transmit gain measurements should be compared with the standards set at acceptance testing. Any changes that exceed those limits should be reported.

Geometric Accuracy (Three Axes)

Geometric accuracy, also referred to as *spatial linearity*, refers to the amount of geometric distortion in the image due to displacement or improper scaling of the distance between points being displayed on the image (Fig. 13-2). This is affected primarily by the homogeneity of the main magnetic field and the linearity of the magnetic field gradients. Other factors contributing to geometric inaccuracies are: low receive bandwidth, poor eddy current compensation, and gradient miscalibration. When using the ACR MRI accreditation phantom, geometric accuracy measurements are considered acceptable when they are less than or equal to 2 mm of the true values when measured over a 25-cm field of view (FOV). The greatest amount of distortion is typically seen near the edges of the FOV, or increasingly distorted as you move farther from the magnet isocenter. Although these edge distortions are commonly expected, consideration should be given to procedures guided by the MR image such as surgical and treatment planning, in which distance measurements are critical. The results of this test also can be used to verify reported FOV and the accuracy of the scanner's distance-measuring tools.

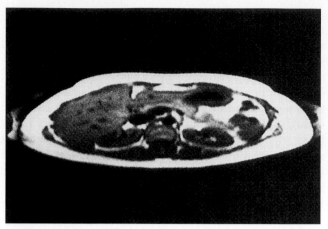

FIGURE 13-2 Example of gradient amplitude falloff resulting in A-P minification of a T1-weighted (T1W) axial image of the upper abdomen. *(From Ros PR, Bidgood WD: Abdominal magnetic resonance imaging, St Louis, 1993, Mosby. Courtesy GE Medical Systems, Milwaukee, Wis.)*

Site engineers often perform geometric accuracy tests on systems when they perform the regularly scheduled preventive maintenance. If you find there have been changes in geometric accuracy, simply reshimming the magnet or removing lost ferromagnetic objects (e.g., paper clips, coins, bobby pins) from the magnet bore may improve the system's performance.

High-Contrast Resolution (Spatial Resolution)

High-contrast resolution is the MR system's ability to resolve small objects. The phantom used for this test is unlike those previously discussed. It should consist of an array of pegs, bars, rods, or holes of known sizes. A typical spatial resolution phantom may have an array of varying element sizes. The ACR MR accreditation phantom has inserts with arrays of holes varying in diameter of 0.9 mm, 1 mm, and 1.1 mm.

The scanning sequence can be any multislice sequence, as long as the SNR parameters are chosen to minimize noise. The testing parameters are those that affect the pixel size, slice thickness, matrix, and FOV. A two-dimensional pixel size can be determined by dividing the acquisition matrix into the FOV.

Example:

FOV: 200 mm FOVp × 240 mm FOVf

Matrix: 192 phase encodings × 256 frequency encodings

200 mm FOVp divided by 192 phase encodings = 1.04 mm

240 mm FOVf divided by 256 frequency encodings = 0.93 mm

Therefore the pixel size or in-plane resolution would be 1.04 mm by 0.93 mm.

PROCEDURE

1. Seven measurements of known lengths are made from the scans acquired from the ACR phantom using the MR system's length measurement tools for on-screen display. Follow the ACR requirements for setting the window width and window level for display of the phantom images for the purposes of taking length measurements.
2. Using the sagittal localizer image, measure the end-to-end length of the phantom along a line near the center of the phantom (Fig. 13-3). Use slice 1 and measure the diameter of the phantom in the top-to-bottom and left-to-right directions (Fig. 13-4). Use slice 5 and measure the phantom in four directions: top-to-bottom, left-to-right, and both diagonals (Fig. 13-5).
3. The length measurements are compared with the known values of the distances within the ACR phantom, which are inside end-to-end length = 148 mm and inside diameter is 190 mm.
4. All measurements should be within ± mm of their true values.

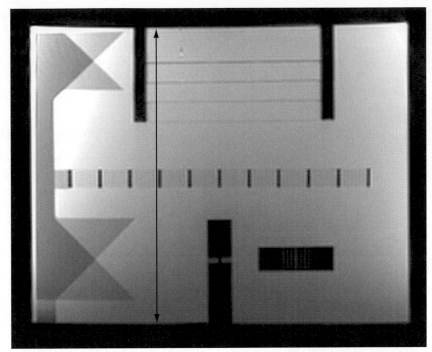

FIGURE 13-3 Sagittal localizer with end-to-end measurement shown *(arrow). (Courtesy St. Luke's Health System.)*

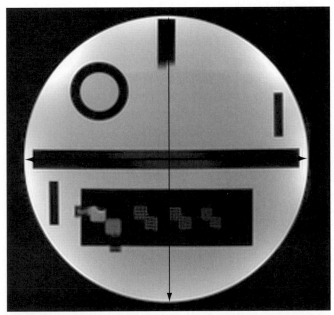

FIGURE 13-4 Slice 1 from ACR T1 series with diameter measurements shown *(arrows). (Courtesy St. Luke's Health System.)*

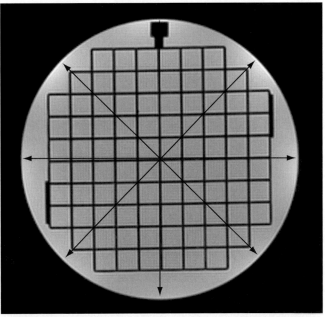

FIGURE 13-5 Slice 5 from ACR T1 series with diameter measurements shown *(arrows). (Courtesy St. Luke's Health System.)*

1. Use slice 1 acquired with the ACR phantom using the T1 and T2 axial series test protocols (Fig. 13-6).
2. Keeping the resolution insert visible, magnify the image by a factor between 2 and 4 (Fig. 13-7).
3. Adjust the window level and width to best demonstrate the insert.
4. Identify and record the smallest hole size that can be resolved in both the right-to-left and top-to-bottom directions.
5. The ACR test protocol uses a field of view and matrix size for the axial series that should produce a resolution of 1.0 mm in both directions.

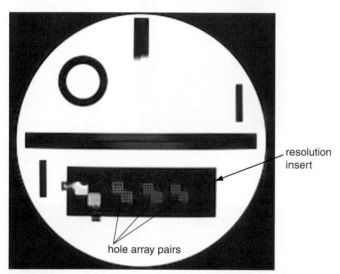

FIGURE 13-6 Slice 1 from ACR T2 series demonstrating resolution insert and hole array pairs. *(Courtesy St. Luke's Health System.)*

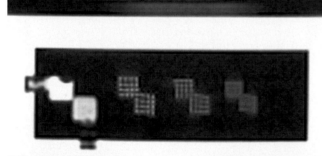

FIGURE 13-7 Magnified portion of slice 1 displayed for visual assessment of high-contrast resolution. *(Courtesy St. Luke's Health System.)*

The ACR standard is a measurement of 1 mm or better in both directions.

Although resolution is traditionally known as *lines pairs per millimeter*, here it is determined by the pixel size and what the human eye can resolve on the image. Resolution is determined by the smallest array element (e.g., a bar or rod) visible that is completely separated by distance from the adjacent element. The calculated pixel size is then compared with the smallest resolvable element.

This quality control test may be routinely performed by the site engineer during the preventive maintenance of the system. This test is likely to fail in conjunction with the failure of the geometric accuracy test. The gradient amplitude, the gradient duty cycle, and reconstruction filters can easily affect the spatial resolution.

Low-Contrast Resolution (Detectability)

Low-contrast resolution is a measure of the MR system's ability to differentiate between adjacent tissues having minimal differences in signal intensities. Several factors can influence low-contrast resolution, including increased noise, ghosting artifacts, improper phantom positioning, RF coil malfunctions, and improper use of image filters.

Typically, low-contrast resolution is expressed in one of two ways: the smallest diameter of an object with a specific contrast that can be detected or the smallest difference in signal intensity that can be discriminated for an object of a specific diameter. A phantom that contains objects of varying size and contrast should be selected. The ACR MRI accreditation phantom consists of three rows of low-contrast objects that radiate from the center in a circular arrangement. Each row contains 10 holes of varying diameters (from 7 mm to 1.5 mm). Slices acquired from four locations within the phantom provide contrast values of 1.4%, 2.5%, 3.6%, and 5.1%.

1. When using the ACR phantom, measurements for this test are made by counting the number of complete spokes seen in each of the images
2. Use slices 8–11 from the ACR phantom test series.
3. Starting with slice 11, adjust the window width and level display settings for best visibility of the objects (typically a narrow window width) (Fig. 13-8).
4. Begin counting the number of complete spokes starting with the spokes with the largest diameter disks (positioned at 12 o'clock or just slightly to the right of 12 o'clock). Count clockwise from spoke 1 until a spoke is reached where 1 or more of the disks is not distinguishable from the background. The number of complete spokes counted is the score for the slice. Repeat the counting procedure with slices 8–10.
5. MR systems with field strengths less than 3T should have a total score of at least 9 spokes for each ACR series, and there should be a score of 37 spokes for MR systems with field strengths of 3T.
   Note: A spoke can only be counted as complete if all 3 of its disks are discernible.

According to the action limits of the ACR, an MR scanner with a field strength less than 3T should be able to display nine spokes of holes from the low-contrast inserts and 3T MR systems should be able to display 37 spokes. The ACR requires that a MR scanner pass on both of the ACR T1 and T2 series or on both of the site's T1 and T2 series.

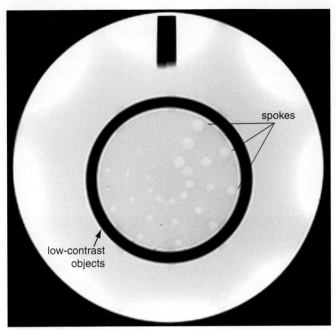

FIGURE 13-8 Slice 2 of ACR T1 series with the circle of low-contrast objects displayed. *(Courtesy St. Luke's Health System.)*

Artifact Analysis

Various artifacts can occur during the routine QC testing procedures. Artifacts can vary according to imaging conditions, pulse sequence parameters, choice of RF coils, and with individual patients. The presence of artifacts can be an early indication of equipment failure. The MR technologist should become familiar with the common appearances of artifacts that are due to particular subsystems of the MR scanner. These include the radiofrequency system, gradient system, image and data processing, and magnetic field homogeneity.

During each QC test, the MR technologist should be evaluating each image for signs of ghosting, geometric distortion, discrepancies in signal intensities and any other interference with the known parameters of the image. The ACR requirement for assessment of image artifacts follows the following procedure:

1. Use the image slices from the ACR T1-weighted slices.
2. Adjust the display window width and window level to show the full range of pixel values for each image.
3. On each image validate the following: the phantom appears circular and is not distorted, there are no ghost images of the phantom, there are no streaks or spots, and there are no abnormal or new elements in the image.

Film Quality Control

Any digital modality is challenged to provide hard-copy images that match the gray-scale display of the system's monitor. One way to verify accurate representation of the gray scale between the monitor and hard copy is with a Society of Motion Picture and Television Engineers (SMPTE) test pattern.

ACR control limits for the SMPTE test pattern:

SMPTE Test Pattern	Control Limits
0	± 0.15
10%	± 0.15
40%	± 0.15
90%	± 0.8

Visual Checklist

The visual checklist is a method to quantitatively and qualitatively verify that all equipment is available and working properly. The checklist can be scanner specific depending on the use of the equipment. Items that are typically included in a visual check are patient table, alignment lights, RF coil/cable integrity, monitors, and emergency cart. Items that are missing or malfunctioning should be repaired or replaced as soon as possible.

ANNUAL TESTS

As stated previously, all quality control measurements are considered essential for overall system performance. Box 13-1 lists abbreviated definitions of tests that should be performed by a medical physicist or system engineer. They should be performed on a regular schedule and also whenever there are changes to the site scanner and environment such as hardware and software upgrades, magnet quench, or facility construction. The ACR requires that the following tests be performed on an annual basis to meet the ACR MRI Accreditation Standard.

Magnetic Field Homogeneity

The homogeneity of a system's magnetic field is an indication of the quality or uniformity of its field. Homogeneity is usually expressed in parts per million within a given spherical volume. A spherical volume is given as the diameter of a spherical volume (DSV). MRI system manufacturers provide specifications for their magnets, and values obtained from QC tests should be compared to those specified. The medical physicist can choose from a couple of methods for

BOX 13-1 | Quality Control Tests Performed by a Medical Physicist or System Engineer

Receiver Gain (Attenuation): The receiver setting is the amount by which MR signals are amplified before digitization.

Transmitter Setting: The transmitter setting is a number expressed in decibels that influences the flip angle of each RF pulse.

Coil Q: Known as the quality factor, coil Q describes the performance of a coil used to receive MR signals.

Ghost Intensity: Ghost intensity is an expression of the intensity of background ghosts relative to the intensity of a phantom.

RF Shielding Effectiveness: The RF shielding effectiveness test verifies that the RF shield is attenuating radiowaves originating from outside the scan room.

Surface Coil Performance: For the surface coil performance to be checked, a separate test is done on each surface coil to determine the SNR and image uniformity.

Slice Thickness: Slice thickness is the FWHM of a slice profile, the region from which MR signals are emitted.

Maximum Gradient Strength: The maximum gradient strength determines if gradients are still achieving the maximum amplitude specified by the manufacturer and originally measured.

Specific Absorption Rate Monitor: The SAR monitor verifies that the imaging procedures do not cause excessive RF power to be deposited into a patient.

MR, Magnetic resonance; *RF,* radiofrequency; *SAR,* specific absorption rate; *SNR,* signal-to-noise ratio.

measuring the magnetic field homogeneity. The spectral peak method uses a uniform, spherical phantom to measure the full width at half maximum (FWHM) of the spectral peak over the imaging volume. The other method uses a phase difference map to calculate the magnetic field inhomogeneity. Using phase-contrast images, a medical physicist can calculate the change in phase across images acquired from a uniformity phantom as proportional to the inhomogeneity of the magnetic field. For a superconducting magnet, typical values are 2 ppm over a 30- to 40-cm DSV. For MR systems with spectroscopy capabilities, the suggested value is less than or equal to 0.5 ppm at 35 cm DSV.

Poor homogeneity can result in poor image quality and artifacts. Changes in homogeneity can be due to ferromagnetic objects located within the bore of the magnet and external ferromagnetic structures that may be neighboring the magnetic field. Sometimes magnetic inhomogeneities can be improved with gradient adjustments or shimming.

Slice Position Accuracy

The slice position test is performed to ensure that the land-marking location is actually centered to the magnet bore. Misalignment can simply be due to mechanical problems with the table, positioning devices, or alignment light beams. Other causes of poor performance include operator error, gradient miscalibration, magnetic field inhomogeneities, and table positioning shift.

PROCEDURE

1. Use slices 1 and 11 of the ACR T1 and T2 phantom test series and magnify the images by a factor of 2 to 4, making sure to keep the vertical bars of the crossed wedges within the displayed image (Figs. 13-9 and 13-10).
2. Using a fairly narrow display window width, measure the difference in length between the left and right bars of the cross wedges in each image.

Note: Since the crossed wedges have a 45° slope, the measured bar length difference is really twice the actual slice displacement meaning that if the measurement of the bar length difference is 6.0 mm, the slice is displaced superiorly by 3.0 mm (Fig. 13-11).

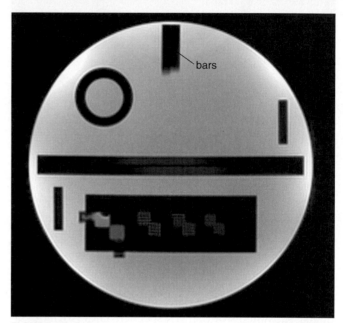

FIGURE 13-9 Slice 1 of ACR T1 series with pair of dark vertical bars from the 45° crossed wedges indicated. *(Courtesy St. Luke's Health System.)*

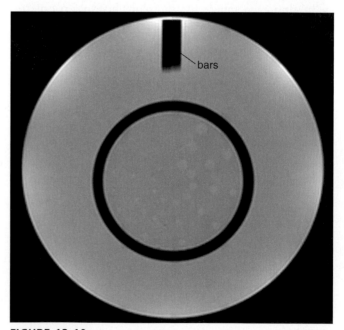

FIGURE 13-10 Slice 2 of ACR T1 series with pair of dark vertical bars from the 45° crossed wedges indicated. *(Courtesy St. Luke's Health System.)*

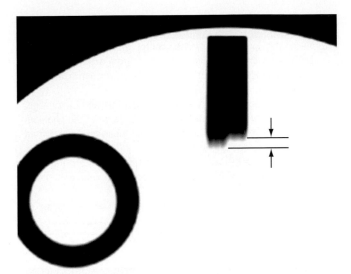

FIGURE 13-11 Magnified portion of slice 1 showing measurement for slice position error. The arrows indicate the difference in bar length. *(Courtesy St. Luke's Health System.)*

The ACR MR accreditation phantom uses crossed-wedges from slices 1 and 11 as a reference. On slices 1 and 11, the crossed wedges appear as a pair of dark bars at the top of the phantom. The ACR criterion is the absolute bar length difference should be equal to or less than 5 mm.

Slice Thickness Accuracy

Slice thickness is an important image-quality parameter. The accuracy of slice thickness is especially important for stereotactic and interventional procedures. The thickness of each slice is determined by both the transmit RF bandwidth and the amplitude of the slice select gradient. Factors that influence slice thickness include gradient calibration and the RF pulse profile. Inaccuracies in slice thickness can cause interslice interference (crosstalk) in multislice acquisitions and can alter the validity of SNR measurements in all pulse sequences.

When the ACR MRI Accreditation phantom is used to perform this test, the lengths of 2 signal ramps located within the slice thickness insert in slice 1 are measured. To meet the ACR criteria, the measured slice thickness should be 5.0 mm ± 0.7 mm.

Radiofrequency Coils (Fig. 13-15)

The performance of the RF coils used to generate MR images is critical to the overall performance of the MR system as a whole. Currently, the ACR requires 3 different measurements for volume coils and 1 measurement for surface coils. The QC tests required for volume coils provide measurements of image uniformity, SNR, and percent signal ghosting. The QC test used for surface coils measures only the maximum SNR.

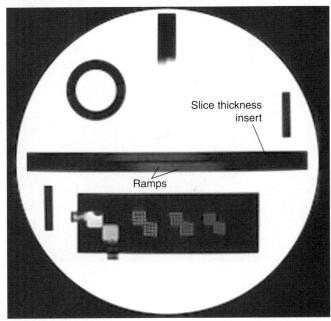

FIGURE 13-12 Slice 1 from ACR T2 series demonstrating the slice thickness insert and signal ramps. *(Courtesy St. Luke's Health System.)*

1. Use slice 1 of the ACR T1 and T2 phantom test series and magnify the images by a factor of 2 to 4, making sure the keep the slice thickness insert visible within the displayed image (Fig. 13-12).
2. Display the images with a narrow window level and window width to provide optimal visualization of the signal ramps.
3. Place a rectangular ROI at the middle of each signal ramp and note the mean signal values for both ROIs, then average the 2 values together (Fig. 13-13).
4. Lower the window level of the display to half of the average of the ramp signal calculated in step 3.
5. Measure the length of the top and bottom ramps and record their lengths (Fig. 13-14).
   Note: The following formula is used to calculate slice thickness:

   slice thickness $= 0.2 \times (\text{top} \times \text{bottom})/(\text{top} + \text{bottom})$

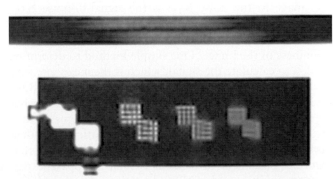

FIGURE 13-13 Magnified portion of slice 1 showing placement for rectangular ROIs to measure average signal in the ramps. *(Courtesy St. Luke's Health System.)*

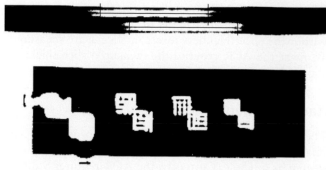

FIGURE 13-14 Magnified portion of slice 1 showing measurements for the slice thickness signal ramps. *(Courtesy St. Luke's Health System.)*

PROCEDURE

1. Place the phantom in the center of the magnet and perform a typical multislice acquisition, from a commonly used clinical protocol, with a slice thickness of 10 mm in the axial plane.
2. Select an image and place an ROI over the center of the image. The ROI should cover at least 10% of the area of the phantom or 100 pixels, whichever is greater. The mean pixel value from the ROI represents the signal.
3. Place the same ROI over the background and record the standard deviation, which represents the noise inherent in the system.
4. The formula for calculating the SNR is 1.41 × (Mean ÷ Standard deviation).

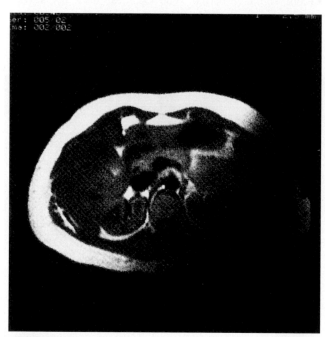

FIGURE 13-15 Nonuniformity of image intensity produced by radiofrequency (RF) field inhomogeneity. Note the region of hypointensity in the left flank. The cause in this case is improper setting of active shim coil current; an unwanted focal gradient is produced in the main magnetic field. *(From Ros PR, Bidgood WD: Abdominal magnetic resonance imaging, St Louis, 1993, Mosby. Courtesy GE Medical Systems, Milwaukee, Wis.)*

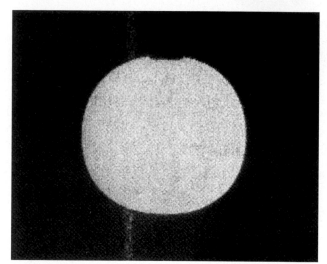

FIGURE 13-16 Radiofrequency (RF) interference from a steady carrier frequency source. A strong signal from the nitrogen fill–monitor circuit is detected within the pass-band of the magnetic resonance imaging (MRI) receiver. It is displayed as a full vertical column perpendicular to the *x* coordinate that corresponds to the frequency of the spurious signal. The overall receiver performance is degraded by intermodulation distortion, which causes the background noise level to rise in comparison with the signal of the phantom. *(From Ros PR, Bidgood WD: Abdominal magnetic resonance imaging, St Louis, 1993, Mosby. Courtesy Siemens Medical Systems, Iselin, N.J.)*

Signal-to-Noise Ratio. The ratio of signal intensity in the image to the noise level is the signal-to-noise ratio (SNR). Although some describe it in complicated mathematical calculations, others simplify it as a measure of the graininess of the image. One simple method to determine SNR is to calculate the signal, which is the mean intensity within a uniform phantom region of interest (ROI), divided by the noise, which is the standard deviation within an ROI in the background. Most MR systems have a means to calculate the SNR automatically. When performing tests to measure SNR, one must be aware that incorrect placement of ROIs can result in apparent artifacts that will impede SNR calculations. Several factors can influence SNR; resonance frequency, RF shielding, scanning parameters, field strength, RF coil performance, and general system calibration (Figs. 13-16 and 13-17).

Image Intensity Uniformity. Image intensity uniformity is a parameter that describes the spatial sensitivity of RF coils. An image intensity uniformity test measures the image intensity over a large uniform area of a homogeneous phantom lying in the sensitive region of a volume RF coil (see Box 13-2).

Percent Signal Ghosting (PSG). Artifacts that appear as a faint copy of the imaged object or as multiple replications of the object smeared along the phase encode direction are called phase-encode ghosts. Ghost artifacts are created as a result of signal instability between pulse cycle repetitions. The percent signal ghosting test assesses the level of ghosting in the images.

The following procedure uses the ACR MRI accreditation phantom to measure the SNR, percent image uniformity, and percent signal ghosting of volume coils:

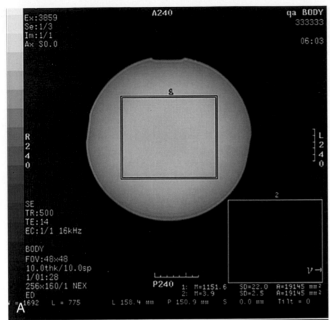

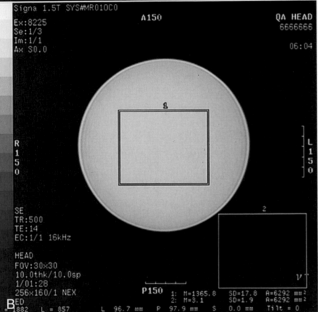

FIGURE 13-17 A, A signal-to-noise ratio (SNR) test performed with the body coil phantom. **B,** An SNR test performed with the head coil phantom. Note that the head coil yields a higher SNR.

FOV, Field of view; *ROI,* region of interest.

Interslice Radiofrequency Interference. Interslice RF interference tests can be used to determine how close slices can be before adjacent slices interfere with each other. The effects of interslice RF interference can be due to miscalibrated transmit modulators or a poor RF slice profile, or both. The ACR recommends that the SNR should not be reduced more than 20% when comparing images acquired with 100% gap to images acquired with 0 gap.

Soft-copy Display Devices

More and more radiology services are providing primary readings from soft-copy display devices. Soft-copy display has, in fact, replaced film in many institutions. As a primary diagnostic tool, soft-copy devices should be tested at acceptance testing and at regular intervals thereafter for maximum and minimum luminance, luminance uniformity, resolution, and spatial accuracy. The ACR's suggested performance criteria for soft-copy display devices are as follows:

- Maximum luminance should exceed 90 Cd m-2, and minimum luminance should be less than 1.2 Cd m-2.

(Continued)

PROCEDURE—CONT'D

7. Determine the noise standard deviation as the root mean square value of all the pixel intensities in the "noise ROI." Record the value on the data form.

8. Place 4 elliptical ROI's outside the phantom along the 4 edges of the field of view. The elliptical ROIs should have a length-to-width ratio of 4:1 and a total area of about 10 cm. Record the mean value for each ROI and label them according to position: left, right, top and bottom.

9. The SNR is calculated by dividing the mean signal by the standard deviation.

10. The percent image uniformity (PIU) is calculated using the following formula:

$$PIU = 100 \times [1 - (\text{maximum signal} - \text{minimum signal})/ (\text{maximum signal} + \text{minimum signal})]$$

11. The percent signal ghosting (PSG) is calculated using the following formula, which gives the value for ghosting as a fraction of the primary signal:

$$\text{ghost ratio} = \{[(\text{top} + \text{bottom}) - (\text{left} + \text{right})]/ [2 \times (\text{mean signal})]\}$$

The ACR criteria for SNR, PIU, and PSG are

SNR: no significant change from baseline

PIU $\geq$ 87.5% for MR systems with field strengths less than 3T and $\geq$ 82.0% for 3T MR systems

ghosting ratio: $\leq$ 0.025

• Luminance uniformity should be within 30% of the maximum brightness measured in the center of the screen.

• Resolution: The monitor should display a resolution bar pattern of 100% contrast when the spatial frequency of the bar phantom is equal to half the monitor line frequency in vertical and horizontal directions.

• Spatial accuracy: Lines displayed on the monitor should be straight to within + 5 mm.

OPTIONAL TESTS

Signal-to-Noise Ratio Consistency

The repeatability of an RF coil's performance can be tested during the annual testing of the RF coil's performance. This is done by conducting SNR tests on a specific coil several times separated by a few hours. Variations of more than a few percentage points can reflect intermittent system or noise problems.

Magnetic Fringe Field

Periodically checking the magnet's fringe field is a good idea to ensure that all spaces over 5 gauss have appropriate warning signs. Many instances of a magnet's fringe field exceeding the posted 5 gauss line have occurred. This violates the Food and Drug Administration requirements and could present a potential source of liability.

SUMMARY

Quality control procedures for MRI are becoming more prevalent because of the introduction of the MR Site Accreditation program by the American College of Radiology (ACR) in the spring of 1997. The ACR has a dedicated quality control component to the application for the accreditation process. A specific phantom must be used;

information about the entire process can be obtained by contacting the ACR (www.acr.org). Like all quality management and accreditation processes, documentation of all quality control testing and maintenance of all records is imperative for program success. Many imaging facilities where quality control was not routinely performed now have to be educated on the various testing methods and quality factors. Although some facilities do just what is necessary to get by, others with dedicated quality assurance departments likely have a comprehensive program for each imaging modality. In MRI this can include assessment of the placement of a warning sign, fire alarms and extinguishers, magnet quench procedures, computer room air conditioners, the patient/technologist intercom, the resetting of halon systems, the start-up and shutdown of MR systems, and even jam clearing in the camera and processor.

Training and competency assessment of new and existing MR personnel help maintain the overall quality of the facility. With a limited operating budget, MR technologists often are required to do a considerable amount of error troubleshooting before calling for service. Ironically, productivity issues may drive quality assurance programs, whereas quality assurance should be thought of as enhancing productivity.

Refer to the Evolve website at https://evolve.elsevier. com for Student Experiment 13.1: Magnetic Resonance Scanners.

REVIEW QUESTIONS

1. Phantoms for MRI quality control tests are made with which material?
   a. Aluminum
   b. Copper
   c. Manganese
   d. All of the above

2. Daily quality control tests should be performed by which employee?
   a. Medical physicist
   b. MR technologist
   c. Service engineer
   d. System specialist

3. When the SNR test is performed, changing the imaging parameters does not affect the resulting SNR.
   a. False
   b. True

4. Which equation is used to calculate the system's resonance frequency?
   a. Bloch
   b. Fourier
   c. Larmor
   d. Plank

5. Between which of the following should image uniformity values range?
   a. 20% and 40%
   b. 40% and 60%
   c. 60% and 80%
   d. 80% and 100%

6. The phantom used for the spatial linearity test can be the same as the phantom for the resonance frequency test.
   a. False
   b. True

7. Which of the following terms identifies the quality control test performed to ensure that the landmarking location is at the isocenter?
   a. Slice position
   b. Slice thickness
   c. Slice uniformity
   d. Spatial localization

8. An acquisition with a 20-cm FOV and a 1282 matrix yields a pixel of what size?
   a. 0.78 mm^2
   b. 1.56 mm^2
   c. 1.92 mm^2
   d. 2.56 mm^2

9. What term is used to describe the quality factor of the coil used to receive signals?
   a. Coil Q
   b. Receiver setting
   c. Resonance frequency
   d. SNR

10. Which of the following personnel are considered key to a good quality control MR program?
    a. Medical physicist
    b. MR technologist
    c. Service engineer
    d. All of the above

Ultrasound Equipment Quality Assurance

James A. Zagzebski and James Kofler

OBJECTIVES

At the completion of this chapter the reader will be able to do the following:
- Discuss the importance of quality assurance for ultrasound equipment
- Describe the various phantoms used in ultrasound quality assurance
- Identify the basic quality control tests for ultrasound
- Explain the importance of documentation of quality assurance testing
- Describe the basic quality control testing for Doppler color flow equipment

In an imaging facility, quality assurance is a process carried out to ensure that equipment is operating consistently at its expected level of performance. During routine scanning each sonographer is vigilant for equipment changes that can lead to suboptimal imaging and might require service. Thus in some ways, ultrasound equipment quality assurance is carried out every day, even when it is not identified as a process itself.

Quality assurance steps to be discussed here go beyond judgments of scanner performance that are made during routine ultrasound imaging. They involve prospective actions to identify problem situations, even before obvious equipment malfunctions occur. Quality assurance testing provides confidence that image data such as distance measurements and area estimations are accurate and that the image is of the best possible quality from the imaging instrument.

COMPONENTS OF AN ULTRASOUND QUALITY ASSURANCE PROGRAM

Quality Assurance and Preventive Maintenance

Various approaches are used by ultrasound facilities when setting up a quality assurance program for their scanners. Sometimes these programs include both preventive maintenance procedures performed by trained equipment service personnel and in-house testing of scanners with phantoms and test objects. Some facilities rely on only one of these measures. For preventive maintenance, emphasis is usually given to invasive electronic testing of system components such as voltage measurements at test points inside the scanner. Sometimes preventive maintenance also involves an assessment of the imaging capability by scanning a phantom.

In-house scanner quality assurance programs usually involve imaging phantoms or test objects and assessing the results. In-house tests may be performed by sonographers, physicians, medical physicists, clinical engineers, or equipment maintenance personnel. Detailed recommendations from professional organizations and experts in ultrasound on establishing an in-house quality assurance program are available elsewhere (ACR Ultrasound Accreditation Program, 2001; Goodsitt et al., 1998; Zagzebski, 2000).

Tissue-Mimicking Phantoms

In-house scanner quality assurance tests most often are performed with tissue-mimicking phantoms. In medical ultrasound a **phantom** is a device that mimics soft tissues in its ultrasound transmission characteristics. Phantoms represent "constant patients," and images can be taken at different times for close comparison. Image penetration capabilities, for example, are readily evaluated for changes over time when images of a phantom are available for comparison. Phantoms also have targets in known positions, so images can be compared closely with the region that is scanned. Examples include simulated cysts, echogenic structures, and thin "line targets."

Tissue Properties Represented in Phantoms

Tissue characteristics mimicked in commercially available phantoms are the speed of sound; ultrasonic attenuation; and, to some degree, echogenicity (i.e., the ultrasonic scattering level). Phantoms cannot exactly replicate the acoustic properties of soft tissues. This is partially due to the complexity and variability of tissues. Instead, phantom manufacturers construct these objects to have acoustic properties that represent the average properties of many different tissues. Sometimes the term *tissue-equivalent* is used when phantoms are described; however, this term should not be interpreted literally because most phantom materials are not acoustically equivalent to any specific tissue.

Typical Quality Assurance Phantom Design

An example of a general purpose ultrasound quality assurance phantom is shown in Figure 14-1. Such phantoms are examined with scanner settings that are similar to those used when patients are being scanned. The phantom images have gray-scale characteristics that are analogous to characteristics of organs, although the actual structures are not anatomically represented.

Figure 14-1, *B* shows the internal structure of this phantom. The tissue-mimicking material within the phantom consists of a water-based gelatin in which microscopic particles are mixed uniformly throughout the volume (Burlew et al., 1980; Madsen et al., 1978). The speed of sound in this material is about 1540 m/sec, the same speed assumed in the calibration of ultrasound instruments. The ultrasonic attenuation coefficient versus frequency is one of two values: either 0.5 dB/cm per megahertz or 0.7 dB/cm per megahertz (Box 14-1). Some users prefer the lower-attenuating material because they find it easier to image objects in the phantom. However, standards groups recommend the higher attenuation because it challenges machines more thoroughly (Zagzebski, 2000).

Attenuation in the gel-graphite material in the phantom is proportional to the ultrasound frequency and mimics the behavior in tissues (Lu et al., 1999; Madsen et al., 1978; Maklad et al., 1984). Other types of materials have been used in phantoms, but only water-based gels laced with powder have both speed of sound and attenuation with tissuelike properties (Madsen et al., 1978; Zagzebski, 2000).

Small scatterers are distributed throughout the tissue-mimicking material; therefore, the phantoms appear echogenic when scanned with ultrasound imaging equipment (see Fig. 14-1, *C*). Many phantoms have simulated "cysts," which are low-attenuating, nonechogenic cylinders. These should appear echo free on B-mode images and should exhibit distal echo enhancement. Some tissue phantoms provide additional image contrast by having simulated masses or test objects of varying echogenicity. Such objects are evident in Figure 14-1, *C*.

Most quality assurance phantoms also contain discrete reflectors such as nylon-line targets to be used mainly for evaluating the distance measurement

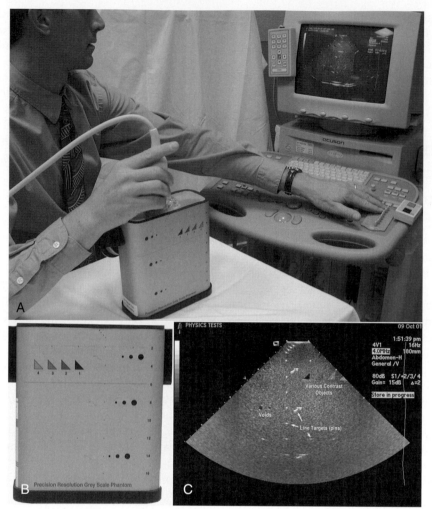

FIGURE 14-1 Example of a general-purpose quality assurance phantom. **A,** Phantom being imaged with an ultrasound scanner. **B,** Close-up of phantom, with diagram of interior contents. **C,** B-mode image of the phantom.

BOX 14-1 | Tissue Attenuation Coefficients

Attenuation coefficients are normally specified in decibels per centimeter. To include the dependence of attenuation on frequency, phantom manufacturers divide the attenuation coefficient by the frequency at which the measurement is done. This yields units of decibels per centimeter per megahertz. Strictly speaking, this approach should be used only when attenuation is directly proportional to the frequency, as we often assume for tissues. The value of 0.7 dB/cm per megahertz is representative of the attenuation coefficient in difficult-to-penetrate fatty liver.* The depth that structures can be visualized within tissue-mimicking material having this amount of attenuation more closely correlates with clinical penetration.

*Lu ZF, Lee FT, Zagzebski JA: Ultrasonic backscatter and attenuation in diffuse liver disease, *Ultrasound Med Biol* 25:1047, 1999.

accuracy of a scanner. Tests of the accuracy of distance measurements rely on the manufacturer of the phantom to have filled the device with a material with a sound propagation speed of 1540 m/sec or at least close enough to this speed that no appreciable errors are

introduced in calibrations. These phantoms also rely on the manufacturer having defined the reflector positions accurately. With the correct speed of sound (1540 m/sec) and precisely known distances between pointlike reflectors, it is easy to check the accuracy of distance measurements with calipers, as described later.

Phantoms often contain a column of reflectors, each separated by 1 or 2 cm, for vertical measurement accuracy tests. One or more horizontal rows of reflectors are used for assessing horizontal measurement accuracy. Additional sets of reflectors may be found for assessing the axial resolution and the lateral resolution of scanners.

Cautions About Phantom Desiccation

When a phantom made of water-based gels is used, loss of water (desiccation) may become a problem as the phantom ages. If this occurs, the speed of sound in the phantom may have changed. A scanning surface that has become concave is an indication of severe

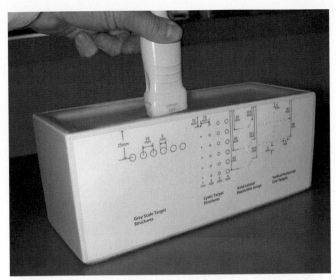

FIGURE 14-2 A phantom with rubber-based, tissue-mimicking small parts. Although the acoustic properties are not as precise as the water-based phantoms, less care is required during manufacturing and with on-site storage to minimize changes over time.

desiccation. Occasionally, water losses become so problematic that air entering the phantom window leads to the inability to image the phantom effectively. Users should follow the instructions given by the phantom manufacturer to avoid significant desiccation. For example, some manufacturers recommend storage in a humid, airtight container, and this practice should be adhered to if so stated.

Desiccation is not a problem with rubber-based phantom materials (Fig. 14-2) produced by some manufacturers. Storing these phantoms with the tissue-mimicking material directly exposed to the environment can be an advantage compared with water-based gels. The main disadvantages of rubber materials are that their speed of sound is lower than 1540 m/sec ($\approx$1450 m/sec in some rubber-based phantoms) and that their attenuation is not proportional to the ultrasound frequency (Zagzebski, 2000). Therefore, they may not be as effective as water-based gel phantoms when imaging over a large frequency range.

BASIC QUALITY CONTROL TESTS

A recommended set of instrument quality control tests includes checks for the consistency of instrument sensitivity; evaluation of image uniformity; assessment of gray-scale photography or image workstation brightness levels; and, where necessary, checks of both vertical and horizontal distance measurement accuracy (ACR Ultrasound Accreditation Program, 2001; Goodsitt et al., 1998; Zagzebski, 2000). This group of tests can be performed by a sonographer in 10 to 15 minutes, which includes the time for recording the results on a worksheet or in a notebook.

Visual Inspection

The visual inspection is used to evaluate the physical condition of the scanner's mechanical components, along with a few quick scan tests. This should be performed monthly or according to the user manual provided by the manufacturer. A checklist for documentation of the visual inspection is found on the enclosed CD-ROM. Some of the items to check during the visual inspection are described as follows.

Transducers: Cables, housings, and transmitting surfaces should be checked for cracks, separations, and discolorations. Any bent or loose prongs on the plug should be fixed.

Power cord: The cable and plug should be checked for any cracks, discoloration, and damage.

Control panel: Check for dirty or broken switches and knobs, as well as any burnt-out indicator lights.

Video monitor: The video display monitor should be clean and free of scratches. The brightness and contrast controls should be set at proper levels.

Wheels and wheel locks: All wheels should be checked to ensure that they rotate freely and that the unit is easy to maneuver. The wheels also should be seated securely, and wheel locks should be checked to ensure they lock securely.

Dust filters: Dust filters should be inspected and free of lint and clumps of dirt. Otherwise, overheating of the internal electronic components can occur and shorten the life span of the unit.

Scanner housing: The unit should be inspected for dents or other "cosmetic" damage, which could indicate events that might have caused damage to the internal components.

Transducer Choice

Results of some test procedures depend on which transducer/frequency combination is used with the instrument. On systems in which several transducers are available, tests should be done with two transducers (ACR Ultrasound Accreditation Program, 2001). Choose the most common transducer that is used in most examinations; additionally, it is preferable to test another transducer that has a different frequency range and a different scan format. For example, with a general-purpose scanner, a low-frequency (2 to 5 MHz) curvilinear or phased array and an intermediate-frequency (5 to 8 MHz) or even a high-frequency linear array are appropriate. This transducer combination should be used for all subsequent test procedures. All necessary transducer assembly identification information should be checked including the frequency, size, and serial number so that future tests will be conducted with the same probe. If several identical scanners are available, the same transducer/scanner pairs should be used for all subsequent testing.

System Sensitivity

The **sensitivity** of an instrument refers to the weakest echo signal level that can be detected and displayed clearly enough to be discernible on an image. Most scanners have controls that vary the receiver amplification (gain) and the transmit level (e.g., output or power). These are used to adjust the sensitivity during clinical examinations. The *maximum sensitivity* of the instrument occurs when these controls are at maximum practical settings. Often the maximum sensitivity is limited by electrical noise that appears on the display when the receiver gain is at maximum levels. The noise may be generated externally, for example, by electronic communication networks or by computer terminals. More commonly the noise arises from within the instrument itself, such as in the first preamplification stage of the receiver amplifier.

Concerns during quality assurance tests are usually centered on whether notable variations in sensitivity have occurred since the last quality assurance test. Such variations might result from a variety of causes such as damaged transducers, damaged transducer cables, or electronic drift in the pulser-receiver components of the scanner. Questions related to the sensitivity of a scanner sometimes occur during clinical imaging; a quick scan of the quality assurance phantom and comparison with results of the most recent quality assurance test help determine whether there is cause for concern.

A commonly used technique for detecting variations in maximum sensitivity is the measure of the maximum **depth of visualization** for signals from scattered echoes in the tissue-mimicking phantom (ACR Ultrasound Accreditation Program, 2001; AIUM standard methods for measuring performance of ultrasound pulse-echo equipment, 1990; Carson and Goodsitt, 1995; Goodsitt et al., 1998; Zagzebski, 2000). The technique includes the following:

1. Adjust the output power transmit levels and receiver sensitivity controls so that echo signals are obtained from as deep as possible into the phantom. Now the output power control is positioned for maximum output, and the receiver gain is adjusted for the highest values without excessive noise on the display. (Experience helps in establishing these control settings; they should be recorded in the quality control worksheet, which is described later.)
2. Scan the phantom and estimate the maximum depth of visualization of texture echo signals (Fig. 14-3).
3. File a digital or hard copy image of the phantom.

In the examples in Figure 14-3, the maximum depth of visualization is 16.8 cm at 4 MHz. With a 2-MHz mode, the maximum depth of visualization is at least as deep as the length of the phantom, so it cannot be measured with this phantom. The lower frequency results in a lower attenuation and therefore greater maximum depth of visualization.

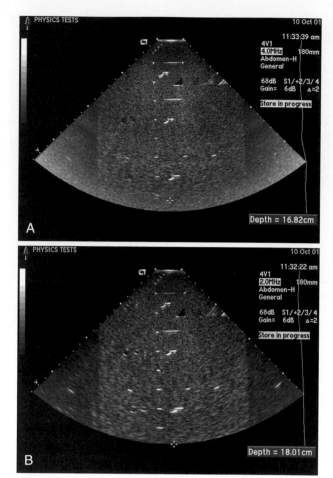

FIGURE 14-3 Images obtained for the maximum depth of the visualization quality assurance test with a multifrequency array transducer. The phantom has an attenuation coefficient of 0.7 dB/cm per megahertz. **A,** At 4 MHz the maximum depth of visualization is 16.8 cm. **B,** At 2 MHz the maximum depth of visualization cannot be determined with this phantom because visualization remains excellent all the way to the bottom of the phantom.

For the test results to be interpreted, a comparison is made with maximum visualization results from a previous test, perhaps 6 months earlier. Results should agree within 1 cm. Normal trial-to-trial variations in scanning and interpretation prohibit closer calls than this. However, with digital or hard-copy images and records of maximum depth of visualization tests, ascertaining whether a scanner/transducer combination has drifted significantly over time in echo detection capabilities should be possible.

In addition to this measurement being made with the standard transducer, occasionally performing the test with different transducers is useful. For example, the test can be performed with all of the transducers that are available for each instrument when quality control tests are first established and semiannually thereafter. This method helps pinpoint the source of any decrease in the maximum sensitivity. If the maximum depth of visualization decreases on all of the transducers tested on a specific scanner, the problem is most likely associated with the scanner and not the transducer assemblies.

Photography and Gray-Scale Hard Copy

Perhaps the most frequent source of ultrasound instrument variability over time is related to image photography. Too often, drift in the imaging instrument, in the hard-copy cameras, or in film processing reduces image quality to the point that significant amounts of detail related to echo signal amplitude variations are lost on hard-copy B-mode images. However, if image viewing monitors and recording devices are set up properly and if sufficient attention is given to photography during routine quality control, these problems can be reduced. The advent of laser printers with automatic (or semiautomatic) calibration has greatly reduced much of the variability of producing a hard-copy image. However, even laser printers have problems.

Monitor Setup and Recording Devices. Most instruments provide both an image display monitor, which is viewed during scan buildup, and an image recording device. As a general rule the display monitor should be set up properly first, and then adjustments should be made, if necessary, to the laser printers or other hard-copy recording devices to produce acceptable gray scale on hard-copy images. The establishment of proper settings is expected only during the installation of a scanner, during major upgrades, or during the detection of image problems. Changes made to the display settings are not automatically reflected in the printed image. Changing the display settings requires adjustment of the hard-copy device to properly match the printed image to the displayed image; therefore, image display settings should not be shifted routinely. Many facilities go so far as to remove the control knobs on image monitors once the contrast and brightness are adjusted to an acceptable level; thus, the temptation to change settings casually is removed.

An effective method for setting up both viewing and hard-copy devices has been described by Gray (1985).

It is recommended that adjustments be done with an image that contains a clinically representative sampling of gray shades.

1. First, attend to the display monitor viewed during scanning. With the contrast settings of the monitor initially set at minimum settings, adjust the brightness to a level that just allows television raster lines to be discernible.
2. After the adjustment, increase the monitor contrast until just before the text on the display begins to become distorted (the text, which is typically displayed at a maximum brightness, begins to smear to the left and right if the contrast is too high). Verify that the settings are adequate with a clinical image.

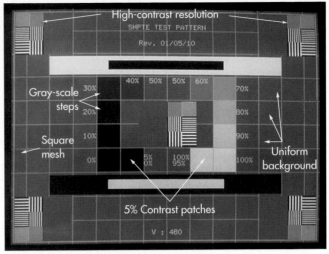

FIGURE 14-4 A test pattern of the Society of Motion Picture and Television Engineers (SMPTE). The pattern contains a gray-scale range in increments of 10% video level. There are also 5% contrast patches at the 0% *(black)* and 100% *(white)* levels, a mesh pattern to check for spatial distortions, and several resolution patterns.

After the viewing monitor is properly adjusted, make provisions to prevent casual changes in settings by department personnel.

3. Adjust the image recording device to obtain the same gray shades that appear on the display monitor. This adjustment may require several repetitions, varying the contrast and the overall brightness, until satisfactory results are obtained. Many manufacturers provide gray-scale test patterns such as a pattern by the Society of Motion Picture and Television Engineers (SMPTE) (Fig. 14-4) that can be displayed on the scanner. These patterns are useful for matching the hard-copy image to the display image. If such a pattern is unavailable, a small gray-scale bar is usually presented on the real-time image.

Routine Quality Assurance of Image Recording. Routine checks should be performed on the quality of gray-scale photography or other hard-copy recording media. Detailed analysis performed in some installations includes film sensitometry and film-emulsion batch crossovers. These processes are well established and documented (Goodsitt et al., 1998) and are not explained in detail. Images of a tissue-mimicking phantom, along with the gray-bar pattern that appears on the edge of most image displays, can be used for routinely assessing photography settings. In photography and processing, all brightness variations in the viewing monitor image should be successfully recorded on the hard-copy image.

A quick check of gray-scale recording can be done as follows:

1. On an image of a tissue-mimicking phantom (or of a patient), check to see whether weak echo signal dots appearing on the viewing monitor are successfully recorded on film.

2. Determine whether the entire gray bar is visible and whether all gray levels are distinguishable. For example, for a scanner with a gray bar including 15 levels of gray, along with the background, the hard-copy image should portray distinctions among all of the different levels. Continuous gray bars are more of a visual challenge when display bars are compared with printed gray levels. In this case, focus attention on the light and dark ends of the patterns and compare the differences in the extent of white and black areas on the bars. The suggested action level is any optical density that is greater than or equal to 0.2 optical density units from the baseline.

3. The entire length of the gray bar pattern displayed on the viewing monitor should be visible on the final image (see Fig. 14-3, *B*). For multiple images on a single sheet of film or paper, all of the images should have the same background brightness and should display the gray-bar pattern in the same manner. These images can be verified from clinical images taken on the same day the quality assurance tests are taken or from the quality assurance films themselves.

4. Some laser printers offer features for setting other characteristics of the printed image such as border width and background density. These settings should be decided, usually by trial and error, by all of those involved in reading the images. Once a conclusion has been reached, the settings should be installed in all printing devices used for ultrasound and documented for future reference.

Many imaging facilities now use digital images archived on computer systems and image workstations, rather than film recording. Workstation displays require periodic evaluation to ensure optimum performance. The displays should be cleaned periodically and before any quality assurance testing. Ideally, a lint-free cloth should be used for wiping the surface of the display. Cleaning solution should be applied to the cloth and not sprayed directly on the display. Some displays, especially flat-panel displays, may require specific cleaning products because of antiglare or other special coatings on the screen surface, so the manufacturer's cleaning instructions should be checked before applying any chemical product to the display. Storing a cloth and cleaner solution next to the workstation display is a convenient practice to promote a dust-free, clean display screen.

The SMPTE pattern (see Fig. 14-4) is useful for the routine quality assurance of displays. The large squares on the SMPTE pattern are used to note any distortions caused by the display; they should appear as an array of perfect squares over the entire screen. Degradation of monitor resolution can be noted by viewing the high-contrast resolution patterns and the text on the SMPTE pattern. These should appear well-defined, not blurry or smeared. The 5% contrast patches should be visible in the 100% video *(white)* and 0% video *(black)*

squares. The gray background of the SMPTE pattern should be uniformly gray across the entire display.

The following characteristics should be noted when performing display quality assurance (Groth et al., 2001):

- *Monitor cleanliness.* The display screen should be free of dust or other markings (e.g., pen markings and fingerprints).
- *Spatial distortion.* The display should be serviced if the squares on the SMPTE pattern are distorted at the corners or if their aspect ratios (width/height) are not correct (e.g., a square shape that appears to be rectangular). Some displays provide controls that allow the user to correct minor spatial distortions.
- *Monitor resolution (edge definition).* Any high-contrast boundary such as white text on a dark background should be well-defined.
- *Gray-scale uniformity.* The intensity on the display should be consistent over the entire screen. This requires a test pattern that contains a constant gray level over the entire screen or at least at all four sides and in the center. Moving a small uniform image from one side of the screen to the other is typically an ineffective alternative to a single large image.
- *Low-contrast visibility.* The 5% difference in video level (on black and on white) of the SMPTE pattern should be noticeable on the display. Room lighting should be minimal when viewing low-contrast objects. Alternatively, the entire gray bar pattern seen on the scanner monitor should be visualized on the workstation monitor.
- *Display artifacts.* The display should not contain streaks, lines, or dark/light patches. If a test pattern of uniform brightness is unavailable, the brightest pattern available should be used. In this case, the observer must "look through" the test objects at the background of the image. A few nonfunctioning (dropped) pixels, which appear as small black dots, may be tolerable. However, a group of dropped pixels or several dropped pixels scattered over the screen warrants replacement of the display.

Scan Image Uniformity

Ultrasound phantoms typically contain a background material that is distributed throughout the phantom. However, with most phantoms it is impossible to acquire a view that does not contain any test objects. In these cases, **scan image uniformity** can be assessed by focusing attention solely on the background material of the phantom. Ideally, when a region within a phantom is scanned and the machine's gain settings are adjusted properly, the resultant image has a uniform brightness throughout (Fig. 14-5, *A*). Nonuniformities caused by the ultrasound imager can occur because of the following situations:

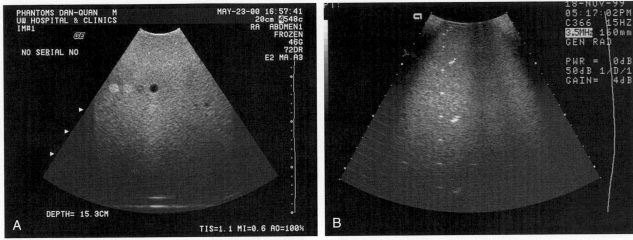

FIGURE 14-5 Image uniformity tests. **A,** Good uniformity. **B,** Results with a transducer that should be repaired or replaced. Note the vertical streaks that are evidence of element dropout for this linear array transducer.

- Bad elements in a linear or curved array or loose connections in beam former board plug-ins can lead to vertically oriented nonuniformities (see Fig. 14-5, *B*). (Boards can be loosened if the scanner is wheeled over bumps or if it is transported by a van to other hospitals or clinics.)
- Inadequate side-to-side image compensation in the machine can lead to variations in brightness from one side of the image to another.
- Inadequate blending of pixel data between transmit and receive focal zones can lead to horizontal or curved streaks parallel to the transducer surface. Quality assurance testing is an ideal time to assess whether such faults are noticeable. An image is taken of a uniform region in the quality assurance phantom, and the image is inspected for these problems.

A uniformity image is useful in the detection of subtle artifacts that may not be readily evident on the clinical images. Care should be taken to inspect the image thoroughly for any streaks, any dark or light patches, or any gray-scale gradients in the axial or lateral directions. Occasionally a swirling pattern with the background texture may be noticed. However, this pattern is typically a result of the phantom manufacturing process, which can be verified by comparison with uniformity images from other transducers. The suggested action level would be nonuniformity greater than or equal to 4 dB or any consistent measurable change from the baseline.

Distance Measurement Accuracy

Instruments used for measuring structure dimensions, organ sizes, and areas can be tested periodically for accuracy of distance indicators. However, many individuals think that routine distance measurement accuracy checks are not useful because digital measurement

systems on scanners exhibit satisfactory stability over time (ACR Ultrasound Accreditation Program, 2001; Goodsitt et al., 1998).

Distance indicators usually include 1-cm-deep markers on M-mode and B-mode scanning displays and electronic calipers on B-mode scanning systems. Calipers on workstations that are part of computer archiving systems also should be checked for accuracy. The principal distance measurement tests are separated into two parts: one part is for measurements along the sound beam axis, which is referred to as the **vertical distance measurement** test, or the *axial distance measurement test,* and the other part is for measurements taken perpendicular to the sound beam axis, which is called the **horizontal distance measurement** test.

Vertical Distance Measurements. Vertical distance measurement accuracy also is called *depth calibration accuracy* in some texts.

1. To evaluate a scanner's vertical distance measurement accuracy, scan the phantom, ensuring that the vertical column of reflectors in the phantom is clearly imaged (Fig. 14-6).
2. Position the digital calipers to measure the distance between any two reflectors in this column.
   - Correct caliper placement is from the top of the echo from the first reflector to the top of the echo from the second reflector or from any position on the first reflector to the corresponding position on the second reflector.
   - When testing general-purpose scanners, choose reflectors positioned at least 8 to 10 cm apart for this test. Most laboratories also measure a smaller spacing such as 4 cm. For small-parts scanners and probes, use a distance of 1 or 2 cm. In general, the largest separation allowed by the transducer/frequency combination and the target placement in the phantom is appropriate for the distance accuracy test.

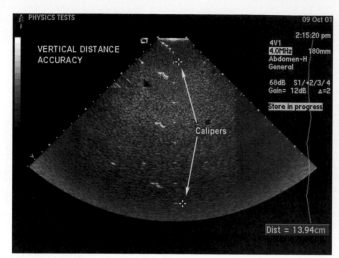

FIGURE 14-6 Vertical distance measurement check. The caliper reading (13.94 cm) is compared with the actual separation (14 cm) between pins positioned along a vertical column in the phantom. Shorter distances should be used when high-frequency transducers are evaluated.

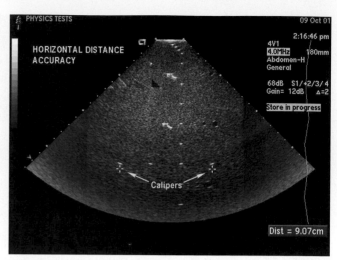

FIGURE 14-7 Horizontal distance measurement check. The caliper reading (90.7 mm) is for a measurement taken horizontally on the image and compared with the actual pin separation (90 mm).

3. Determine that the measured distance agrees with the actual distance given by the phantom manufacturer to within 1 mm or 1.5%, whichever is greater. If a larger discrepancy occurs, consult with the ultrasound scanner manufacturer for possible corrective measures.

Horizontal Distance Measurements. Horizontal measurement accuracy should be checked in a manner similar to vertical distance measurement. Measurements obtained in this direction (Fig. 14-7) are frequently less accurate because of beam width effects and scanner inaccuracies. Nevertheless, results should agree with the phantom manufacturer's distances to within 3 mm or 3%, whichever is greater. Correct caliper placement for this test is from the center of one reflector to the center of the second reflector. For the example in Figure 14-7, measurement results are within 1 mm of the actual distance between the reflectors examined. This is well within the expected level of accuracy.

Other Important Instrument Quality Assurance Tasks

During routine performance testing it is a good idea to perform other equipment-related chores that require occasional attention. These include cleaning air filters on instruments that require this service (most do); checking for loose and frayed electrical cables; looking for loose handles or control arms on the scanner; checking the wheels and wheel locks; and performing recommended preventive maintenance of photography equipment, which may include dusting or cleaning of photographic monitors and maintenance chores on cameras.

DOCUMENTATION

An important aspect of a quality assurance program is keeping track of the test results. Most laboratories want to adopt a standardized worksheet on which to write the test results. The worksheet helps the user carry out the tests in a consistent manner by having enough information to assist recall of transducers, phantoms, and machine settings. It also includes blank spaces for recording the results. An example is shown in Box 14-2.

SPATIAL RESOLUTION TESTS

Some laboratories include spatial resolution in their quality assurance testing. Measurements of spatial resolution generally require more exacting techniques to achieve results that allow intercomparisons of scanners; therefore, many centers do not do such performance tests routinely but may do so only during equipment acceptance tests (Carson and Goodsitt, 1995). Common methods for determining axial resolution and lateral resolution are discussed in this section.

Axial Resolution

Axial resolution is a measure of how close two reflectors can be to one another along the axis of an ultrasound beam and still be resolved as separate reflectors. Axial resolution also is related to the crispness of the image of a reflector arranged perpendicularly to the ultrasound beam.

Axial resolution can be estimated by measuring the thickness of the image of a line target in the quality assurance phantom. Alternatively, some phantoms contain sets of reflectors for axial resolution testing. Figure 14-8 shows both approaches. The axial separations between successive targets in this phantom are 2 mm,

BOX 14-2	Ultrasound Quality Control Results

Machine: Acuson 128   Room: E3 315
Transducer assembly: I.D.: V4   Serial no: 555–1212
Date: 9/09/97   Phantom: RMI 403GS
Instrument settings: Power 0 dB
                Dynamic range: 50 dB
                Pre 0/Persis 3/Post 0
                Gain: 12 dB
                Transmit focus: 16 cm
                Image magnification: 18 cm

1. Depth measurement accuracy
   Electronic calipers
        Measured distance . . . . 98.8 mm
        Actual distance . . . . 100 mm
        Error . . . . 1.2 mm
2. Horizontal measurement accuracy
   Electronic calipers
        Measured distance . . . . 30.5 mm
        Actual distance. . . . . 30 mm
        Error . . . . 0.5 mm
3. Depth of penetration (4 MHz)
        Measured distance . . . . 152 mm
        Baseline distance . . . . 150 mm
        Variation from baseline . . . . 2 mm
4. Image uniformity
   Significant   Excellent
   Nonuniformity   Uniformity
   1   2   3   ④   5
5. Photography
   Gray bars
        Number of gray bars visible 13
        Number of gray bars visible on baseline 15
        Variation 2
   Low-level echoes
        All echoes displayed on viewing monitor also seen on
        film: Yes X_____ No_____
   Contrast and brightness
   Level of agreement between contrast and brightness on
   viewing monitor and film:
   Poor   Excellent
   1   2   3   4   ⑤
6. Filters
   Clean _____   Dusty X_____

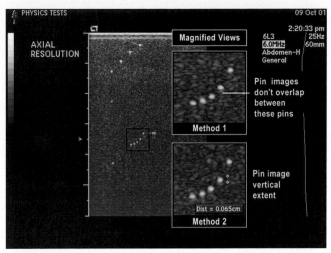

FIGURE 14-8 Axial resolution measurement. The thickness of the pin target is 0.65 mm. In the axial resolution target set (vertical separation 2 mm, 1 mm, 0.5 mm, and 0.25 mm), the 1-mm pair is separated a sufficient distance vertically so that there is no vertical overlap of the images of these two targets, whereas the 0.5-mm pair overlaps if the two targets are on a vertical line. The axial resolution is just over 0.5 mm, in agreement with the estimate made from the thickness of the single target image.

1 mm, 0.5 mm, and 0.25 mm. The targets are offset horizontally to minimize the effects of shallow targets shadowing the deeper ones. The pair most closely spaced yet clearly distinguishable in the axial direction indicates the axial resolution. This implies that to be considered resolved, the axial extent of one-pin depiction does not overlap with that of the next one below, even though the two pins may be distinguishable because of their lateral separation. Often, as in this phantom, the target pair separations are not finely spaced enough to allow a good measure of axial resolution; that is, the 0.25-mm pair in this example is not clearly resolved, whereas the 1-mm pair certainly is and the 0.5 mm is almost

resolved. The vertical thickness of a single target (0.6 mm in this case) is sometimes used (Burlew et al., 1980) to obtain more detailed indication of the axial resolution (*Method 2* in Fig. 14-8). The suggested action level is 1 mm (or 2 mm if transducer frequency is < 4 MHz) or any consistent measurable change from the baseline value.

Lateral Resolution

Lateral resolution is a measure of how close two reflectors can be to one another, be perpendicular to the beam axis, and still be distinguished as separate reflectors on an image. One approach that is used for lateral resolution tests is to measure the width on the display of a point-like target such as a line target inside a phantom. For example, Figure 14-9 shows such a measurement. The cursors indicate that the displayed width is 0.7 mm for this case. The displayed response width is related to the lateral resolution at the depth of the target. Through the imaging of targets at different depths, it is easy to see that the lateral resolution usually varies with depth for most transducers. Additionally, the lateral resolution measurement is sensitive to any focal zone placement. The suggested action level is any change greater than 1 mm from the baseline value.

Cautions About Resolution Tests with Discrete Targets

The lateral and axial dimensions of the displayed image of a point-like target depend on the power and gain settings on the machine. Such dependency is one of the

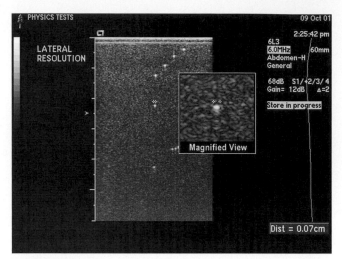

FIGURE 14-9 Lateral resolution measurement. The horizontal size of the pin target is 0.7 mm.

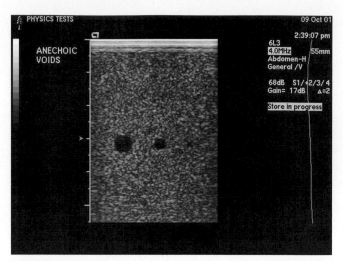

FIGURE 14-10 B-mode image of a phantom containing 3 anechoic cylinders of different sizes (6, 4, and 2 mm diameter) acquired with a 4-MHz linear transducer. Some echoes are evident within the voids, and the edges are well-defined. The smallest void is easily detectable.

difficulties of adopting such tests in routine testing. Quantitative results for axial and lateral resolution have been obtained by measuring the dimensions of point-like targets when they are imaged at specified sensitivity levels above the threshold for their display (AIUM standard methods for measuring performance of ultrasound pulse-echo equipment, 1990; Carson and Goodsitt, 1995). The procedure is as follows:

1. Obtain an image with the sensitivity of the scanner set so that the target is barely visible on the display.
2. Next, obtain a second image, with the scanner sensitivity increased 20 dB above the setting for display threshold.
3. Set the calipers to measure the lateral resolution at this scanner setting. Additional information is available elsewhere (Goodsitt et al., 1998; Zagzebski, 2000).

OTHER TEST OBJECTS AND PHANTOMS

Most general-purpose phantoms contain additional objects for the evaluation of image performance. Although these tests are not considered as essential to a routine quality assurance program, they may be useful for testing or optimizing specific imaging configurations. These tests are subjective; therefore, the comparison of results with those acquired previously is essential.

Anechoic Voids

Many phantom designs include cylindrical anechoic voids (Fig. 14-10). These voids appear as dark circular objects on an ultrasound image and can yield a wide range of information about the performance of a scanner. The void depictions can be inspected for spatial distortions; the voids should not be elliptical.

The edges of the voids should be relatively sharp, and the interior of the voids should be echo free. If voids of different sizes are available, the smallest visualized void can be noted.

Objects of Various Echogenicity

Many phantoms also include a set of objects with different inherent contrasts (Fig. 14-11). These objects can be visually assessed as a means of comparing one scan configuration with another or the performance of a specific scan configuration over time. For example, these objects may be useful to demonstrate the effect of changing the log compression. However, there must be

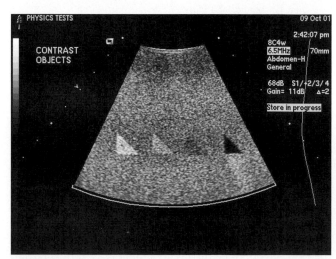

FIGURE 14-11 Image of a phantom containing four triangular-shaped objects of different contrast values acquired with a 6.5-MHz curvilinear transducer. The higher contrast objects (the outer two) are clearly visualized. The second object from the right is barely visible. The corners of the two inner objects are poorly defined.

caution when the impressions obtained by the set of various contrast objects are extrapolated into the clinical environment because the entire clinical range of inherent object contrasts may not be completely represented by the test objects. As with the anechoic voids, the perimeter of the objects can be inspected for edge definition.

Spherical Object Phantom

Another phantom becoming increasingly popular for spatial resolution tests is one that has simulated focal lesions embedded within echogenic tissue-mimicking material (AIUM standard methods for measuring performance of ultrasound pulse-echo equipment, 1990; Madsen et al., 1991). Different simulated lesion sizes and different object contrast levels (e.g., relative echogenicity) have been tried (Madsen et al., 1991). An example is shown in Figure 14-12, in which the phantom imaged contained 4-mm-diameter, low-echo masses. The centers of the masses are coplanar and distributed in a well-defined matrix.

A test of the ultrasound imaging system is used to determine the "imaging zone" for detection of masses of a given size and object contrast (Madsen et al., 1991). The 5-MHz phased array used for Figure 14-12 can successfully detect the masses over a 5- to 12-cm depth range. The **slice thickness** (Goodsitt et al., 1998) is too large for this transducer to pick up these structures at more shallow depths.

A particularly useful aspect of spherical mass phantoms is that they present realistic imaging tasks that readily demonstrate resolution capabilities in terms of resolution. For spherical targets the resolution is a combined, effective resolution composed of axial, lateral, and slice thicknesses.

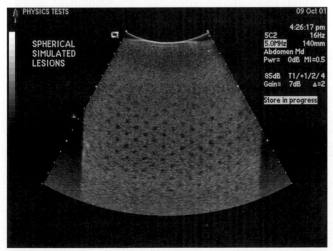

FIGURE 14-12 B-mode image of a phantom containing 4-mm low-scattering spheres that mimic cysts. The spheres are centered in a regular array within a plane, and the scanning plane is carefully aligned to coincide with the plane containing the spheres. They can be visualized from depths of 5.0 through 12.0 cm with this transducer.

If cylindrical objects are used as phantoms, only two dimensions, usually axial and lateral, are involved in their visualization. Because slice thickness is usually the worst measure of spatial resolution with array transducers, cylindrical objects can be misleading in terms of translating minimum sizes resolved into resolution of actual focal masses. The spherical lesion phantom is superior in this regard.

DOPPLER TESTING

Limited evaluations of Doppler and color flow equipment also can be made in the clinic. A number of devices including string test objects, flow velocity test objects, and flow phantoms are available to clinical users for carrying out tests of Doppler equipment (Hoskins et al., 1994; Performance criteria and measurements for Doppler ultrasound devices, 1993; Zagzebski, 1995).

String Test Objects

String test objects consist of a thin string wound around a pulley and motor-drive mechanism. The string is echogenic, so it produces echoes that are detected by an ultrasound instrument. The drive moves the string at precise velocities, either continuously or after a programmed waveform. This provides a way to evaluate the velocity measurement accuracy of Doppler devices. String test objects also may be used to evaluate the lateral and axial resolution in Doppler mode and can be used to determine the accuracy of gate registration on duplex Doppler systems (Hoskins et al., 1994).

The advantage of the string test object is that it provides a small target moving at a precisely known velocity. The disadvantages are that the echogenic characteristics of the string are not the same as those of blood and that actual blood flow, with its characteristic distribution of velocities across the vessel, is not mimicked.

Doppler Flow Phantoms

Doppler flow phantoms (Figs. 14-13 and 14-14) consist of one or more hollow tubes coursing through a block of tissue-mimicking material. A blood-mimicking fluid is pumped through the tube(s) to simulate blood flowing through vessels in the body. Usually the blood-mimicking fluid is a solution of water and glycerol that has small plastic particles suspended in it. The blood-mimicking material should provide the same echogenicity as whole human blood at the ultrasound frequencies of the machine, and reasonable representative blood-mimicking materials are now available for use in these phantoms. If the tissue-mimicking material in the body of the phantom has a representative amount of beam attenuation, the depth-dependent echogenicity of the fluid within the phantom is representative of signal levels from actual vessels in vivo.

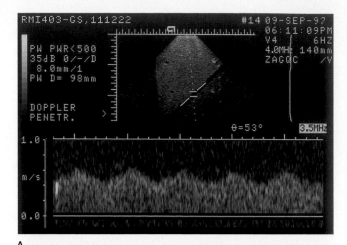

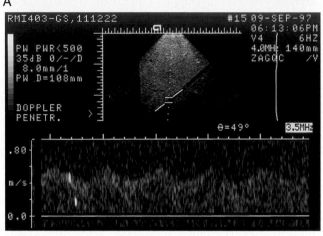

FIGURE 14-13 B-mode and spectral Doppler display of a flow phantom for evaluating Doppler penetration. **A,** A strong Doppler signal and a good signal-to-noise ratio is obtained when the sample volume is at a depth of 9.8 cm. **B,** The Doppler signal is just detectable above the electronic noise when the sample volume is at a depth of 10.8 cm. The maximum depth of detection of the Doppler signal in this case is 10.8 cm.

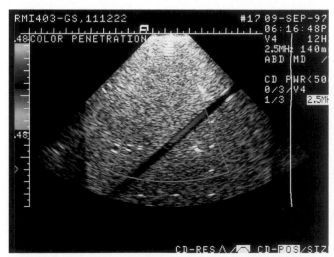

FIGURE 14-14 An example of a color flow image of a Doppler flow phantom used to determine the maximum penetration in color.

Doppler flow phantoms are used for the following types of tests of Doppler and flow imaging equipment (Hoskins et al., 1994; Zagzebski, 1995):

- *Maximum detection depth.* The maximum depth at which flow waveforms can be detected in the phantom has been used to assess whether the Doppler sensitivity has varied from one quality assurance test to another.* This is shown in Figure 14-13. Penetration in this case is 10.8 cm.
- *Alignment.* The phantom can be used to evaluate whether the pulsed Doppler sample volume is aligned with the volume indicated on the B-mode image.
- *Volume flow accuracy.* Some Doppler flow phantoms have precise volume flow measuring equipment. A flow phantom can thus be used in assessments of the accuracy of flow measuring algorithms on Doppler devices.
- *Velocity accuracy.* If the velocity of the fluid within the phantoms can be determined accurately, then this can be used to evaluate velocity displays on Doppler and color flow machines.
- *Color flow penetration* (see Fig. 14-14). System sensitivity settings are at their maximum levels without excessive electronic noise. The maximum depth at which color data can be recorded in the flow phantom is noted. Any changes over time such as greater than 1 cm indicate a change in the sensitivity of the instrument.
- *Alignment of color flow image with B-mode image* (image congruency test). This test checks whether the color flow image and B-mode image are aligned so that they agree spatially. Color images of vessels should be completely contained within the B-mode image of the vessel. Sometimes bleeding out occurs, and this can be corrected by equipment service personnel.

ELECTRONIC PROBE TESTS

A frequent cause of nonuniformity on B-mode images is nonfunctioning elements in ultrasound transducer arrays. We previously saw that nonfunctioning elements in a transducer array often result in dark "shadow-type" regions emanating from the transducer as seen on a B-mode image.

Quantitative tools for assessing transducer integrity now are becoming available. One of these is a mode on a scanning machine for testing transducers. Although

---

*This measurement may be useful for consistency checks, which are an essential part of quality assurance, in attempting to verify that equipment is operating at least as well as when it was delivered or last upgraded. As an absolute measure of Doppler sensitivity, it is controversial because many factors are involved in the concept of Doppler sensitivity (Performance criteria and measurements for Doppler ultrasound devices, 1993).

not available generally, such modes would greatly facilitate routine QA in the clinic and would allow operators to do tests quickly and routinely. Beta versions of the transducer test mode separately address each element in the transducer and channel in the machine. The test mode excites the element with the system pulser and measure the resultant ringdown signal. Criteria are then applied to the signal to judge whether the element is operating normally or is faulty. In this way, a profile of the array functionality can be obtained. Although such modes are not yet available on scanners, manufacturers are encouraged to provide this information to enable more convenient assessment of transducer integrity than can be done at the present time.

An alternative, more sensitive means to evaluate transducer function is to use an electronic probe tester. Special purpose transducer testers, such as the Aperio by Sonora (Longmont, CO, USA) (Figure 14-15) are available. Analogous to the probe testing mode just described, the function of the probe tester is to evaluate each element in an array transducer, testing its transmission and echo detection capability and its acoustic and electrical properties.

The transducer to be tested is immersed in water and oriented to transmit waves toward a specular interface. (Fig. 14-15) Users select a planar interface for testing linear arrays (Fig. 14-15, *B*) and phased arrays, while a concave shaped interface is selected for testing curvilinear arrays. Transducer data provided by the probe tester manufacturer guide placement of the transducer, and a screen that displays the echo amplitude and exact distance between selected elements and the reflector aids users to achieve the correct transducer orientation. When alignment is satisfactory, users switch the software into test mode. In this mode each element is isolated, a short electrical pulse is applied to it, and the resultant echo from the interface is detected and analyzed. Information including the amplitude of the signal produced by the element, the frequency content of this echo, and the electrical capacitance is provided.

Graphs that depict the amplitude of the signal from each array element (Fig. 14-16) are used to evaluate the condition of the transducer. The top record in this figure shows this transducer has 8 elements that are compromised in some way, as seen by the relative amplitudes of their signals. The electrical capacitance test in the lower figure helps engineers pinpoint whether the problem is likely caused by electrical malfunctions or by mechanical problems, such as delaminations of the matching layers that exist between the transducer and the medium. This transducer was operating poorly enough to warrant replacement following the test.

Advantages of the probe tester include the following:

1. This is a more sensitive test than use of images of uniform phantoms for establishing whether a transducer is functioning well or not.
2. Users can readily establish objective pass-fail criteria for a transducer. For example, the test manufacturer suggests that if there are 3 or more nonfunctioning elements in a typical 128 element transducer, the probe should be replaced.
3. Often the data provided by the electronic probe tester enable users to determine the cause of any dead elements and consider whether repair is possible. An auxiliary test of the electrical capacitance of transducer elements helps pinpoint whether a dead or weak element is a result of a disconnect in the

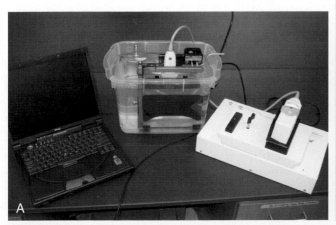
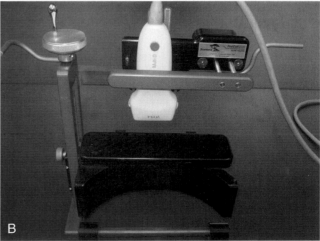

FIGURE 14-15 A, Arrangement for testing transducers using an electronic probe tester. The transducer is connected to the tester through its port. The tester may have various special ports to adapt to different manufacturer's transducer connectors. The face of the probe is immersed in water and directed towards a smooth reflector. A computer controls the tester and produces printouts of test reports. **B,** Typical arrangement for testing a linear array transducer. Positioners on the holder enable users to orient the transducer so that beams are perpendicular to the smooth reflecting surface. The mount is immersed in a water bath so that the path from the transducer to the reflector is water.

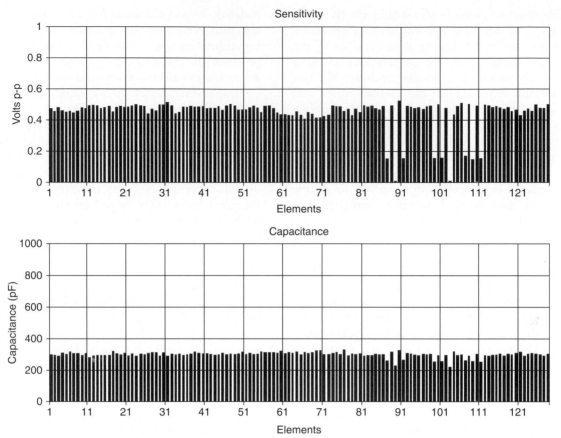

FIGURE 14-16 Typical probe test result for a transducer with 8 dead elements. "Volts p-p" in the top record indicates the relative amplitude of the echo signal detected by each element from the specular reflector. For 8 of the elements the signal clearly is much weaker than for the other elements. The lower record displays the electrical capacitance of each element and its electric lead.

electrical path between the probe cover and the transducer housing or whether the flaw is caused by delaminations between the element and the lens material or matching layers.

Disadvantages of the system include the following:

1. The system is costly. Besides the basic test unit and target fixture, individual transducer adapters are needed for different manufacturer's transducers.
2. Not all transducers are testable. The pin connection of transducer connectors are not standardized in the probe industry, requiring extensive testing by the electronic probe tester manufacturer to provide "probe definition files" that apply to each transducer.
3. New transducers such as multidimensional and 2-dimensional arrays are less likely to have probe definition files available because of the complicated nature these transducers must operate.

In spite of these shortcomings, many large imaging centers where dozens of transducers are available and must be evaluated in a QA testing environment, find electronic probe testers essential to their routine ultrasound quality management program.

Refer to the Evolve website at https://evolve.elsevier. com for Student Experiment 14.1: Ultrasound System Visual Inspection.

REVIEW QUESTIONS

1. Which term best describes routine tests done to determine that an ultrasound scanner is operating at its expected level of performance?
   a. Equipment acceptance tests
   b. General equipment maintenance
   c. Quality assurance
   d. Instrument upgrades
2. Which one of the following statements is true about quality assurance tests of ultrasound scanners?
   a. They require expertise of a hospital engineer or physicist.
   b. Quality assurance for each scanner takes approximately 2 hours per week.
   c. Good record keeping is an essential component.
   d. Quantitative results generally are not necessary.

3. In-house quality assurance programs usually involve all but which of the following?
   a. Tests with phantoms
   b. Inspection and cleaning of air filters
   c. Records and worksheets with test results
   d. Voltage measurements at specified points

4. Material making up the body of a typical quality assurance phantom is "tissuelike" in terms of its _____ properties.
   a. attenuation and perfusion
   b. sound speed and attenuation
   c. sound speed and reflector location
   d. echogenicity and reflector location

5. To be used for tests of geometric accuracy, the _____ and _____ in a phantom must be precisely specified.
   a. echogenicity; reflector location
   b. sound speed; reflector location
   c. attenuation; reflector location
   d. echogenicity; attenuation

6. What is the percentage error in the caliper readout if the actual distance between two reflectors in a phantom is 4 cm but the digital caliper readout indicates it is 3.8 cm?
   a. Less than 1%
   b. 1.5%
   c. 5%
   d. 10%

7. Which of the following tests does not need to be performed routinely as part of a quality assurance program?
   a. Uniformity
   b. Distance accuracy
   c. Axial resolution
   d. Maximum depth of visualization

8. What is a string phantom useful for measuring?
   a. The maximum depth of Doppler signal detection
   b. Velocity accuracy on a spectral Doppler display
   c. Axial resolution in B-mode
   d. Vertical distance measurement accuracy

9. What are Doppler flow phantoms useful for determining?
   a. The maximum depth of Doppler signal detection
   b. The vertical distance measurement accuracy
   c. The acoustic output during color flow imaging
   d. The horizontal distance measurement accuracy

10. For echo signals to be produced that are of a similar magnitude as blood in the body, what two factors in a Doppler phantom must be comparable to human tissues?
   a. Phantom material attenuation and mimicking material blood echogenicity
   b. Phantom material density and mimicking material blood attenuation
   c. Mimicking material blood viscosity and attenuation
   d. Mimicking material blood velocity and acceleration

REFERENCES

ACR Ultrasound Accreditation Program, Reston, VA, 2001, American College of Radiology.

AIUM standard methods for measuring performance of ultrasound pulse-echo equipment, Committee Report, Laurel, MD, 1990, American Institute of Ultrasound in Medicine.

Burlew M, et al: A new ultrasound tissue-equivalent material with a high melting point and extended speed of sound range, *Radiology* 134:517, 1980.

Carson P, Goodsitt MM: Acceptance testing of pulse-echo ultrasound equipment. In Goldman L, Fowlkes B, editors: *Medical CT and ultrasound: current technology and applications*, Madison, WIS, 1995, Advanced Medical Publishers.

Goodsitt M, et al: Real-time B-mode ultrasound quality control test procedures. Report of AAPM Ultrasound Task Group No 1, *Med Phys* 25:1385–1406, 1998.

Gray J: Test pattern for video display and hard copy cameras, *Radiology* 154:519, 1985.

Groth D, et al: Cathode ray tube quality control and acceptance program: initial results for clinical PACS displays, *Radiographics* 21:719, 2001.

Hoskins PR, Sheriff SB, Evans JA, editors: *Testing of Doppler ultrasound equipment*, Rep no 70, York, UK, 1994, The Institute of Physical Sciences in Medicine.

Lu ZF, Lee FT, Zagzebski JA: Ultrasonic backscatter and attenuation in diffuse liver disease, *Ultrasound Med Biol* 25:1047, 1999.

Madsen EL, et al: Tissue mimicking material for ultrasound phantoms, *Med Phys* 5:391, 1978.

Madsen EL, et al: Ultrasound lesion detectability phantoms, *Med Phys* 18:1771, 1991.

Maklad N, Ophir J, Balara V: Attenuation of ultrasound in normal and diffuse liver disease in vivo, *Ultrason Imaging* 6:117, 1984.

Performance criteria and measurements for Doppler ultrasound devices, Committee Report, Laurel, MD, 1993, American Institute of Ultrasound in Medicine.

Zagzebski J: Acceptance tests for Doppler ultrasound equipment. In Goldman L, Fowlkes B, editors: *Medical CT and ultrasound: current technology and applications*, Madison, WIS, 1995, Advanced Medical Publishers.

Zagzebski J: US quality assurance with phantoms. In Goldman L, Fowlkes B, editors: *Categorical course in diagnostic radiology physics: CT and US cross-sectional imaging*, Oak Brook, Ill, 2000, Radiological Society of North America.

CHAPTER

15

Quality Assurance in Nuclear Medicine

Joanne Metler

KEY TERMS

American College of Radiology
bioassay
center of rotation
chemical impurity
chi-square test
chromatography
collimator
count rate
counts per minute
disintegrations per minute
dose calibrator
energy resolution
field uniformity
gamma camera
gas-filled detector

Geiger-Müller meters
hydrolyzed reduced technetium
molybdenum-99
multichannel analyzer
Nuclear Regulatory Commission
Occupational Safety and Health
   Administration
photomultiplier tubes
photon
photopeak
pixel size
positron emission tomography
pulse height analyzer
radionuclide impurity
scintillation crystal

scintillation detectors
sensitivity
single-photon emission computed
   tomography
spatial linearity
spatial resolution
spectrum
standardized uptake value
technetium-99m
technetium-99m pertechnetate
The Joint Commission
thermoluminescent dosimeter
uniformity correction flood

OBJECTIVES

At the completion of this chapter the reader will be able to do the following:

- Describe the principles of radiation detection and measurement
- Describe the scintillation crystal
- Describe the basic principles of the gamma camera
- Describe the scintillation camera performance characteristics of image linearity, image uniformity, intrinsic spatial resolution, detection efficiency, and counting rate problems
- Describe the design and performance characteristics of commonly used collimators
- Describe planar camera quality control testing methods of calibration, gamma energy spectrum, window determination, daily floods (intrinsic and extrinsic), weekly resolution (intrinsic and extrinsic), counting efficiency and sensitivity, and multiwindow spatial registration

- Describe gamma camera single-photon emission computerized tomography (SPECT) systems
- Describe SPECT quality control (i.e., flood uniformity, center of rotation, attenuation correction, and pixel size)
- Describe positron emission tomography and its quality control
- Describe nuclear medicine nonimaging equipment and related quality control procedures (i.e., gas-filled detectors such as dose calibrators, survey meters, Geiger-Müller (GM) meters, and scintillation detectors such as the multichannel analyzer and thyroid probe)
- Describe quality control procedures in a radiopharmacy and radionuclide generator quality control evaluation of contaminant such as molybdenum, aluminum, and hydrolyzed reduced technetium

OUTLINE

Nuclear medicine technology is a scientific and clinical discipline involving the diagnostic, therapeutic, and investigative use of radionuclides. The nuclear medicine professional performs a variety of responsibilities in a typical day including formulating, dispensing, and administering radiopharmaceuticals; performing in vivo and in vitro laboratory procedures; acquiring, processing, and analyzing patient studies on a computer; performing all daily equipment testing; preparing the patient for the studies; operating the imaging and nonimaging equipment; and maintaining a radiation safety program. Because of the variety of responsibilities in the nuclear medicine department, **The Joint Commission** (TJC) has recognized the necessity for an established quality assurance program in nuclear medicine. TJC states that "There shall be quality control policies and procedures governing nuclear medicine activities that assure diagnostic and therapeutic reliability and safety of the patients and personnel (Accreditation manual for hospitals, 1993)." The **American College of Radiology** (ACR) also offers accreditation of nuclear medicine departments and mandates that certain quality assurance procedures be performed. This chapter discusses the many quality assurance procedures routinely performed in nuclear medicine. In the summer of 2008, Congress passed the Medicare Improvements for Patients and Providers Act of 2008 (MIPPA), which mandates that any nonhospital institution performing advanced diagnostic services (such as nuclear medicine and PET) must be accredited (by January 1, 2010) in order to receive federal funding (Medicare reimbursement). The CARE bill (discussed in Chapter 1) if passed, would make similar requirements for hospital-based facilities; therefore, accreditation programs are becoming mandatory for nuclear medicine departments to succeed.

THE SCINTILLATION GAMMA CAMERA

The scintillation **gamma camera** was first developed by Hal Anger in 1958 and has undergone many changes in design and electrical sophistication since its inception.

However, the basic components of the gamma camera remain the same (Fig. 15-1) (Anger, 1958). The camera consists of a circular or rectangular detector mounted on a gantry, which allows flexible manipulation around a patient, and electronic processing and display components. In addition, the camera system is interfaced to a computer to control study acquisition, analysis, and display. The detector head contains a thallium-activated sodium iodide (NaI[T1]) crystal, **photomultiplier tubes** (PMTs), preamplifiers, a position energy circuit, a pulse height analyzer, and a display mechanism.

Because radiation is a random process, gamma rays are not easy to control. The energy of the ionizing gamma radiation is too high to be deflected like visible light. However, the gamma **photon** can be directed through holes in a **collimator** while it blocks tangential or

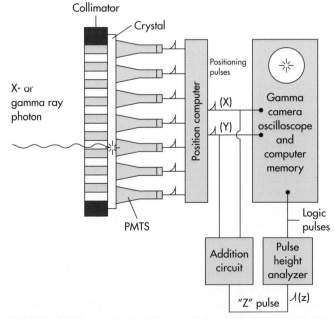

FIGURE 15-1 Basic scintillation camera detector components. *PMTS*, photomultiplier tubes. *(From Thrall JH, Ziessman HA:* Nuclear medicine: the requisites, *St Louis, 1995, Mosby.)*

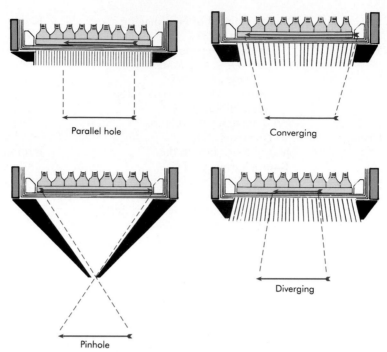

FIGURE 15-2 Four common types of collimators used on gamma cameras. *(From Bernier DR, Christian PE, Langan JM: Nuclear medicine: technology and techniques, ed 3, St Louis 1994, Mosby.)*

scattered photons. For a resolving image to be obtained, the collimator must be placed on the face of the detector head; this placement allows the desirable gamma photons to pass through to the NaI(T1) crystal. A collimator is a lead-filtering device that consists of holes through which a gamma photon can pass. These holes are separated by lead septa (Fig. 15-2). The photons that are not absorbed or scattered by the lead septa pass straight through to the NaI(T1) crystal and subsequently create an image of the isotope distribution from the patient. With high-energy photons, thicker lead septa are required to prevent scatter from degrading the image.

Collimators are available from several manufacturers. The collimator chosen for a patient study depends on the isotope energy and resolution required for the specific diagnostic procedure. Collimators commonly used in nuclear medicine include low-, medium-, and high-energy parallel hole; high-resolution parallel hole; high-sensitivity parallel hole; general all-purpose parallel hole; pinhole; and converging and diverging collimators (Early and Sodee, 1995). Because collimators are made specifically to operate within a gamma photon's energy range, a nuclear medicine department must have collimators suitable for several types of applications. The most common type used for diagnostic studies is the parallel-hole collimator. The parallel-hole collimator is preferred because it directs photons from a patient onto the scintillation crystal without varying the image. Once the photon passes through the collimator, it reaches the NaI(T1) **scintillation crystal** and is converted to light. The number of light photons produced is directly proportional to the energy of the gamma photon. Typically, 30 photons are produced

per kiloelectron volt (keV) of energy (Murray and Ell, 1994). The NaI(T1) crystals vary in diameter, shape, and thickness. Changing the parameters of the crystal affects sensitivity or resolution (i.e., if sensitivity is increased by the use of a thicker crystal, then the resolution is compromised and vice versa). The NaI(T1) crystal is hygroscopic and extremely sensitive to sudden temperature changes. The environment of the gamma camera must remain stable, and precautions must be taken to prevent moisture from entering the NaI(T1) crystal and sudden temperature shifts (Early and Sodee, 1995). In addition, an accidental impact may cause the crystal to crack.

The scintillation, or light, photon interacts with the PMT. The light generated in the NaI(T1) crystal is then converted to electrical signals. The electrons produced are amplified and accelerated a millionfold in the PMT system. After conversion to an electrical pulse, a position circuit produces X and Y position signals, which are directly related to the location of the photon interaction on the NaI(T1) crystal. Because of the high potential of ionizing radiation interacting with matter, not all of the gamma photons detected by the NaI(T1) crystal are the original primary gamma photons of interest. The interactions with matter from the patient and through the camera system can cause scatter radiation. Too much scatter radiation can cause degradation in the resolution of the final image. It is therefore possible to electronically exclude undesirable photons by only accepting the gamma ray photons above a certain energy.

The discrimination and selection of the gamma photon are performed with a **pulse height analyzer** (PHA). The PHA can be preset to accept only specific energy signals from the detector. The gamma photon energy required is specified by creating an energy "window" in the PHA. The energy window designates lower and upper limits of the gamma photon energy of interest. The model and age of equipment determine how a window is set; three different methods can be used. A threshold window may be set with a window reading above it; the reading is usually expressed in a percentage of total kiloelectron volts of the gamma energy in question. A midline energy may be set at the energy of the gamma ray or at the maximum count position of the voltage or gain adjustment. The percent window is then applied above and below this midpoint or peak. Finally, some instruments allow setting window thresholds at any position including overlapping energies and multiple discrete windows for multiple isotope studies. Multiple windows also may be set up for those radionuclides that emit more than one gamma ray (e.g., thallium-201, indium-111, gallium-67). The signal is then sent to a display controller to produce a numeric display and an image. The display can occur simultaneously on a cathode-ray tube, a scalar, a film, and a computer screen. Many camera systems can display an analog or a digital image, or both. An analog camera allows the image to be displayed directly onto film in a cassette with or without the use of a computer. The analog camera also may be interfaced to a computer that simultaneously collects the image in the computer and displays it digitally. Finally, a digital camera digitizes the output of each PMT to create a digital image.

Various gamma camera configurations are available. The gamma camera detector may have a small or large field of imaging capability. The detector also may be circular or rectangular. In addition, the gamma camera system may hold one, two, or three detectors. These configurations are better known as single-, dual-, or triple-head cameras. In addition, some gamma cameras are fixed, whereas others are mobile. The scintillation gamma camera system is a complex mechanism accompanied by a variety of components that are crucial to producing a reliable and factual clinical image. The quality of the nuclear medicine image is determined by a variety of parameters. These parameters must be perpetually evaluated to guarantee that the image the physician is interpreting is accurate and truly diagnostic of the patient's pathologic condition.

According to the National Electrical Manufacturers Association (NEMA), 12 acceptance test standards are performed at the factory on all gamma cameras (Murphy, 1987; National Electrical Manufacturers Association, 1980, 1986). Box 15-1 lists the tests that are performed. The quality control measures taken at the factory ensure the good working condition of the new system. However, once the gamma cameras are in the nuclear medicine department, it is impractical and sometimes impossible for all of the NEMA standard acceptance tests to be performed (Sorenson and Phelps, 1987). However, the

BOX 15-1	NEMA Acceptance Tests for Scintillation Cameras (SPECT)

Intrinsic Spatial Resolution
Intrinsic Energy Resolution
Intrinsic Field Uniformity
Intrinsic Count Rate Performance
Intrinsic Spatial Linearity
Multiple Spatial Registration
Sensitivity
Angular Variation of Spatial Position
Angular Variation of Flood Field Uniformity and Sensitivity
Reconstructed System Spatial Resolution
Spatial Resolution with and without Scatter
System Count Rate Performance with Scatter

From the National Electrical Manufacturers Association: *NEMA standards for performance measurements of scintillation cameras*, Pub No NUI-1986, Washington, DC, 1986, The Association.
NEMA, National Electrical Manufacturers Association; *SPECT*, single-photon emission computerized tomography. Intrinsic Spatial Resolution

TABLE 15-1	Gamma Camera Quality Control	
Quality Control Procedure	**Frequency**
Peaking	Daily and before each new radionuclide used
Counting rate limits	Daily
Field uniformity	Daily, after repair
Spatial resolution	Weekly, after repair
Spatial linearity	Weekly, after repair
Sensitivity	Quarterly

quality control procedures listed in Table 15-1 are required by TJC (Accreditation manual for hospitals, 1993) and regulatory agencies and are to be performed routinely (Rao et al., 1986). The quality control procedures performed on all imaging equipment ensure that the patient's diagnostic study is safe and accurate.

QUALITY CONTROL PROCEDURES FOR IMAGING EQUIPMENT

Energy Resolution and Photopeaking

Before any quality control or patient procedure, the correct energy setting for the radionuclide being used must be selected and the primary gamma ray energy, or **photopeak**, centered around an energy window. The quality control is performed daily, either manually or automatically, depending on the manufacturer's specifications. The PHA is centered about the photopeak(s) of the radionuclide of interest, usually with a 5% to 10% window. This is generally referred to as "peaking" the camera. It is accomplished by adjusting the baseline window setting of the PHA around the specific energy of the gamma ray.

For example, **technetium-99m** (^{99m}Tc) is used daily in a nuclear medicine department. The primary gamma ray of ^{99m}Tc has an energy of 140 keV. The window generally used for imaging is 20% around 140 keV; therefore, resetting a 20% window "tells" the PHA to accept only gamma photons with energies from 126 to 154 keV and to center the photopeak at 140 keV. The camera must be peaked before any radionuclide is used.

Because radioactive decay is random, each step in converting the radiation to an electrical current is subject to random error. The **spectrum** (curve) of the radionuclide of interest is not a straight line representing complete absorption of the gamma ray, but a Gaussian distribution resulting from random error, Compton scattering, or material attenuation (Fig. 15-3). The light photons emitted by the NaI(T1) crystal are given off in all directions with random probability. The **energy resolution** can then be expressed as the spread, or width, of the spectrum divided by the center photopeak. The spread of the spectrum or the full width at half maximum (FWHM) measurement is the energy range of the widest width of the spectrum, which is halfway down from the photopeak (Fig. 15-4). The energy resolution is calculated as follows:

$$\text{Percent energy resolution} = \frac{\text{FWHM at half maximum}}{\text{Photopeak center}} \times 100$$

The narrower the curve, the better is the energy resolution of the detector. A good energy resolution is between 8% and 12% and enables the camera system to better discern gamma rays with close energies. A reliable energy resolution is significant because it represents the system's ability to accurately depict two separate events in space,

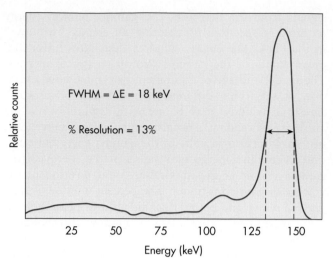

FIGURE 15-4 Energy spectrum of technetium-99m (^{99m}Tc). The full width at half maximum (FWHM) is 18 kiloelectron volts (keV). The energy resolution is 13%. ΔE, Change in energy. *(From Thrall James JH, Ziessman HA: Nuclear medicine: the requisites, St Louis, 1995, Mosby.)*

time, or energy. The ability of a system to detect separate radiation events becomes clinically relevant, especially when used for in vitro or in vivo counting, which potentially leads to a patient's clinical diagnosis. Performing a test of energy resolution also verifies that scatter rejection is sufficient to provide optimal contrast in clinical studies.

Counting Rate Limits

The sensitivity (counting ability) of a gamma camera generally decreases with increased amounts of activity. If the activity is too high, the detector is "paralyzed" and cannot count. The system's inability to count is referred to as *dead time*. Dead time describes the duration the detector requires to process the ionizing events as they occur in the NaI(T1) crystal. The manufacturer's specification of the **count rate** limit per second states that the observed count rate through a 20% window should not exceed 20% of the counts lost as a result of dead time (Greer et al., 1985). The electronic circuitry of most contemporary gamma cameras reaches counting limits of 120,000 to 150,000 counts per second before experiencing a 20% loss because of dead time (Henkin et al., 1996). Before any quality control procedure is performed, the count rate of the radioactive point or flood source must be determined to ensure that the counts per second do not exceed the manufacturer's specifications. Once the count rate is determined to be within the counting rate limits for that gamma camera, only then can the quality control testing continue. The procedures to determine count rate are simple: The radioactive source is placed at the appropriate location necessary for quality control, and the time/count scalar continuously displays the counts per second. Count rates that exceed the gamma camera's design limits can result

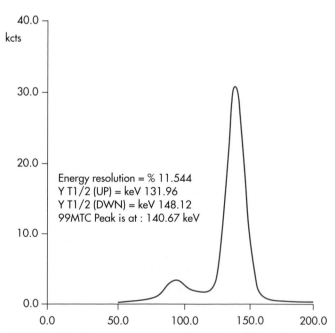

FIGURE 15-3 Energy spectrum of the radionuclide technetium-99m (^{99m}Tc). *kcts,* kilocounts; *keV,* kiloelecron volt.

Energy resolution = % 11.544
Y T1/2 (UP) = keV 131.96
Y T1/2 (DWN) = keV 148.12
99MTC Peak is at : 140.67 keV

in degradation of the images and loss of counts (Henkin et al., 1996). If the counts-per-second rate is too high and it is necessary to decrease the count rate, the radioactive source is repositioned at an increased distance, or the amount of radioactivity in the source is decreased.

Field Uniformity

Field uniformity refers to the gamma camera's ability to detect a uniform source of radiation and respond exactly the same at any location within the imaging field. The uniform response of the gamma camera results in an image with an even distribution of radioactivity (Fig. 15-5). The uniformity of the gamma camera depends on the uniform response of the NaI(T1) crystal and the PMTs. The response of each PMT must match that of all the other PMTs. In addition, the counting window must be centered around the photopeak. Mispositioning the photopeak may alter the field uniformity (Fig. 15-6). Nonuniformity also may arise because of, for example, the use of the incorrect photopeak for a specific radionuclide, a malfunctioning PMT, a cracked NaI(T1) crystal, and total system malfunction (Fig. 15-7). Because the uniformity of the camera ultimately determines the accuracy of a patient's image and, ultimately, the diagnosis, it is imperative that the field uniformity or flood be performed daily. This quality control procedure must be performed before any patient studies.

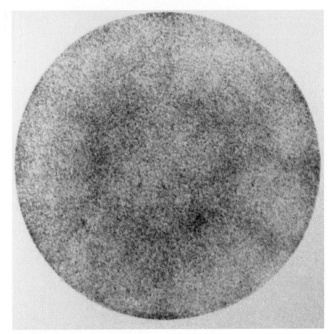

FIGURE 15-6 Mispositioned photopeak resulting in a nonuniform flood.

The measurement of the daily field uniformity can be performed intrinsically or extrinsically. Intrinsic uniformity is the measurement of the uniformity of the gamma camera detector with no collimator in place. The procedure is generally performed with a point source of radioactivity placed at a distance equivalent to 4 to 5 diameters of the detector's field of imaging (Scintillation camera acceptance testing and performance evaluation, 1980) cautions should be taken that the counts-per-second rate does not exceed that particular system's limits. The intrinsic uniformity determines the integrity of the NaI(T1) crystal and its electronic components. The phenomenon known as *edge packing* can show up as a bright rim of activity around the perimeter of the flood. To prevent edge packing, most manufacturers provide a lead-shielded ring that masks the effect when attached to the edge of the camera head.

Extrinsic uniformity testing is also the measurement of the camera's field uniformity; however, it is performed with the collimator (which is used for imaging) in place. A uniform flood source of radioactivity is placed directly on the collimated camera (Fig. 15-8). The two commonly used extrinsic radioactive sources are (1) an acrylic plastic (Plexiglas) container filled with water and generally 1 to 10 millicurie (mCi) of ^{99m}Tc and (2) a solid-sealed 10 mCi cobalt-57 sheet (Steves, 1992). The ^{99m}Tc liquid-filled acrylic plastic (Plexiglas) source does have some disadvantages. It must be manually filled with technetium and thoroughly mixed to secure even distribution of the radionuclide. The procedure increases the risk of radioactive contamination to the technologist and equipment; thus, the technologist's risk of radiation exposure is increased. The extrinsic

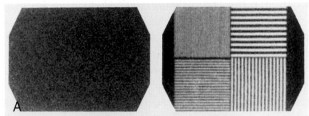

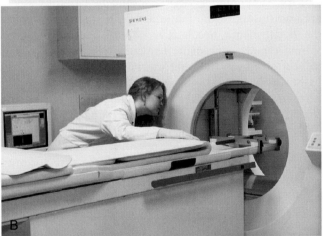

FIGURE 15-5 **A,** Field uniformity flood and resolution pattern. **B,** Nuclear medicine technologist preparing to obtain a field flood uniformity on a dual-head camera system. (**B,** *Courtesy Northwest Community Hospital, Arlington Heights, Ill.*)

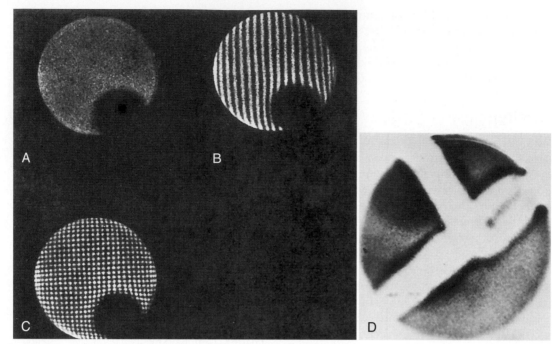

FIGURE 15-7 Example of a nonfunctioning photomultiplier tube (PMT) seen in the flood field **(A)**, the orthogonal hole resolution pattern **(B)**, and the parallel-line equal space (PLES) phantom **(C)**. **D,** Examples of nonuniform flood fields caused by a cracked crystal. *(A, from Rollo FD: Nuclear medicine physics, instrumentation, and agents, St Louis, 1997, Mosby; B, from Early PJ, Sodee BS: Principles and procedures of nuclear medicine, ed 2, St Louis, 1995, Mosby.)*

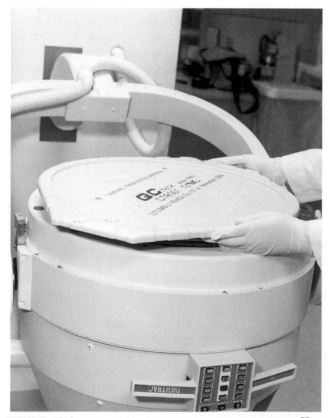

FIGURE 15-8 Extrinsic flood uniformity with a cobalt-57 (^{57}Co) sheet source.

uniformity, in addition to evaluating the NaI(T1) crystal and electrical components, allows visualization of a defect or damage to the collimator. Annual inspection of collimators with extrinsic field uniformity testing is recommended and should become a routine part of any quality assurance program. A defect in a collimator will visualize in an image as photopenic areas (Fig. 15-9).

A flood field image of 1 to 3 million counts is generally acquired whether the intrinsic or extrinsic method is used. However, it is recommended that the quality control for each gamma camera should be carefully evaluated according to the manufacturer's specifications and the department's needs. The quality control test used should remain consistent. The consistency allows visual inspection of any nonuniformity of the camera system to be easily monitored. The uniformity flood must be performed daily on every piece of imaging equipment. Visual inspection of the flood and comparison with that of the previous days reveal any subtle changes in uniformity that are not always apparent by looking at one image. Any areas of nonuniformity of the detector must be noted and repaired before clinical use. In addition to the performance of daily floods, the TJC quality assurance program recommends that every piece of equipment also have a preventive maintenance program performed biannually (Accreditation manual for hospitals, 1993).

Gamma cameras of the late 1970s through the present have been developed to correct some of the nonuniformities

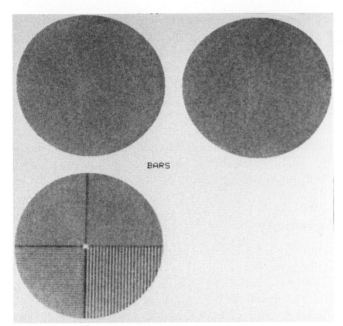

FIGURE 15-9 Note the photopenic area in the flood field and the resolution bar pattern. These are due to collimator damage.

seen in older images. A microprocessor built into the gamma camera generates a correction factor for each pixel of the matrix, according to the variation in counts of different pixels (Saha, 1993). Figure 15-10 demonstrates the difference between an uncorrected and corrected uniformity flood. Subsequently, when patient images are generated, the correction factors are applied to each pixel; thus, non-uniformity is reduced (Saha, 1993).

Spatial Resolution and Spatial Linearity

Spatial resolution is the gamma camera's ability to reproduce small details of a radioactive distribution (Greer et al., 1985). The smaller the details that a camera can reproduce, the better is the spatial resolution of that system. ❻ *The spatial resolution quality control procedure is required to be performed a minimum of once a week on every imaging system.* The quality

control determines the camera's ability to detect and image fine differences of a radioactive distribution that exist in closely spaced areas. In essence, the gamma camera detects the small abnormalities of different radioactive concentrations that may subsequently be seen on patient images. For the exact spatial resolution of a gamma camera system to be determined, one of the following resolution test pattern transmission sources must be used: four-quadrant bar phantom with varying size bars, parallel-line equal space (PLES) bar pattern with constant bar and spacing sizes, or an orthogonal hole phantom with varying sizes of holes (Bernier et al., 1997; Eisner, 1985).

The manufacturer of every gamma camera system determines the intrinsic spatial resolution specific for the gamma camera. This is important when choosing the type and size of a transmission resolution pattern. For example, if the manufacturer specifications say that gamma camera 1 has an intrinsic spatial resolution of 3 mm, then the four-quadrant bar phantom used must have bars between 2 and 5 mm. The resolution pattern is placed on the collimator or camera for an intrinsic resolution quality control test and on the collimator for an extrinsic resolution quality control test. The resolution pattern is placed in the center of the field of view (FOV) in such a way that the center of the pattern is directly over the center of the detector. A ^{99m}Tc or ^{57}Co sheet source is then placed on the resolution pattern so that the radioactivity is transmitted through the resolution pattern. It is recommended that when the four-quadrant bar pattern is used, four images should be obtained at 90 degrees between positions (Bernier et al., 1997; Henkin et al., 1996). This allows verification of the spatial resolution in the X and Y positions and allows the bars barely resolved to be evaluated in each quadrant of the FOV (Fig. 15-11).

The PLES bar resolution pattern is sometimes preferable to the four-quadrant pattern. A PLES pattern is preferable for testing spatial resolution because it is specifically designed to minimize the number of images that are actually required to evaluate resolution (Henkin et al., 1996). Only two images are required to evaluate the camera spatial resolution because the size of the bars and the spacing between the bars are constant (Fig. 15-12). The orthogonal hole phantom is a hexagonal lead sheet containing holes of equal diameter at right angles to each other. Only one image is required to determine the resolution and uniformity over the entire FOV of the camera detector.

Regardless of which resolution test pattern is used routinely for a gamma camera system, it is important to visually inspect each image to detect any fluctuation in resolution. This inspection is made by the comparison of the weekly resolution image with the previous ones. A change in the resolution can be caused by several factors. If there is a change in resolution, the photopeak, window, source, source distance, gamma photon,

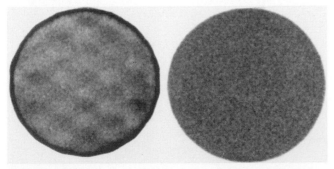

FIGURE 15-10 An uncorrected and a microprocessor-corrected uniformity flood.

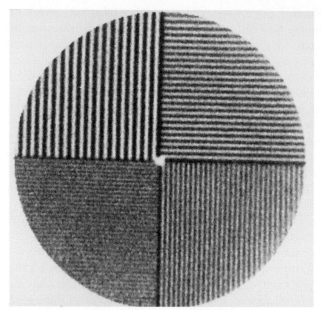

FIGURE 15-11 Spatial resolution with a four-quadrant bar pattern. Four images are obtained 90 degrees apart.

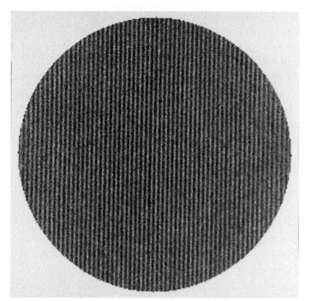

FIGURE 15-12 Parallel-line equal space (PLES) bar resolution pattern.

energy, and type of collimator used should all be verified. Any malfunction or misposition of these factors can detrimentally affect the spatial resolution. If all of the factors are properly functioning and are in proper position, the crystal must then be evaluated for damage or degradation.

The **spatial linearity** of a gamma camera system is its ability to produce a linear image with straight lines corresponding to the same straight lines of the bar pattern. Most modern gamma camera systems have circuits that correct for nonlinearity. Linearity is generally

assessed and can be seen by visual inspection of any of the spatial resolution test pattern images. This is done by carefully inspecting the linearity of the bars or holes in both the X and Y positions and comparing the results with the acceptance test results and the results from previous weeks. Any nonlinearity can cause extreme image artifacts, especially in reconstructed tomographic images. A nonlinear image indicates that the gamma camera should be serviced and reevaluated before further clinical use. The service and reevaluation ensure the accuracy of the diagnostic images, both planar and tomographic.

Sensitivity

Sensitivity is another quality control procedure performed to determine the gamma camera detector's ability to detect the ionizing events that occur in the NaI(T1) crystal. The events recorded as **counts per minute** (cpm) are calculated and expressed as counts per minute per microcurie (μCi) of activity present. The sensitivity quality control is performed biannually. It is performed by placing a sealed point source such as ^{57}Co at different locations (center and at least four peripheral locations) on the camera head and by counting for a set time (Fig. 15-13) (Eisner, 1985; National Electrical

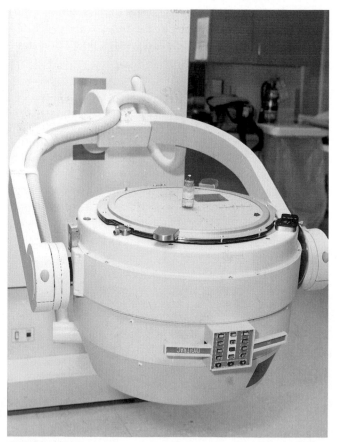

FIGURE 15-13 Sensitivity testing with a known cobalt-57 (^{57}Co) source.

Manufacturers Association, 1980). The sensitivity is equal to the net counts per time divided by the actual activity of the sealed source:

$$\text{Sensitivity} = \frac{\text{Net counts/time}}{\text{Activity of the sealed source in } \mu\text{Ci (on that day)}}$$

The sensitivity is compared with the previous documented sensitivity tests and the manufacturer's specifications to ensure there is no change in the ability of the gamma camera to detect ionizing events.

Multiple-Window Spatial Registration

Gamma cameras are equipped with multiple PHA windows to use with photons of different energies. The multiplicity capability must be evaluated for spatial registration. The position of the X and Y signals must be the same for each energy window. If a study is performed with a radionuclide that has multiple gamma photons of different energies, the photons must be received by their perspective windows and positioned on the cathode-ray tube in the same locations. If they are received in different locations, the resolution of that image is compromised. NEMA recommends that a ^{67}Ga source be used with a bar pattern phantom and sequential images acquired with the three imaging gamma peaks of ^{67}Ga (93 keV, 184 keV, and 296 keV). The individual images are then acquired with each peak individually, and the final images are made with combinations of two peaks. The images are then evaluated for best time and best resolution. In addition, the three floods are superimposed on each other to evaluate the match (Fig. 15-14) (Early and Sodee, 1995).

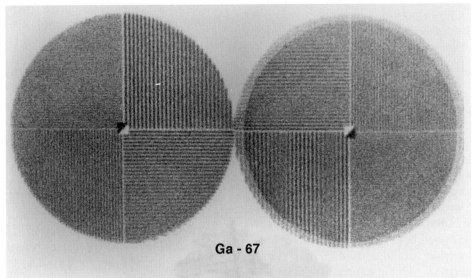

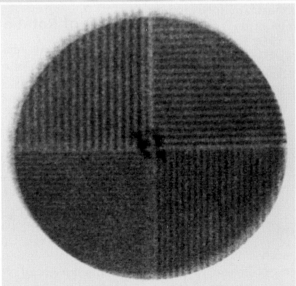

Ga - 67

FIGURE 15-14 Multiwindow spatial resolution testing. *Ga-67*, Gallium 67. *(From Henkin RE, Boles MA, Dillehay GL, et al: Nuclear medicine, vol 1, St Louis, 1996, Mosby.)*

QUALITY ASSURANCE OF SPECT CAMERAS

Tomographic techniques have been developed in nuclear medicine for both **single-photon emission computed tomography** (SPECT) and **positron emission tomography** (PET) (Eisner, 1985; English, 1995; Esser et al., 1983). The research and development of various tomographic systems have given way to the rotating gamma camera. The rotating system, with the aid of a computer and reconstruction software, has the ability to perform true transaxial tomography. Rotational SPECT, computed tomography (CT), and PET all share the characteristic that using only data that arise in the particular image plane in the reconstruction of the tomographic image allows higher image contrast (Bernier et al., 1997). SPECT systems are commercially available with single, dual, triple, and quadruple heads. The multiple-head SPECT systems are becoming the preferred model because more information with increased resolution can be obtained in a given period.

The camera head(s) are attached to a mechanical gantry that allows them to rotate 360 degrees in a circular or elliptical orbit about the patient. The gantry unit is designed to enable the camera head to come as close to the patient as possible to ensure the best resolution at the face of the detector head. Some cameras also are designed to follow the patient's body contour in a noncircular orbit (whole body scanner capability). SPECT systems also require a computer to control the gantry, acquire the data, and reconstruct the tomographic images. The quality assurance of a SPECT system requires stricter controls. SPECT quality assurance procedures are not as tolerant as those for planar imaging. For example, a $\pm 5\%$ field uniformity is acceptable for planar imaging; however, variations in uniformity for SPECT cannot exceed $\pm 1\%$ (Henkin et al., 1996; National Electrical Manufacturers Association, 1980). In addition, the camera coordinates must be properly aligned with the axis of rotation of the gantry and the computer image matrix. The SPECT system must adhere to the required quality control procedures of the scintillation gamma camera as recently discussed (i.e., energy calibration, field uniformity, spatial resolution and linearity, sensitivity, and multiple window registration). However, additional procedures must be performed to ensure maximum SPECT camera performance (Graham et al., 1996; Greer et al., 1985). Table 15-2 lists the required and recommended quality control procedures of a SPECT system (Graham et al., 1996).

Uniformity Correction Flood

Field uniformity corrections are much more critical in SPECT imaging than in other forms of imaging. Small changes in extrinsic uniformity may alter the reconstructed images. Acquiring the 1 to 3 million counts needed in a planar system is just not adequate for the

TABLE 15-2	SPECT Gamma Camera Quality Control*	
Quality Control Procedure	**Frequency**
Uniformity correction flood	Weekly
COR	Weekly for every collimator used for tomography
Pixel size	Monthly
Cine to detect patient motion	After each patient acquisition

COR, Center of rotation; *SPECT*, single-photon emitting computerized tomography.
*Quality control procedure in addition to routine gamma camera quality control procedures.

SPECT. Acquiring fewer than 30 million counts for a **uniformity correction flood** may result in a ring artifact (Fig. 15-15). The 30-million-count figure used for uniformity correction is acquired so that there are about 10,000 counts per pixel in a 64×64 matrix. The system's manufacturer requires that a camera with a collimator in place must have uniformity with variations of less than 1%. In addition, some internal software programs are used to verify a 1% standard deviation (SD). Acquiring 10,000 counts per pixel is necessary to obtain the recommended percent relative SD of 1%.

$$\text{Percent SD} = \frac{100}{\sqrt{10,000}} = 1\%$$

A uniform ^{99m}Tc or ^{57}Co source is placed on the collimator. The uniformity correction flood of 30 to 60 million counts with a 64×64 matrix is acquired weekly for each collimator used. The image is stored in the computer and later used to correct raw data used in reconstruction of the tomographic images.

Center of Rotation

No misalignment must exist between the physical or mechanical **center of rotation** (COR) of the SPECT system and the COR in the reconstruction computer matrix. The pixel matrix that forms the projection images of the SPECT acquisition is a function of the computer, not the camera. The alignment of the computer matrix may not be perfectly aligned with the camera head or gantry, or both. The basic mechanical parts of the SPECT system such as the gears and bearings, as well as patient diversity, prevent a consistent symmetry. In addition, daily use and wear and tear of the system could cause rotational discrepancies (English, 1995; Greer et al., 1985). The COR is important to all SPECT systems, from single- to quadruple-head systems. However, multiple-head systems also require software to guarantee synchronization between the heads.

The COR is properly calibrated if a point source placed in the center of the detector head orbit projects

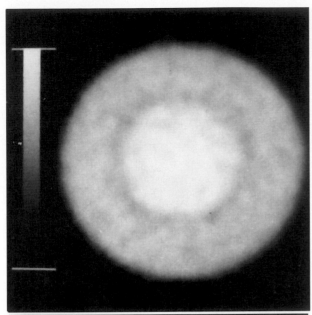

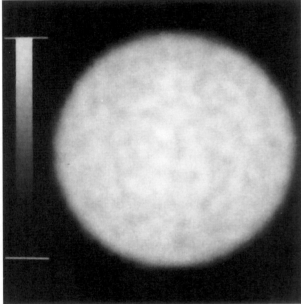

FIGURE 15-15 *Top,* Ring artifact. *Bottom,* Normal image without the artifact. *(Reprinted by permission of the Society of Nuclear Medicine from Greer K et al: Quality control in SPECT, J Nucl Med Technol 13:76, 1985.)*

processing to construct a linear representation to ensure stability. If there is a deviation or a misalignment, the computer generates a straight line with areas appearing outside the line.

Pixel Size

Pixel size of the matrix must be calibrated properly because pixels take on the three-dimensional characteristic of depth in SPECT. Any variation in the pixel size changes depth or distance and subsequently alters attenuation correction factors used in the tomographic reconstructed images. The sizes of the pixels should be monitored monthly for any fluctuations. The pixel size can be adjusted by setting analog-to-digital converters and should be checked in both the X and Y directions (Thrall and Ziessman, 1995). The pixel width should be the same in both directions. Any difference in the pixel dimensions causes problems in reformatting of the image data. In addition, a shift in the analog-to-digital converter also can move the COR matrix.

SPECT Quality Control During and After Patient Procedures

SPECT quality control of the camera and computer systems is important to ensure accurate and optimal image quality for the patient. However, in addition to the quality control of the mechanics of the SPECT system, quality assurance must be practiced during a patient study. It is important to remove any materials from the patient's body that might attenuate the radioisotope being imaged or interfere with image acquisition and reconstruction. This is especially crucial when imaging myocardial perfusion. Examples of external attenuators on a patient are metal coins left in a shirt pocket, a necklace with a hanging metal, an electrocardiogram (ECG) lead left on, or a prosthesis. Breast tissue also may attenuate data and should be noted. Many software programs are able to correct such attenuation. The patient also must be closely monitored for motion. Any vertical or horizontal motion can create artifacts in the reconstruction. In addition, the camera head must be level when the acquisition begins and remain level throughout the study. Once the study acquisition is completed, patient motion can be detected on the computer. The computer programs used today allow inspection for patient motion by summed projection, sinograms, or cine displays. In a summed projection, patient motion appears as a change in the height of the organ imaged. A sinogram is a plot of each projection. If the patient does not move during the acquisition, the plot appears as a bright line. A break in the line indicates patient motion from left to right. A cine display, a raw motion picture of the acquired projections, is a simple way to detect patient motion. If the motion is significant, the study is invalid and must be repeated (Fig. 15-16).

to the center of the 64 × 64 computer matrix, or pixel 32. The COR discrepancies of most SPECT systems are less than 2 mm from the center of the matrix, but the goal is to be no more than 1 mm from pixel 32 (English, 1995; Greer et al., 1985). A point source of ^{57}Co or ^{99m}Tc is used to calculate the COR and the pixel size. A SPECT study is performed on the point source, and the images are reconstructed. A misaligned COR shows the point source to appear larger, blurred, or containing a ring artifact. A COR shift of 3 mm or more can affect the quality of the reconstructed images. The COR quality control must be performed weekly on all SPECT systems. Many SPECT systems now use computer

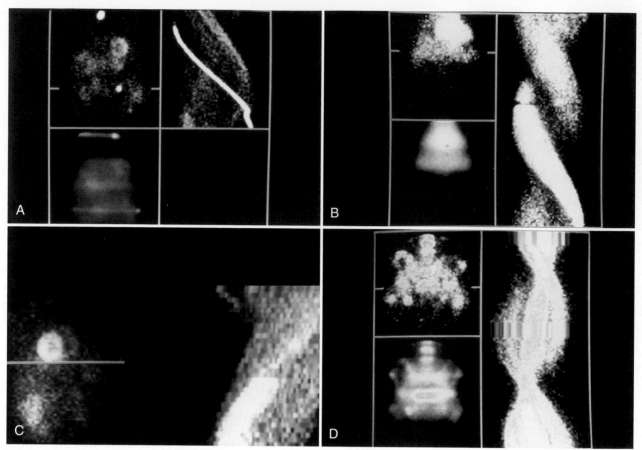

FIGURE 15-16 Problems identified with the patient motion quality control displays. **A,** Single-photon emission computerized tomography (SPECT) catches patient's bed during rotation. **B,** Patient sits up during acquisition. **C,** Patient's bed translates axial during acquisition. **D,** Gantry stops before completion of study. *(From Henkin RE, Boles MA, Dillehay GL, et al: Nuclear medicine, vol 1, St Louis, 1996, Mosby.)*

POSITRON EMISSION TOMOGRAPHY

Positron emission tomography (PET) is a fast-growing imaging modality of nuclear medicine that produces tomographic images of the distribution of positron-emitting radiopharmaceuticals. The excitement surrounding PET technology is that the images depict both physiologic and biochemical processes of the human body. According to the study of nuclear physics, positrons are emitted from proton-rich nuclei that only travel a short distance before encountering an electron; this encounter results in annihilation of both particles. On annihilation, two gamma rays of 511 keV are produced and travel 180 degrees apart in opposite directions. A great quantity of energy is required for positron emission to occur. The radionuclides that emit positrons must be artificially produced in a linear or cyclotron accelerator. Examples of the more common radioisotopes used for PET are carbon-11, oxygen-15, nitrogen-13, and fluorine-18. In addition, generator-produced positron-emitting radioisotopes rubidium-82, copper-62, germanium-68, and gallium-68 also are used. The chemical characteristics of the radioisotopes used for PET enable the synthesis of molecules that are used in tissue metabolism.

The metabolic radiopharmaceuticals currently being studied and researched entail diagnostic applications in tumor biology, neurology, psychiatry, and cardiology.

The PET camera is a system that has many crystal detectors, the most common of which is bismuth germanium oxide (BGO), which is placed in a circular configuration about the patient. Other crystal detector materials now in use are lutetium oxyorthosilicate (LSO) and gadolinium oxyorthosilicate (GSO). The system hardware configuration looks similar to the CT; however, the operation has no similarity. A positron-emitting radiopharmaceutical is administered to the patient. The crystal detectors are paired off 180 degrees apart to count simultaneously, and the 511-keV photons are detected (Esser et al., 1983). The PET system then establishes where the event occurred simultaneously and acquires the data (Esser et al., 1983). The computer software then manipulates the data and reconstructs tomographic slices of the original images.

The PET system is a complicated detection device that can have literally thousands of crystals. Specific quality control testing varies according to scanner manufacturer, but some common requirements include the following:

- Adjustments of PMT gain—daily
- Crystal and energy map—a crystal map converts the analog position of a detected event to a specific crystal within the detector block (daily)
- Coincidence timing calibration—adjusts for timing delays so that events from each block are time-stamped equivalently (daily)
- Detector drift check—based on change in sonogram (visual or numeric comparison) or drifts of baseline or peaks (daily)
- Blank scan—used with the transmission data in the computation of attenuation correction factors to monitor system stability. These are acquired daily using transmission rod sources.
- Normalization—compensates for the variation in efficiency in each line of response (LOR) in the sonogram and for axial sensitivity variation in some scanners (monthly or as required)
- Calibration—used to convert the reconstructed image pixel values into activity concentration (monthly or as required)
- Phantom image evaluation—allows for evaluation of tomographic uniformity, region of interest, spatial resolution, noise, and the **standardized uptake value** (SUV), which is a measure of FDG uptake, contrast and scatter/attenuation.

The quality control tests required at installation and thereafter and described and outlined in depth by Karp and colleagues (Karp et al., 1991) and NEMA (National Electrical Manufacturers Association, 2001) are radial resolution, tangential resolution, axial resolution, sensitivity, linearity, uniformity, attenuation accuracy, scatter determination, and dead time corrections (National Electrical Manufacturers Association, 2001).

POSITRON EMISSION TOMOGRAPHY/ COMPUTED TOMOGRAPHY SYSTEMS

Systems combining PET scanning capability and computed tomography (CT) scanning into the same machinery are rapidly becoming commonplace in diagnostic imaging departments. With these systems, quality control testing of the PET scanning circuitry and the CT circuitry must be performed separately using procedures discussed here and in Chapter 12. Additional quality control testing such as spatial coregistration between CT and PET image data also must be performed. Check with the manufacturer's quality control manual for your particular system for further details.

QUALITY CONTROL OF NONIMAGING EQUIPMENT

In addition to the variety of imaging systems used in nuclear medicine, nonimaging equipment is essential for the function and safety of all nuclear medicine departments. Nonimaging devices are used daily in radiation protection, in vitro studies, and all radiopharmacy procedures. A radiation protection quality assurance program is essential and required by TJC (Accreditation manual for hospitals, 1993) and the **Nuclear Regulatory Commission** (NRC) (USNRC Title 10, 1987). A radiation protection program ensures that the workplace, employees, and patients are safe and not needlessly exposed to any ionizing radiation. A quality assurance program is also crucial in the radiopharmacy of any nuclear medicine department. Radionuclides must be produced and radiopharmaceuticals prepared and subsequently dispensed and administered to the correct patients. In addition, the procedure of Universal Precautions, enacted into law and enforced by the **Occupational Safety and Health Administration** (OSHA) (Strasinger and Di Lorenzo, 1996), must be an integral component of any nuclear medicine quality assurance program to secure a safe environment for both the patient and the healthcare worker. This is especially important to all individuals who may come in contact with needles and blood products.

For the guarantee of safe and accurate diagnostic and therapeutic studies, it is imperative to have quality control procedures in place from the moment a radionuclide is produced or received until the patient study is completed.

Gas-Filled Detectors

Many radiation detection devices not only detect radiation but also quantitate the amount of ionizing radiation present. The **gas-filled detector** is one type of radiation detection device. The gas-filled detector is a mechanism that consists of a chamber filled with a gas, an anode, a cathode, an external voltage source, and a display meter. The operation of gas-filled detectors is based on the principle that the ionization-induced electrical currents are produced within the gas chambers of these detectors. As radiation passes through the gas chamber, ions are produced, and the positive ions migrate to the cathode, while the electrons migrate to the anode. The amount of ion pairs collected is a function of the voltage applied and is directly proportional to the energy and quantity of gamma rays entering the chamber. The detector then responds to the presence of radiation by discovering the ionization-induced electrical currents and displaying the current to read in radiation units. Ionization chambers and **Geiger-Müller** (GM) **meters** are the most common gas-filled detectors used in nuclear medicine. ❻ *The NRC regulation Title 10 Code of Federal Regulations Part 35.50* (USNRC Title 10, 1987) *(10 CFR 35.50) requires that nuclear medicine departments must assay all radionuclides administered to patients in a dose calibrator, a specialized ionization chamber.* **Ion-Detecting Radiation Detectors.** Three types of ion-detecting radiation detectors are commonly used in nuclear medicine. The ionization survey meter, which includes the "cutie-pie"* type, measures radiation exposure rates (roentgens [R] per hour); the dose calibrator measures the quantity of the radiation dosage in microcuries to curies (Ci); and the GM survey meter and room monitor measure qualitative exposure rates. ❻ *The NRC requires that nuclear medicine departments possess all three types of radiation detectors* (Henkin et al., 1996).

The ionization survey meter is generally battery operated and portable. The ionization survey meter is commonly used in the nuclear medicine department to secure radiation safety of the personnel and the work environment. ❻ *The NRC states in section 35 of the CFR* (USNRC Title 10, 1987) *that any licensee using radioactive materials or radiopharmaceuticals is required to possess a portable radiation survey meter* (Henkin et al., 1996). *In addition, the NRC regulations state that a daily area survey must be performed in any area where radioactive materials are used and stored. Unrestricted areas must not exceed 2 millirem (mrem) in any 1 hour* (USNRC Regulatory Guide, 1977). *The NRC requires that the survey meter be capable of detection of dose rate from 0.1 to 100 milliroentgen (mR)/hr* (Henkin et al., 1996; USNRC Regulatory Guide, 1977).

The radiation monitoring equipment must function accurately and properly to ensure that all monitoring and daily survey radiation exposure readings are true values and conform to the NRC regulations. ❻ *The NRC requires that all survey meters undergo an annual calibration and a daily reference check before use.* The survey meter must be calibrated; otherwise, the values it produces when exposed to radiation have no meaning. The survey meter must be calibrated against a point source that is traceable to a standard certified within 5% accuracy by the U.S. National Institute of Standards and Technology (NIST) (Thrall and Ziessman, 1995). The survey meter is adjusted if necessary to read the calculated value of the standard (i.e., cesium-137). ❻ *The survey meter should be calibrated on three to five scales (0.1, 10, 100). The procedure and requirements of the NRC can be found in 10 CFR 35.51* (USNRC Title 10, 1987).

The reference check is a simple procedure. It requires that the instrument measure a standard, long-lived, radioactive source at the same geometry. The readings obtained in the reference check must be within 20% of the exposure rate checked at calibration, which must always be posted on the side of the instrument (USNRC Title 10, 1987). The reference check of the survey meter ensures that the instrument is maintaining calibration. In addition, because the survey meter is battery operated, it is good practice to perform a battery check on the instrument before each use.

Geiger-Müller Meters. The GM meter is a survey meter used mainly for radiation protection purposes as a survey instrument and an area monitor. One of its uses is as a room monitor. The audible mechanism allows a quick and inexpensive way to determine the presence of ionizing radiation and is a reminder to work quickly. The intensity of the sound increases with the intensity of the ionizing radiation field. However, the GM meter is not capable of accurately measuring and quantitating radiation exposure caused by diverse energy photons commonly found in a nuclear medicine department. The GM meter cannot accurately measure radiation exposure or dose rate, although it is calibrated in milliroentgens per hour or counts per minute. It can only indicate the presence of ionizing radiation. ❻ *The NRC requires that all GM meters undergo the same quality control as the ionization survey meters. The GM meter must be calibrated annually, and the reference and battery checked before use* (USNRC Title 10, 1987).

Dose Calibrator

A **dose calibrator** is an ionization chamber that is used to verify radioactivity measurements of all radionuclides, radiochemicals, and radiopharmaceutical doses subsequent to their administration to the patient. Confusion of the terminology used in the radiopharmacy can be avoided by knowing the following definitions of the "radio" terms:

- *Radionuclide:* any radioactive atom
- *Radiochemical:* a radionuclide that has combined with a nonradioactive chemical molecule
- *Radiopharmaceutical:* a radionuclide combined with a biologically active molecule

Radioactive material may require the addition of stabilizers, reagents, or buffering agents. In addition, a radiopharmaceutical requires approval by the Food and Drug Administration (FDA) before clinical use (Thrall and Ziessman, 1995). ❻ *The four NRC-required quality control tests performed on a dose calibrator are accuracy, constancy, geometry, and linearity.*

The accuracy test evaluates the ability of the radionuclide dose calibrator to accurately measure the activity of standard sources such as ^{57}Co, cesium-55, and barium-133. These reference sources must be traceable to the NIST. The accuracy test, performed annually, compares the actual activity of the standard sources with the observed readings of the dose calibrator. ❻ *If the dose calibrator readings vary from the reference sources by more than 10%, then the instrument must be recalibrated, repaired, or replaced* (Fig. 15-17).*

---

*The "cutie-pie" is considered more accurate and linear over all of its ranges compared with the GM tubes.

*Note: The 10% variance refers to the NRC regulations. The accepted variance is 5% in most agreement states. Please check with your individual state's regulations for the correct value.

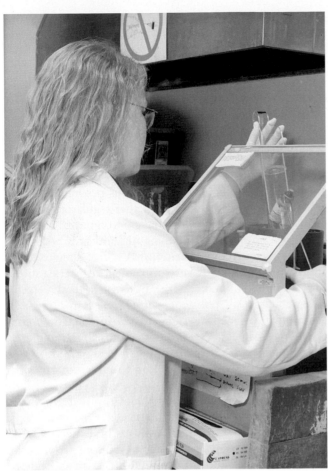

FIGURE 15-17 Nuclear medicine technologist performing the quality control tests on a dose calibrator.

The constancy test assesses and verifies the precision of the dose calibrator. A long-lived sealed reference source such as ^{57}Co, ^{137}Cs, or radium-226 is assayed daily on all commonly used radionuclide settings, and the readings are compared with the standard reference source. ⊕ *The dose calibrator readings must not vary from the reference source activity by more than 10%.* *

There may be significant variation in measured values versus actual radioactivity present as a result of a variation of sample volume. For example, 10 mCi (370 megabecquerels [MBq]) contained in the volume of a 1-mL syringe or a 20-mL syringe or vial might vary significantly. ⊕ *If the geometric variations cause the actual measurements to vary by more than 10% from the true value, correction factors are calculated and used for that specific volume.* * The geometric variation test is required on installation of the dose calibrator and after any repair.

Radionuclide dose calibrators should display the actual radioactivity of a sample. A linearity test determines the accuracy of the dose calibrator's response to measure a wide range of activities. The dose calibrator should be able to measure a full range of activities from microcuries to millicuries. ⊕ *Two methods are readily used and accepted by the NRC.* The first linearity test

requires assaying a decaying source of ^{99m}Tc sequentially over 3 to 5 days. The readings are compared with the actual decay of ^{99m}Tc at the same time intervals. The second method involves the use of precalibrated lead sleeves that are placed sequentially over the same source. The advantage of using the lead sleeves is that the procedure only takes about 5 minutes and results in a much lower level of radiation exposure to the technologist. The linearity test is performed at installation, at 3-month intervals, and after any repair. ⊕ *The observed values in either method must be within 10% of the actual calculated activities.* *

Nonimaging Scintillation Detectors

Along with the scintillation gamma camera systems mentioned previously, there are also nonimaging systems found in nuclear medicine that use the NaI(T1) crystal and detect radiation with the same basic principle of scintillation. The **scintillation detectors** used in nuclear medicine have many functions. The single-channel or **multichannel analyzers** (well counters) are scintillation detectors that are used to count blood and urine samples obtained from in vitro procedures such as red cell mass and plasma volume determinations and Schilling tests. In addition to in vitro patient studies, well counters are used to count the quality control **chromatography** strips required to evaluate radionuclides and radiopharmaceuticals (Zimmer, 1991). The advantage of the multichannel over the single-channel analyzer is that samples with multiple radioisotopes presenting low to high energy can be analyzed simultaneously. In addition, because the spectrum display is directly proportional to the radio-nuclide energy, it is possible to determine the unknown radiation that might be present in some contamination. It is also possible to see at a glance the whole spectrum and proper peaking over the energy of interest. This is important when performing NRC-required, daily, area-wipe surveys to locate, identify, and quantitate any contamination. The quality control procedures required for a scintillation detector are listed in Table 15-3.

Calibration is performed to determine and preset the correct operating voltage that is necessary for the detector to place the gamma energy peak in the center of the spectrum window. This results in achieving the highest and most accurate count rate. Generally, a long-lived radionuclide such as ^{137}Cs, with a gamma photon energy of 662 keV, is used. The voltage is adjusted so that the pulse height of 662 keV is at the center of the spectrum and the window is spaced equally above and below 662 keV.

Because the scintillation detectors count a variety of radionuclides (e.g., ^{99m}Tc, iodine-123, iodine-125, iodine-131, and ^{57}Co), the detector must be photopeaked before each new radionuclide is counted. Once this is accomplished, the detector's high voltage is adjusted properly for that specific radionuclide. When environmental samples are counted for contamination, windows are set wide to

TABLE 15-3	Scintillation Detector Quality Control
Quality Control Procedure	**Frequency**
Energy calibration	Daily
Peaking	Daily and before each new radionuclide used
Background	Daily and before each new radionuclide used
Constancy	Daily
Instrument calibration	Annually, after repair
Energy resolution	Annually, after repair
Efficiency	Annually, after repair
Chi-square test (reproducibility)	Quarterly, weekly recommended

capture the gamma rays of all radionuclides that may be potentially released as contaminants. Matching the photopeaks on the spectrum to specific energies allows identification of the radionuclide in the sample.

A background measurement with no radionuclide present is taken to ensure that no contaminating radioactivity will affect the true counts. The background is taken for the same period that the sample is counted. The background counts must be subtracted from each sample's gross counts to obtain the true, or net, counts (i.e., net counts = gross counts − background counts). A new background count must be taken for each radionuclide and for each separate procedure to obtain accurate clinical data.

A constancy test is performed daily to verify the stability of the detector. A long-lived source such as ^{137}Cs is counted, and the counts per minute per microcurie are determined and compared with the counts per minute per microcurie at the time of calibration. A change of more than 10% indicates that repair is necessary (Graham et al., 1996).

An annual calibration is performed to regulate the gain and high-voltage settings in such a way that dial settings of the channels read directly to the energy kiloelectron volt of the radionuclide. A ^{137}Cs source is used in the detector, and the energy peak is set on 662 keV with a 5% window. The voltage and gain are adjusted until the center, or photopeak, is exactly centered on 662 keV.

The energy resolution can be thought of as the ability of the scintillation detector to accurately discern two different energies as separate. Energy resolution quality control is discussed in the section on quality control of imaging equipment. To review, the energy resolution can then be expressed as the spread or width of the spectrum divided by the center photopeak. The spread of the spectrum or the FWHM is the energy range of the widest width of the spectrum, which is halfway down from the photopeak. The energy resolution is calculated as follows:

$$\text{Percent energy} = \frac{\text{FWHM at half maximum}}{\text{Photopeak center}} \times 100$$

The energy resolution of most scintillation systems that use ^{137}Cs is between 8% and 12% (Bernier et al., 1997).

The efficiency of a counting detector is measuring the sensitivity of the detector. It is expressed as the observed count rate divided by the disintegration rate of a radioactive sample (Sorenson and Phelps, 1987).

$$\text{Percent efficiency} = \frac{\text{Counts per minute}}{\text{Disintegrations per minute}}$$

This concept is important because counts per minute must be converted into **disintegrations per minute** (dpm) for the technologist to know whether regulatory requirements are being met for keeping environmental contamination within specific contamination limits for both fixed and removable contamination. For the same sample activity and geometry, every instrument registers a different count per minute on the basis of several detector design factors; therefore, an efficiency factor must be determined for each instrument used to count in counts per minute and convert to disintegrations per minute.

Radioactive decay of an atom is a random process, so when a radioactive source is said to undergo a number of disintegrations per second, the value represents only the average. Because the number of disintegrations per unit time varies, it can be expected that the counts obtained also vary. The variation to be expected when counting the same sample is due to random error. A statistical test called the **chi-square test** is used to evaluate the reliability of the detector. The results of the chi-square test indicate whether the error that exists in counting is due to randomness. If the error is due to some other problem such as a technical or mechanical error, the detector must be serviced before clinical use. The chi-square quality control test is easy to perform. A radioactive sample is counted 10 times for 1 minute each time. The sample must be placed at a distance from the detector that results in a minimum of 10,000 counts. The 10,000 counts are necessary to obtain good statistical data within 1% SD. The data are then used to determine the chi-square value:

$$\text{Chi} - \text{square} = \frac{\text{Sum}(x_i - \text{mean})^2}{\text{Mean}}$$

where x_i = individual count rates

The result is then located on the table of chi-square values to determine the probability that the discrepancy between the observed and expected frequency is due to random error. Most scintillation detectors are computer driven and maintain the statistical programs that automatically calculate the chi-square values.

Another NaI(Tl) scintillation detector used in nuclear medicine is the thyroid uptake probe. The thyroid probe is used clinically to determine the function of the patient's thyroid. A percent uptake of an ingested radioisotope of iodine is calculated. The thyroid uptake probe is a

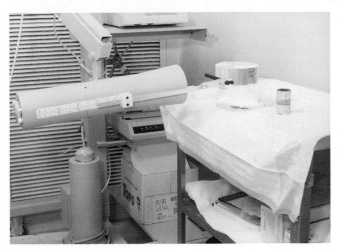

FIGURE 15-18 Thyroid probe quality control with a neck phantom.

multichannel analyzer with a flat-face crystal and PMT encased in an open-field collimator that faces the patient's thyroid during the procedure. The collimator is generally 20 to 30 cm long, which is the length required to obtain the proper counting geometry of the patient's thyroid. All of the quality control procedures required for a scintillation detector are performed on the thyroid probe. However, because distance and geometry are crucial in measuring a patient's iodine uptake, a thyroid phantom is used in all daily quality control procedures (Fig. 15-18). The thyroid phantom has been designed to mimic the location of a thyroid in a patient. The phantom ensures that the quality control procedures are accurate and can be related to the patient study.

QUALITY ASSURANCE IN THE RADIOPHARMACY

Sealed Radioactive Source

The sealed sources used in the previously mentioned calibrations and for calibration of other nonimaging and imaging equipment must be tested for any leakage of radioactive material. ❺ *The NRC requires that all photon-emitting sealed sources containing 100 μCi or more be tested for leakage biannually* (USNRC Regulatory Guide, 1977). *Any sealed sources with more than 0.005 μCi of removable activity per test must immediately be removed, properly stored, and reported to the NRC* (USNRC Title 10, 1987). *In addition, the NRC requires that all sealed sources be inventoried and surveyed quarterly for radiation exposure.*

Molybdenum-99/Technetium-99 Radionuclide Generator

The radionuclide generator system, a long-lived parent yielding to a shorter-lived daughter, allows the production of useful radionuclides for clinical use. The combination of half-lives of the radionuclides in the generator system makes the shipping of radionuclides from a commercial pharmacy to a hospital more cost-effective; deliveries are required once a week rather than daily. Most of the radiopharmaceuticals prepared by the nuclear medicine technologist are labeled with ^{99m}Tc. The most commonly used generator system in hospitals and clinics is the **molybdenum-99/technetium-99m** (^{99}Mo/^{99m}Tc) system. The ^{99}Mo/^{99m}Tc generator is an alumina ion-exchange column onto which ^{99}Mo, the parent, has a high affinity. Subsequently, ^{99m}Tc has a lower affinity to the column; therefore, the separation of ^{99m}Tc from the parent, ^{99}Mo, is simple. When saline solution is pulled through the alumina column by means of an evacuated collection vial, the daughter, Tc^{99m}, is removed, or eluted, from the column. The technetium eluted is in the radiochemical form ^{99m}TcO$_4^-$ (**technetium-99m pertechnetate**), and the ^{99m}Tc is in the valence state of +7. Quality control procedures are essential on the technetium eluent each time the generator is eluted, to ensure that the eluent does not contain any contaminants or impurities including **radionuclide impurity** of ^{99}Mo, molybdate, **chemical impurity** of Al^{+3}, alumina, or radiochemical impurity of **hydrolyzed reduced technetium** (HR-Tc).

A common contaminant found in the generator eluent is the parent, ^{99}Mo. The appearance of ^{99}Mo in the eluent is called *moly breakthrough*. If any ^{99}Mo is injected into a patient, the liver absorbs the ^{99}Mo and receives unnecessary radiation.

Testing for moly breakthrough is simple to perform. A lead container, which absorbs the ^{99m}Tc 140-keV energy but allows the passage of the higher-energy 740- and 780-keV ^{99}Mo photons, is used. The generator eluent vial is placed in the moly lead shield and assayed in the dose calibrator. The amount of ^{99}Mo contamination is calculated by dividing the total amount of ^{99}Mo assayed by the total amount of ^{99m}Tc. ❺ *The NRC allowable limit is 0.15 μCi of ^{99}Mo activity per 1 mCi of ^{99m}Tc activity at the time of injection of the administered dose* (USNRC Title 10, **1987**). *This is critical because the concentration of ^{99}Mo/^{99m}Tc may creep up and exceed limits several hours after elution.*

The chemical impurity that can be present in the generator eluent is alumina, Al^{+3}, which comes from the ion-exchange column. The U.S. Pharmacopoeia (USP) has established that the Al^{+3} concentration limits not exceed 10 μg of Al^{+3} per milliliter eluent. Aurin tricarboxylic acid is used for colorimetric spot testing (Thrall and Ziessman, 1995). The color reaction for a standard alumina sample is compared with the generator eluate. The comparison is qualitative and made by visual inspection. Excessive levels of aluminum can interfere with normal distribution of some radiopharmaceuticals.

In addition, the radiochemical impurity that may exist in the eluent solution is hydrolyzed reduced ^{99m}Tc (HR-Tc). Technetium that is eluted is expected to have a valence state of +7, which is the desired chemical form for most kit preparations. If the ^{99m}Tc is present in other forms, then the distribution of the final radiopharmaceutical product in a patient is altered. Unbound, or free, TcO_4^- accumulates in the stomach, thyroid gland, and salivary gland. ^{99m}Tc-colloidal uptake occurs in the reticuloendothelial system, especially the liver. ❻ *The USP standard for the generator eluent is that 95% or more of the technetium activity be in the +7 valence state* (Klingensmith et al., 1995).

Radiopharmaceuticals

Because radiopharmaceuticals are intended for diagnostic and therapeutic patient procedures, quality control procedures are crucial in ensuring the safety and effectiveness of these preparations (Zimmer, 1991). When a nuclear medicine department uses unit doses provided by a commercial nuclear pharmacy, the preparations undergo extensive quality control procedures by the manufacturer or the commercial nuclear pharmacy. However, many radiopharmaceutical preparations are prepared with lyophilized radiopharmaceutical preparation kits and short-lived radionuclides such as ^{99m}Tc. As a result, the absolute responsibility for the quality assurance of the radiopharmaceuticals lies with the radiopharmacist or the nuclear medicine technologist preparing the kits.

Whether the radiopharmaceuticals are prepared by commercial manufacturers or at the hospital nuclear pharmacy, they must be subjected to physiochemical and biologic testing including physical state examination and osmolality, pH, chemical, radionuclidic and radiochemical purity, sterility, and pyrogenicity testing (Zimmer, 1991).

Sterility represents the absence of metabolic products such as endotoxins in the final product. Sterility testing uses USP standard media such as thioglycollate and soybean casein digest media to determine the presence of bacteria and fungi in the radiopharmaceutical solution (Thrall and Ziessman, 1995). Because many radiopharmaceuticals are prepared just before patient administration, the sterility test must be performed retrospectively. Pyrogens or microorganism metabolites that may exist in the radiopharmaceutical solution can cause a fever if injected into a patient. The pyrogen test uses the USP limulus amebocyte lysate (LAL) test to detect the presence of pyrogens.

The radiochemical and radionuclidic purity of a radiopharmaceutical may be assessed by many different methods including paper chromatography, thin layer chromatography, high-performance liquid chromatography, and gel electrophoresis (Robbins, 1984; Zimmer, 1991; Zimmer and Pavel, 1977; Zimmer and Spies, 1991). Because of the characteristics of short-lived radionuclides used in the preparation of radiopharmaceuticals, time is critical. Miniaturized chromatography procedures are used to evaluate the radiochemical purity

of radiopharmaceuticals because they are rapid and easy to use (Webber et al., 1983; Zimmer and Pavel, 1977). The miniaturized chromatography system developed by Zimmer (Zimmer and Spies, 1991) uses a support medium such as thin-layer chromatography and a developing solvent to routinely evaluate radiopharmaceutical preparations subsequent to patient administration (Taukulis et al., 1979).

The chromatography procedures involve spotting the radiopharmaceutical being tested on the origin line of the respective paper strips and eluting the strips in the designated solvent system (Fig. 15-19). After solvent migration to the solvent front line, the strips are removed, cut at the cut line, and counted for activity with appropriate counting systems such as the dose calibrator or the well counter (Fig. 15-20). The labeling efficiency or the fraction of total radioactivity incorporated into the radiolabeled material is calculated by subtracting the sum of the fraction of the impurities of free technetium and HR-Tc from 100%.

$$\text{Percent labeling efficiency} = 100 - (\text{Sum of all impurities})$$

❻ *The percent labeling efficacy for most radiopharmaceuticals should be more than 98%* (Accreditation manual for hospitals, 1993).

Radiation Protection of Nuclear Medicine Personnel

Through mutual cooperation, several regulatory agencies control the radiation exposure of radiation workers in the

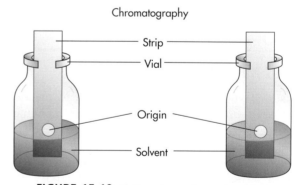

FIGURE 15-19 Eluting chromatography strips.

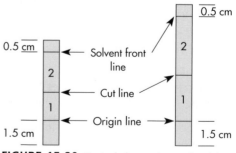

FIGURE 15-20 Typical chromatography strips.

TABLE 15-4	Nuclear Regulatory Commission Dose Equivalent Limits per Year
Anatomic Category	**Dose Equivalent Limit/Yr**
Whole body, head, trunk, blood-forming organs, gonads, and lens of the eyes	5 rem (50 mSv)
Hands, forearms, feet, and ankles	50 rem (500 mSv)
Skin of whole body	30 rem (300 mSv)
Fetus of radiation worker	0.5 rem (5 mSv)*

mSv, Millisievert; *rem*, roentgen equivalent, man.
*Dose equivalent for entire gestation period.

United States. The Department of Transportation (DOT), the Environmental Protection Agency (EPA), OSHA, individual state nuclear safety agencies, and the U.S. Nuclear Regulatory Commission Council on Radiation Protection and Measurements (NCRP) determined and provided the radiation dose exposure recommendations used for establishing the regulations and statutes of the NRC (Bernier et al., 1997). Table 15-4 lists the current acceptable radiation dose limits for occupational radiation workers (USNRC Title 10, 1991).

To ensure that the occupational radiation worker maintains an exposure far below the federal limits, the radiology communities adhere to the philosophy that the radiation dose exposure be "as low as reasonably achievable," or ALARA (Bernier et al., 1997). *The NRC states that the ALARA concept should maintain radiation doses to personnel working in radiation areas of a medical institution to less than 10% of the federal limits of occupational exposure* (Bernier et al., **1997**).

Personnel Monitoring. All radiation workers in the medical institution who may run the risk of exposure to ionizing radiation during routine duties must be provided with and wear a photographic film or **thermoluminescent dosimeter** (TLD) personal radiation detector (Regulatory Guide 8.7, 1992). The detector must be worn on the body part likely to receive the highest radiation exposure. It is recommended that the detector be worn between the shoulders and the waist. Nuclear medicine technologists or others who handle radionuclides or radiopharmaceuticals also must wear a ring or wrist radiation monitor so that radiation exposure of fingers and extremities can be estimated. The average period that a radiation worker routinely wears the radiation detectors is recommended not to exceed 1 month (USNRC Regulatory Guide, 1977). In addition, it is the responsibility of the radiation safety officer to review at least quarterly the results of personnel radiation monitoring and investigate and document any radiation dose exposure exceeding action Level II (30% of the federal limit) (Regulatory Guide 8.7, 1992).

In addition to personnel monitoring, any individual handling certain amounts of radioiodine (USNRC Title 10, 1987) must have a bioassay performed. The

bioassay is performed to determine if any iodine activity in the thyroid is due to ingestion or inhalation. The assay is performed with the thyroid uptake probe. The bioassay must be performed between 6 and 72 hours after handling for any individual dispensing, preparing, or administering a therapeutic dose of sodium iodide-131. Individuals who handle less than 30 mCi of iodine are required to undergo a bioassay each calendar quarter. The NRC recommends that corrective action be taken if the ^{131}I thyroid activity of the radiation worker exceeds 40 nanocuries (nCi).

Area Monitors. In addition to monitoring radiation exposure with personal dosimeters, individuals working in areas with radioactive materials also must monitor themselves before meals and before going home. The individuals can use a portable survey instrument such as a survey meter to determine any contamination to the body or clothing. In addition, each radiation work area must be surveyed daily to ensure that only background levels of radiation are present. If an area exceeds background radiation, it must be decontaminated. *Because the survey meter is the best instrument to detect radiation but not quantitate or identify radionuclide contaminant, a daily wipe test also is required in any radiation areas.* The wipe test is a survey designed to detect any removable radiation contamination by wiping the area to be evaluated with a cotton swab or some other absorbent paper such as filter paper. The wipe sample is analyzed in a scintillation detector such as a well counter or multichannel analyzer to determine the extent of the radionuclidic contamination. *Although the NRC only requires a detector sensitive enough to detect any contamination of 2000 dpm, it recommends that if the wipe sample results are more than or equal to 200 dpm/100 cm², the specific area must be decontaminated and checked again* (USNRC Regulatory Guide, **1977**).

The NRC mandates that areas where radioactive gaseous materials are used such as the nuclear pharmacy, as well as rooms where xenon-133 lung ventilation studies are performed, have negative airflow pressure with respect to surrounding areas (USNRC Title 10, 1987). *With this pressure, airborne activity that might be generated within the room can be removed through the exhaust system. The negative airflow pressure does not permit ^{133}Xe to passively diffuse into any surrounding areas. The exhaust must be a dedicated system and provide enough ventilation to dilute and remove radioactive concentrations that may be released into the room* (USNRC Regulatory Guide, 1977). *The exhaust also must release at a distance away from the public such as the roof top and meet EPA regulations for effluents released.* Quality control procedures must be performed to demonstrate that the airflow at the perimeters of these rooms is toward the room (Regulatory Guide 8.25, 1992). *The airflow must be checked a minimum of every 6 months to demonstrate proper and unchanged ventilation.*

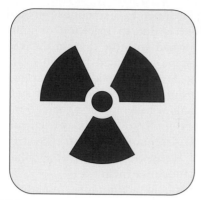

FIGURE 15-21 The three-bladed international warning symbol for ionizing radiation.

Radioactivity Signposting. ❻ *Specific signs are required by the NRC* (Bernier et al., 1997; Early and Sodee, 1995; USNRC Regulatory Guide, 1977). They must be posted near the entrance to any room where radioactive material may be used or stored. This is done to inform anyone entering the area of the potential hazard of radiation exposure. Each sign must bear the three-bladed international warning symbol for ionizing radiation (Fig. 15-21). The three-bladed symbol is magenta on a yellow background. Four different signs are used depending on the amount of potential exposure, as listed in Table 15-5.

Package Shipment, Receipt, and Opening. ❻ *NRC Regulation Part 20 recommends that all radioactive materials be monitored on receipt or within 3 hours if received during normal working hours or within 18 hours if received after normal working hours* (USNRC Title 10, 1987). A good quality assurance program recommends that any radioactive package be handled with disposable gloves, visually inspected, verified for contents, and checked for breakage or leaks. The radiation safety officer is to be notified of any irregularities.

The package must then be monitored with a survey meter at the surface of the package and at 3 feet from the package. In addition, a wipe survey of the exterior surface is performed to determine any removable contamination present. ❻ *Any value in excess of 0.01 $\mu Ci/100\ cm^2$ of surface area tested is a reportable level and must be decontaminated. In addition, exposure levels exceeding 200 mR/hr on the surface or 100 mR/hr at 3 feet from the package require notification of the radiation safety officer* (USNRC Title 10, 1987). *These must be documented daily on receiving forms.*

Infection and Radiation Exposure Control. Protective shielding in a variety of forms must be used when working with radioactive material. Several protective measures must be followed to minimize radiation contamination and exposure. Some examples of shielding protection materials are lead bricks, disposable gloves, leaded glass, shielded bench tops, syringe shields, vial lead containers, lead container "pigs" to transport the dose, lead-shielded containers to transport radioactive materials outside of the nuclear medicine department, and shielded waste receptacles. Use of the gloves and shielding are considered mandatory for the nuclear medicine worker. The department/institution must have a plan in place in case of a spill of radiopharmaceuticals, and training of non-nuclear medicine personnel must be provided and documented.

In addition, OSHA requires that all personnel who work with needles and blood products minimize their chance of exposure to the human immunodeficiency virus (HIV) and the hepatitis virus by practicing universal precautions (Strasinger and Di Lorenzo, 1996). When working with patient procedures that include needles and patient blood products, personnel are now required to wear disposable gloves. The universal precaution guidelines assert the prevention of recapping of needles at all costs. The used syringe must be placed in an approved infectious control needle and syringe receptacle, or sharps container (Fig. 15-22). Because nuclear

TABLE 15-5	Radiation Signs
Type of Sign	**Radiation Exposure Potential**
CAUTION, RADIOACTIVE MATERIALS	Areas in which radioactive material is stored or used in amounts not exceeding 5 mrem in 1 hr
CAUTION, RADIATION AREA	Areas in which an exposure could result in excess of 100 mrem in any 1 hr
CAUTION, HIGH RADIATION AREA	Areas in which an exposure could be > 5 mrem in 1 hr or > 100 mrem in 5 consecutive days
CAUTION, AIRBORNE RADIOACTIVITY AREA	Areas in which the airborne radioactivity level may exceed the restricted limit or may exceed 25% of the restricted area limit when averaged over 1 wk

mrem, Millirem.

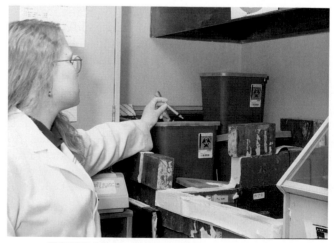

FIGURE 15-22 Following Universal Precautions.

medicine deals with radioactive needles and syringes, the sharps container also must be properly shielded, be decayed, and have stored a minimum of 10 half-lives before disposal to the biohazard department.

Radiopharmaceutical Administration

After preparation and quality control testing, the radiopharmaceutical is ready to be dispensed and administered to a patient. Quality assurance does not stop here. The individual who is dispensing and injecting the radiopharmaceutical should again verify the requisition, the identity of the radiopharmaceutical, the activity, and the patient. The following information must be visually inspected and verified on each request before the nuclear medicine procedure is initiated:

- Patient's name
- Hospital identification number and room number
- Requesting physician's name
- Patient history, condition, and preliminary diagnosis
- Examination agreement with the physician's orders and possible diagnosis of the patient
- Correct radiopharmaceutical for the examination
- Contraindications that can interfere with the radiopharmaceutical biodistribution
- Patient's physical limitations
- Allergies or potential drug interactions
- Potential nuclear medicine radiopharmaceutical interference with other diagnostic or therapeutic procedures
- Patient concerns

After the information has been checked and it is determined that the examination is correct, the person who is administering the radiopharmaceutical must continue to practice good quality assurance. The radiopharmaceutical, the activity, and the volume to be administered must be verified. Before administration, the patient's name and hospital identification number must be verified on the patient's wristband. Finally, if an outpatient is being treated, he or she must be identified through name, birth date, and social security number. If misadministration occurs, the radiation safety officer must be notified immediately. ❻ *The radiation safety officer determines what NRC classification of misadministration has occurred and immediately takes appropriate action (USNRC Title 10, 1991) including notification of ordering physician, medical director, patient, and NRC or agreement state. An investigation must be conducted to determine all factors contributing to the misadministration and a plan made of corrective action including training to prevent future occurrences.*

REVIEW QUESTIONS

1. The scintillation detector is based on the principle that certain crystals _____ after deposition of energy by some ionizing radiation.
   a. vibrate
   b. refract
   c. emit
   d. trap

2. The crystal that is used in most planar and SPECT gamma cameras is the _____ crystal.
   a. cesium iodide (CsI[T1])
   b. cesium fluoride (CsF)
   c. lithium iodide LiI(Eu)
   d. NaI(T1)

3. _____ testing involves performing a quality control performance evaluation of the camera system without the collimator.
   a. Extrinsic
   b. Intrinsic
   c. Phantom
   d. Dead time

4. What are the two most important quality control procedures that must be performed on a scintillation gamma camera?
   a. Intensity; persistence
   b. Counting efficiency; sensitivity
   c. Flood field uniformity; spatial resolution
   d. Linearity; geometry

5. A dose calibrator is an example of an ionization chamber. The following quality control procedures are mandated by the NRC except for which of the following?
   a. Geometry
   b. Chi-square
   c. Linearity
   d. Accuracy
   e. Constancy

6. Which of the following values is the allowable (NRC) limit of molybdenum in the generator eluent of ^{99m}Tc pertechnetate?
   a. 0.0015 μCi/mCi
   b. 0.015 μCi/mCi
   c. 0.15 μCi/mCi
   d. 1.5 μCi/mCi
   e. 1.5 mCi/μCi

7. _____ is the gamma camera's ability to see detail in any image.
   a. Spatial linearity
   b. Spatial resolution
   c. Relative position
   d. Energy resolution

8. In addition to the routine quality assurance procedures required for planar gamma cameras, the SPECT systems require evaluation of its tomographic performances, as well as reconstruction algorithms. Uncorrected center-of-rotation errors greater than ½ pixel can produce significant loss of spatial resolution. The quality control procedure COR aligns the COR projected onto the computer matrix with the center of the _____ used for reconstruction.
   a. camera
   b. patient
   c. computer matrix
   d. camera gantry

9. Evaluating the equipment used in a SPECT system is important, as is evaluating each patient study for artifacts or errors. The sinogram of a selected tomographic slice is a summed image of all the projection data. It is useful in detecting _____, which can degrade the quality of the SPECT study.
   a. patient motion
   b. dead time
   c. correct acquisition time
   d. incorrect radionuclide energy

10. Impurities found in radiopharmaceutical preparations are placed in all of the following categories except which of the following?
   a. Chemical impurities
   b. Nuclidic impurities
   c. Radionuclide impurities
   d. Radiochemical impurities

REFERENCES

Accreditation manual for hospitals, vol 1, Standards, Oakbrook Terrace, Ill, 1993, Joint Commission on Accreditation of Healthcare Organizations.

Anger HO: Scintillation camera, *Rev Scient Inst* 29:27, 1958.

Bernier DB, Christian PE, Langan JM, et al, *Nuclear medicine: technology and techniques*, ed 4, St Louis, 1997, Mosby.

Early PJ, Sodee BD: *Principles and practices of nuclear medicine*, ed 2, St Louis, 1995, Mosby.

Eisner R: Principles of instrumentation in SPECT, *J Nucl Med Technol* 13:23, 1985.

English RJ: *SPECT single-photon emission computerized tomography: a primer*, ed 3, Reston, Va, 1995, The Society of Nuclear Medicine.

Esser PD, Sorenson JA, Westerman BR: *Emission computed tomography*, New York, 1983, The Society of Nuclear Medicine.

Graham SL, Kirchner PT, Siegel BA: *Nuclear medicine: self study program II: instrumentation*, Reston, VA, 1996, The Society of Nuclear Medicine.

Greer K, et al: Quality control in SPECT, *J Nucl Med Technol* 13:76, 1985.

Henkin RE, et al: *Nuclear medicine*, vol 1, St Louis, 1996, Mosby.

Karp JS, et al: Performance standards in positron emission tomography, *J Nucl Med* 2:2342, 1991.

Klingensmith WC III, Eshima D, Goddard J: *Nuclear medicine procedure manual: 1995-1996*, Englewood, CO, 1995, Wick.

Murphy PH: Acceptance testing and quality control of gamma cameras including SPECT, *J Nucl Med* 28:1221, 1987.

Murray IPC, Ell PJ, editors: *Nuclear medicine in clinical diagnosis and treatment*, vol 1, Edinburgh, 1994, Churchill Livingstone.

National Electrical Manufacturers Association: *NEMA standards for performance measurements of scintillation cameras*, Pub No NUI-1986, Washington, DC, 1986, The Association.

National Electrical Manufacturers Association: *NEMA standards for performance measurement of positron emission tomographs*, Publication 2-2001, Washington, DC, 2001.

National Electrical Manufacturers Association: *Performance measurements of scintillation camera*, Washington, DC, 1980, The Association.

Rao DV, Early PJ, Chu RY, et al: *Radiation control and quality assurance surveys: nuclear medicine—a suggested protocol*, Rep No 3, 1986, American College of Medical Physicists.

Regulatory Guide 8.25: *Air sampling in the workplace*, Washington, DC, 1992, US Nuclear Regulatory Commission.

Regulatory Guide 8.7: *Instructions for recording and reporting occupational radiation exposure data*, Washington, DC, 1992, US Nuclear Regulatory Commission.

Robbins PJ: *Chromatography of technetium-99m radiopharmaceuticals: a practical guide*, New York, 1984, The Society of Nuclear Medicine.

Saha GP: *Physics and radiobiology of nuclear medicine*, New York, 1993, Springer-Verlag.

Scintillation camera acceptance testing and performance evaluation, Rep 6, Chicago, 1980, American Association of Physicists in Medicine.

Sorenson JA, Phelps ME: *Physics in nuclear medicine*, ed 2, Philadelphia, 1987, WB Saunders.

Steves AM: *Review of nuclear medicine technology*, New York, 1992, The Society of Nuclear Medicine.

Strasinger SK, Di Lorenzo MA: *Phlebotomy workbook for the multiskilled healthcare professional*, Philadelphia, 1996, FA Davis.

Taukulis RA, et al: Technical parameters associated with miniaturized chromatography systems, *J Nucl Med Technol* 7:19, 1979.

Thrall JH, Ziessman HA: *Nuclear medicine: the requisites*, St Louis, 1995, Mosby.

USNRC Regulatory Guide: *8.18: Information relevant to insuring that occupational radiation exposures at medical institutions will be as low as reasonably achievable*, Washington, DC, 1977, US Nuclear Regulatory Commission.

USNRC Title 10: *Code of Federal Regulation, Part 20: Standards for protection against radiation*, Washington, DC, 1987, US Nuclear Regulatory Commission.

USNRC Title 10: Code of Federal Regulations, Part 20: *Standards for protection against radiation*, Fed Reg 56 (89):23390, 1987.

USNRC Title 10: Code of Federal Regulations, Part 20: *Standards for protection against radiation*, Fed Reg 56(98):23390, 1991.

USNRC Title 10: *Code of Federal Regulations, Part 35: Human uses of byproduct material*, Washington, DC, 1987, US Nuclear Regulatory Commission.

Webber DI, Zimmer AM, Spies SM: Common errors associated with miniaturized chromatography, *J Nucl Med Technol* 11:66, 1983.

Zimmer AM: *Miniaturized chromatography procedures for radiopharmaceuticals*, Chicago, 1991, Northwestern University Medical Center.

Zimmer AM, Pavel DG: Rapid miniaturized chromatographic quality control procedures for Tc-99m radiopharmaceuticals, *J Nucl Med* 18:1230, 1977.

Zimmer AM, Spies SM: Quality control procedure for newer radiopharmaceuticals, *J Nucl Med Technol* 19:210, 1991.

Review of Radiographic Quality

Radiographic imaging is a multistep process in which the x-ray intensity after attenuation inside of the patient is transferred to different types of information carriers (e.g., intensifying screens and film or digital image receptors) along the imaging chain. The imaging chain consists of three components: image acquisition (accomplished by exposing a film/screen combination or digital image receptor to x-rays), image processing (accomplished by placing an exposed film into an automatic film processor or by sending digital image data into a computer for processing), and image display (accomplished by placing a hard-copy film image onto a viewbox illuminator or displaying a soft-copy digital image on a computer monitor). Once the image is created, the radiographic quality must be sufficient to demonstrate the anatomy of the patient.

Radiographic quality is defined as the accuracy with which an anatomic structure is represented in a radiographic image and is determined by four factors in film/screen radiography: optical density, contrast, recorded detail, and distortion.

- *Optical density:* The amount of black metallic silver remaining on a portion of film after processing is complete
- *Contrast:* The differences among optical densities on the processed radiograph
- *Recorded detail:* The sharpness of structure lines or minute details in a radiographic image

- *Distortion:* Any misrepresentation of the true size, shape, or spatial relationship of the part in the radiographic image

OPTICAL DENSITY

The function of optical density is to provide information in the radiographic image. In conventional film/screen radiography, if there is no black silver on the polyester plastic film base, no information about the patient's anatomy is apparent. In digital imaging, optical density is the brightness level of the individual pixels in the image matrix that appears on the monitor. A pixel with a low brightness level is comparable with a greater optical density on a film. When digital images are transferred to a hard copy (film), they appear virtually identical to conventional radiograph images.

Once optical density is produced in a film, it can be measured with a *densitometer,* which measures the amount of light transmission through a portion of film and assigns a numeric value ranging from 0 to 4 with the following equation:

$$O.D. = \log_{10} \text{ incident light/transmitted light}$$

or

$$\log_{10} I_i/I_t$$

Factors That Influence Optical Density

For film/screen radiography, the following factors influence the optical density that is created in the final image:

- *Kilovolt (peak) (kVp):* An increase in kilovolts (peak) increases the optical density because the x-ray beam is more penetrating (so more of it reaches the image receptor) and because a higher percentage of scatter versus absorption occurs. The exponential, or logarithmic, mathematical relationship between optical density and kilovolts (peak) means that just a small change in kilovolts (peak) can have a major change in optical density. This mathematical relationship can be used in practice with the 15% rule: An increase of 15% in kilovolts (peak) doubles the optical density or is the equivalent of doubling the milliampere-second (mAs).

- *mAs:* An increase in mAs increases optical density because a greater quantity of x-rays are being emitted from the x-ray tube. The direct, or linear, mathematical relationship between mAs and optical density makes it the major control of optical density. A 25% to 30% change in mAs is required to cause a visible change in optical density because of limitations of the human eye.

- *Source-to-image-distance (SID):* An increase in SID causes a decrease in optical density because of the divergent effect of the x-ray beam; the number of x-ray photons is reduced per unit area. An inverse square mathematical relationship exists between the SID and optical density, so if the distance were to change by a factor of 2, the optical density changes by 2^2, or 4 times.

- *Part thickness and tissue density:* An increase in either one or both of these factors decreases optical density if no other factors are altered (such as mAs or kilovolts [peak]). This decrease is due to the extra absorption of primary beam x-rays within the part. As a rule, for every 5-cm change in part thickness, the mAs should change by a factor of 2.

- *Development:* A rise in developer time, temperature, pH, concentration, or replenishment rate increases the optical density of a radiographic image and vice versa. This increase occurs because these factors directly control developer activity (i.e., how well the developer functions). Increasing these factors causes more activity and causes more black silver grains to appear, whereas decreasing these factors has the opposite effect.

- *Field size:* A significant reduction in field size decreases image optical density because of less scattered radiation being produced in the patient. Radiographers should notice this effect when performing a lateral view of the lumbar spine (performed with a larger size image receptor) and then a lateral spot view of the L5-S1 joint space (performed with a small field size). The spot view usually requires a 30% to 50% increase in mAs to compensate for the loss of scattered radiation, as compared with the larger image receptor size.

- *Grid ratio:* A higher grid ratio decreases image optical density because of a greater absorption of both primary and scattered x-rays, as compared with no-grid or lower-grid ratio exposures; therefore, exposures performed with a higher-grid ratio require higher mAs to compensate for this effect to maintain the same optical density.

- *Intensifying screen speed:* A faster-speed screen emits more light on exposure to x-rays, as compared with a slower speed screen that is exposed to the same number of x-rays. This additional light causes a film to have a greater optical density after processing because of the additional amount of exposure; therefore, faster speed screens require lower mAs to produce the same optical density, as compared with a slower speed screen. However, the faster-speed screen may result in a poorer image resolution compared with the slower speed screen (discussed later).

- *Film speed:* Faster-speed film emulsions generally produce greater optical density than slower-speed emulsions that are exposed to the same amount of radiation. The reason is that faster-speed emulsions may have larger silver halide crystals, a larger number of silver halide crystals, or chemical impurities added to the silver halide crystals to increase their speed. Film speed and intensifying screen speed are often combined into a single factor known as *image receptor system speed.* This combination is made by taking the film speed values, which are usually indicated as 50 (slow), 100 (standard), and 200 (fast), and joining them with the screen speed values (ranging from 25 to 1500). For example, if a 100-speed film is used, the screen speed value is also the image receptor system speed because 100 is the standard speed of film. If a 100-speed film is used with a 400-speed screen, the image receptor system speed is also 400. If a 50-speed film is used, the screen speed value is cut in half to obtain the image receptor system speed value. For example, if a 50-speed film and a 400-speed screen are used, the image receptor system speed is 200. Finally, if a 200-speed film is used, the screen speed value is doubled to obtain the image receptor system speed. If a 200-speed film is used with a 400-speed screen, the image receptor system speed is 800.

- *Object-to-image-distance (OID):* A significant increase in OID decreases optical density because of the reduction of scattered radiation reaching the film such as in the air gap technique that is used in lateral cervical spine examinations.

- *Fogging:* Fog is defined as non-informational optical density and, if present, increases the overall optical density and reduces the visibility of detail in the resulting image; therefore, fogging of any type should be avoided. In digital imaging, fogging is comparable to *noise* and causes a decrease in pixel brightness.
- *Presence of disease:* Certain pathologic conditions alter the normal tissue density of an anatomic region and therefore alter the optical density of the resulting image. Disease processes that decrease the normal tissue density (known as *destructive or atrophic diseases*) tend to increase image optical density if no other exposure factors are changed. A general rule is to decrease the mAs by 30% to 50% for patients with atrophic diseases (depending on the severity of the disease or condition) from the technique that is normally used for patients without the disease. Osteoporosis and emphysema are two examples of diseases or conditions in this category. Other diseases (known as *additive diseases*) can increase the normal tissue density and tend to decrease the optical density of the resulting images because of the additional absorption of primary x-rays within the part that is being radiographed. The general rule for these patients is to increase the mAs by 30% to 50% from the usual technique. Edema, pneumonia, and Paget's disease are a few examples of diseases or conditions in this category.
- *Voltage waveform:* High-frequency and three-phase x-ray generators emit more x-rays in a given period than single-phase x-ray generators; therefore, the image optical density is increased. These units generally require 50% less mAs for a given exposure compared with a full-wave-rectified, single-phase x-ray unit.
- *Filtration:* An increase in the amount of beam filtration decreases the image optical density of the resulting image because of the additional absorption of primary beam x-rays by the filtering material.

Inherent Densities

Two types of optical densities are inherent in film without prior exposure to radiation.

- *Base density* is a measurable optical density that is caused by the blue tint added to the base of the film to reduce glare from the fluorescent viewbox illuminator. When measured with a densitometer, it has a value of approximately 0.05.
- *Fog density* is the development of silver grains that contain no useful information, and it is caused by age fog, improper storage conditions, improper safelight conditions, and improper development parameters. When fog density is measured with a densitometer, this value can normally vary between 0.05 and 0.15. If these factors are not within specified parameters, this value can exceed this range and corrective action is required.

The base and fog density values are usually combined into a single value known as the base + fog (B + F) density that is used as an indicator of processor performance during sensitometric testing.

Optical Density and Digital Imaging

As mentioned previously, the optical density of images created by digital imaging systems is determined by the brightness level of the pixels in the image matrix. Darker areas of a conventional radiograph (e.g., air) correspond to less bright areas on a computer monitor screen, whereas brighter areas (e.g., bone) correspond to much brighter areas on the monitor. This means that the pixel brightness (optical density) of the resulting image is controlled more by the computer software than by the factors that have just been discussed with the conventional film/screen systems. The optical density can be manipulated by the radiographers' use of the software factors that are incorporated into their respective systems. These controls generally set the window level (the level within the possible shades that is used to create the middle density in the image window). However, these controls are not yet standardized and vary from manufacturer to manufacturer.

CONTRAST

Contrast is defined as the differences between optical densities on a processed radiograph and functions to make details visible. Three types of contrast exist: radiographic, subject, and film or inherent.

Radiographic Contrast

Radiographic contrast is the contrast as it appears on the finished image and is usually classified as either long scale or short scale.

- *Long-scale, or low, radiographic contrast:* A small, gradual change among the different optical densities that yields a relatively large number of gray shades
- *Short-scale, or high, radiographic contrast:* Large or abrupt differences among optical densities that yields an image with a relatively small number of gray shades (image appears more black and white)

Subject Contrast

Subject contrast is the difference in the quantity of radiation transmitted by a particular part because of the different absorption characteristics of the tissues and structures within the part. The subject contrast helps determine the radiographic contrast. Several factors that affect subject contrast are radiation quality, radiographic part, contrast media, scattered radiation, fogging, and presence of disease.

- *Radiation quality:* As the quality (energy) of radiation increases, the subject (and therefore radiographic) contrast decreases because of greater penetration of the structures within the part. Radiation quality is influenced by the kilovolt (peak) selected, voltage waveform of the x-ray generator, and the amount of filtration in the beam.
- *Radiographic part:* The distribution of tissue densities within the anatomic part significantly affects the subject contrast. If similar tissue densities exist within a particular part (e.g., breast), low subject contrast occurs. Widely different tissue densities (e.g., chest) demonstrate a high subject contrast.
- *Contrast media:* The use of contrast media increases the subject contrast of a particular region by changing the tissue density of the structure in which it is located.
- *Scattered radiation:* Scattered radiation always reduces subject contrast; therefore, any device or procedure that reduces the amount of scattered radiation reaching an image receptor always increases subject (and therefore radiographic) contrast.
- *Fogging:* Any amount of fogging reduces subject contrast. Remember, in digital imaging, fogging is comparable to *noise* which also decreases subject contrast.
- *Presence of disease:* Pathologic conditions can alter the normal tissue density distribution within a region and therefore alter the subject contrast. The effect on radiographic contrast usually appears as an increase in contrast.

Film or Inherent Contrast

The contrast that is built into the image receptor system by the manufacturer helps determine the radiographic contrast and subject contrast. This relationship can be demonstrated mathematically by the following equation:

Radiographic contrast = Subject contrast × Inherent contrast

Factors that affect inherent contrast in film/screen imaging are film emulsion, development, and image receptor system speed.

- *Film emulsion:* Faster speed emulsions generally yield higher-contrast images because they turn black quickly.
- *Development:* Any increase in development time, temperature, pH, concentration, or replenishment from the normal values usually decreases image contrast.
- *Image receptor system speed:* Faster-speed systems tend to create higher-contrast images.

In digital imaging, inherent contrast is affected by factors such as the image receptor (CR imaging plate and DR radiation detectors), bit depth of the computer, and pre and post-processing protocols.

Sensitometric Curve

The relationship between the factors just mentioned and inherent contrast can be demonstrated graphically in film/screen imaging with a sensitometric curve (also known as a *characteristic curve, Hurter and Driffield curve [H & D curve], or a D log E curve*). This curve plots the optical density on the y-axis and the log of exposure to the film on the x-axis. The curve is divided into three main portions (Fig. A-1): the toe, straight line portion, and shoulder.

- *Toe:* Indicates the B + F optical density values
- *Straight line portion:* Contains the diagnostically useful optical densities
- *Shoulder:* Indicates the maximum optical density value obtained

The steeper the straight line portion of the curve, the greater the film contrast (Fig. A-2).

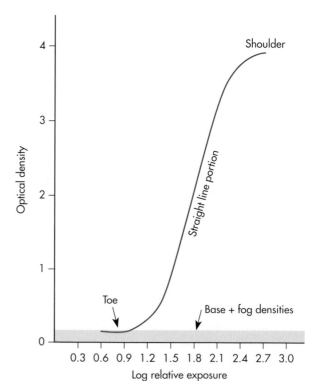

FIGURE A-1 The three main portions of the sensitometric curve.

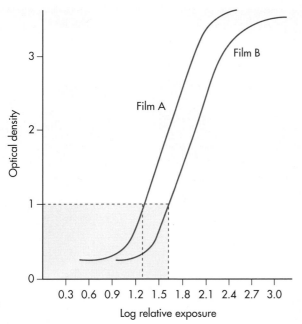

FIGURE A-2 Film A demonstrates a higher contrast and faster speed than film B.

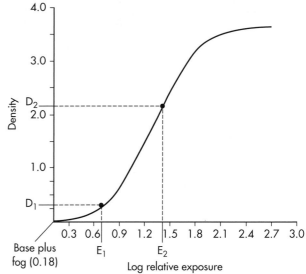

FIGURE A-3 Average gradient determination from a Hunter and Driffield (H & D) curve with the optical density values of 0.25 above base + fog (B + F) and 2.0 above B + F.

The steepness or slope of the straight line portion can be calculated with the following equation:

$$\text{Slope} = \frac{D_2 - D_1}{E_2 - E_1}$$

where D_2 and D_1 correspond to the optical density of the points on the straight line (y-axis) and E_2 and E_1 correspond to the relative log of exposure of the points (x-axis). Two different slope values can be calculated:

- *Film gamma:* This is the slope value measured at the steepest point on the straight line portion.
- *Average gradient:* This is the slope of the straight line between the optical density points of 0.25 above the B + F and 2 above the B + F (Fig. A-3). The average gradient is a better indicator of film contrast than film gamma for radiographic studies and is therefore more commonly used. Most radiographic films have an average gradient value between 2.5 and 3.5.

Other quantities that can be demonstrated with a characteristic curve include film speed or sensitivity, exposure latitude, and solarization or image reversal.

- *Film speed or sensitivity:* The relative exposure needed to produce an optical density of 1 above the B + F. The closer this point is to the y-axis, the faster the speed of the film is (see Fig. A-2).
- *Exposure latitude:* The range of exposures over which the film responds with optical densities in the diagnostically useful range of 0.5 to 2.5. Exposure latitude and contrast are inversely proportional; therefore, high-contrast film has

narrow exposure latitude, and low-contrast film has wide exposure latitude (Fig. A-4).

- *Solarization or image reversal:* A decrease in optical density occurs as the amount of exposure increases beyond the maximum optical density. This process is thought to be caused by a chemical reaction in the film emulsion, known as *rebromination*. This principle is used in duplicating film that has been exposed to the maximum density before purchase (Fig. A-5).

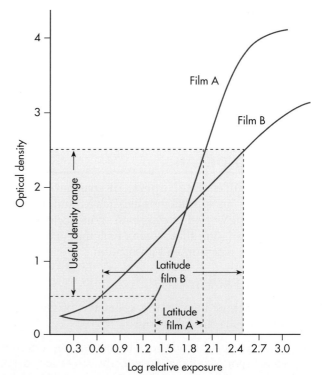

FIGURE A-4 Film A demonstrates a narrower exposure latitude than film B.

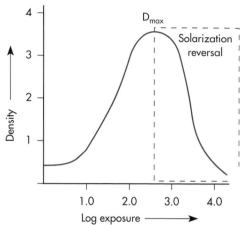

FIGURE A-5 Sensitometric curve demonstrating the effect of solarization. A decrease in optical densities occurs after the maximum density has been achieved.

Image Contrast with Digital Systems

As with optical density, the contrast obtained with digital imaging systems also is controlled mainly by the computer software and is sometimes referred to as *gray scale* instead of contrast. The factors listed previously that affect subject contrast still have a strong influence over the image contrast that is obtained with digital systems, but obviously there is no film or inherent contrast to consider. Instead, radiographers can manipulate the contrast using software factors on the operating console known as dynamic range, window width, or gradational enhancement. When a wider window or dynamic range is selected, the image contrast decreases because there is room for more gray shades to appear (Fig. A-6). The sensitometric curve used to demonstrate inherent contrast in film/screen imaging is replaced by a graph known as a Lookup Table (Fig. A-7) in digital imaging. Contrast in digital imaging also is affected by the bit depth of the computer (the number of gray shades that the computer can create at each pixel location). The greater the bit depth, the more gray shades can be created. Most digital systems use either 10-, 12-, or 16-bit systems.

RECORDED DETAIL

Recorded detail is the sharpness of structure lines or minute details in a radiographic image and is often referred to as *definition* or *sharpness*. Four factors affect recorded detail in film/screen imaging: geometric, motion, image receptor, and absorption.

Geometric Factors

Geometric factors involve the geometry of the x-ray beam and include the following:

- *Effective focal spot size:* The smaller the effective focal spot size, the greater the recorded detail because of the penumbra effect (also known as *geometric unsharpness*). However, a smaller

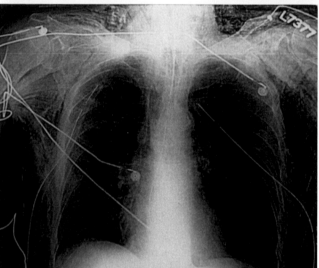

FIGURE A-6 Comparison of image contrast with a conventional image *(top)* and a digital image *(bottom)*.

effective focal spot usually has a decreased heat capacity during an x-ray exposure and should therefore not be used for radiographic examinations of the trunk of the body where higher kilovolt (peak) and mAs combinations may be required.

- *SID:* The greater the SID, the greater the recorded detail because the x-ray photons used for imaging travel more parallel to each other, rather than diverging.
- *OID:* The greater the OID, the poorer the recorded detail because of an increased penumbra effect at the image receptor. The image also is magnified.
- *Heel effect:* The amount of geometric unsharpness or penumbra effect is greater toward the cathode end of the x-ray field, and the result is a poorer recorded detail of structures imaged from this portion of the x-ray beam. This factor must be considered during mammographic procedures in which fine recorded detail is paramount.

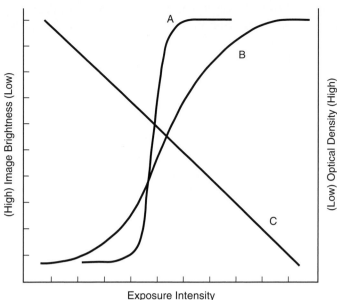

FIGURE A-7 Look-up tables for digital image processing. The curve shape defines the relationship between the intensity of exposure and image brightness (comparable to optical density in film images). **A,** High contrast curve. **B,** Low-contrast (wide latitude) curve. **C,** Linear response curve with a reversed grayscale.

Motion Factors

Any motion of the patient, x-ray source, or image receptor results in poorer recorded detail because of motion blur. This motion can be minimized by proper instructions from the radiographer to the patient, by the use of shorter exposure time during exposures, and by the use of immobilization when appropriate.

Image Receptor Factors

The type of image receptor system that is used to create the image has a significant effect on the level of recorded detail obtained in the resulting image. The ability of an image receptor system to produce recorded detail is known as *resolution* or *spatial resolution*. For film/screen systems, these factors include single screen versus double screen, screen active layer thickness and crystal size, and film speed.

- *Single screen versus double screen:* Single-screen imaging systems and single-emulsion film can demonstrate greater recorded detail than double-screen systems with duplitized film because of the crossover effect. However, this will result in a slower system speed and therefore requires a higher mAs value to obtain the desired optical density.
- *Screen active layer thickness and crystal size:* An increase in active layer thickness or phosphor crystal size (associated with an increase in screen speed) results in poorer recorded detail because of increased light diffusion.

- *Film speed:* In general, fast-speed film emulsions (which tend to have larger silver halide crystals) demonstrate poorer recorded detail than slow-speed emulsions because of the graininess that occurs as a result of larger crystal size.

Absorption Factors

The size or shape of the part being radiographed can decrease the level of recorded detail. In general, larger objects have less recorded detail than smaller objects because structures are farther away from the image receptor.

Recorded Detail or Spatial Resolution with Digital Imaging

The recorded detail or spatial resolution obtained with digital imaging systems depends on geometric, motion, and absorption factors. It also is affected by imaging system parameters such as the size of each detector in the active matrix array (DR systems only), the size of the crystal on the imaging plate (CR systems only), the size of the laser in the image reader device (CR systems only), the computer matrix size, the type of monitor, the bandwidth, and the filtering.

- *Size of each detector in the active matrix array:* Digital radiographic systems (DR) systems incorporate a flat-plate imaging sensor (known as an active matrix array), made up of millions of tiny radiation detectors that send electronic signals directly into the computer. The smaller the size of each detector in the flat-plate imaging sensor, the better the resolution in the final image.
- *Size of the crystal on the imaging plate:* With CR systems, there is an imaging plate that resembles a standard intensifying screen found in a film/screen cassette. The smaller the size of the crystal on the imaging plate, the better the recorded detail because of better spatial resolution.
- *Size of the laser in the image reader device:* Following exposure to x-rays, the CR image plate is scanned with a laser that causes the crystals on the plate to emit light in proportion to the amount of x-ray exposure. The light released by the crystals is then detected by light sensors and these reading are sent to the computer for processing into the final image. The smaller the size of the scanning laser, the better the spatial resolution.
- *Matrix size:* The larger the matrix size of the computer system, the sharper the image resolution. This is because the size of each pixel also must be smaller to accommodate the larger matrix. Most current systems use 2560 × 2048 (CR & DR) or 4096 × 6144 (digital mammography) matrices. The smaller the pixel size, the better the spatial resolution.

- *Type of monitor:* Progressive scanning monitors, which scan all 525 lines in order (standard computer monitor), or a high-resolution monitor, which scans 1050 lines, should be used instead of standard commercial television monitors to view digital radiographic images. The more scan lines in the monitor field, the better the resolution appearing in the image because each scan line is smaller in size. You can have an image stored in the computer memory that has a high spatial resolution, but viewing it on a low resolution monitor will result in poor visibility of this detail.
- *Bandwidth:* This is the frequency response of the incoming electronic signal. The greater the bandwidth (meaning the greater the frequency of the electric current carrying the information), the greater the resolution because more information can be contained in a high-frequency signal. Commercial television is broadcast at approximately 4 MHz, which produces approximately 320 lines of resolution. High-resolution television monitors use a frequency of approximately 20 MHz, which produces about 800 lines of resolution.
- *Filtering:* Digital filtering refers to the computer either accentuating or suppressing certain frequencies in the electronic signal that carries the information. Digital systems use a type of filtering called *high-pass filtering,* or *edge enhancement,* which either amplifies or deletes all but the high frequencies in the electronic signal. As its other name implies, the apparent edges of the structure lines in the image appear enhanced or sharper.

DISTORTION

Distortion is a misrepresentation of the true size, shape, or spatial relationship of an object in a radiographic image. The three types of distortion are size, shape, and spatial.

Size Distortion

Also known as *magnification,* size distortion is the result of the divergence of the x-ray beam from its source. The degree of size distortion chiefly depends on the SID and the OID.

- *SID:* An increase in the SID decreases the degree of size distortion because of a less divergent angle of the x-ray photons within the x-ray beam.

- *OID:* A rise in the OID increases the degree of size distortion because of an increased divergence of the x-ray beam.

Shape Distortion

Shape distortion is caused by improper alignment of the part with respect to the x-ray source and image receptor. The two main types of shape distortion are elongation and foreshortening.

- *Elongation:* With elongation, the object appears longer in the image than it actually is. The main cause of elongation is the central ray not being perpendicular to the image receptor; therefore, any radiographic view that requires a central ray angulation automatically shows elongation in the final image.
- *Foreshortening:* In foreshortening, the object appears shorter in the image because the object is partially superimposed on itself. The most common cause of this shape distortion is that the part being radiographed is not parallel to the plane of the image receptor (such as in the oblique position).

Spatial Distortion

Spatial distortion is a misrepresentation of the true spatial relationship among the various parts of the patient in the radiographic image. It is due to the projection of a three-dimensional object (the patient) onto a two-dimensional image receptor. For spatial distortion to be avoided, two views of the patient are usually taken at 90 degrees apart from each other during most radiographic procedures.

Image Distortion with Digital Imaging

Size, shape, and spatial distortion will occur during digital radiography just as in conventional film/screen radiography and is influenced by the same factors. Size distortion can be manipulated somewhat with digital imaging software because most have some type of zoom or region-of-interest option that can magnify specific areas within the image with the use of cursor control. There is also a minimize and maximize image control much like the software found in personal computers. Shape and spatial distortion appear identical in digital imaging and film/screen imaging.

Agencies, Organizations, and Committees in Quality Assurance

Agency for Healthcare Research and Quality
540 Gaither Road Rockville, MD 20850
www.ahrq.gov

American Association of Physicists in Medicine
One Physics Ellipse College Park, MD 20740
www.aapm.org

American College of Medical Physics
11250 Roger Bacon Drive, Suite 8 Reston,
VA 20190-5202
www.acmp.org

American College of Nuclear Medicine
P.O. Box 175 Landisville, PA 17538-0175
www.acnucmed.org

American College of Radiology
1891 Preston White Drive Reston, VA 20191-4397
www.acr.org

American Institute of Ultrasound in Medicine
14750 Sweitzer Lane Suite 100 Laurel,
MD 20707-5906
www.aium.org

American Society of Radiologic Technologists
15000 Central Avenue S.E. Albuquerque, NM
87123-3917
www.asrt.org

Conference of Radiation Control Program Directors
205 Capital Avenue Frankfort, KY 40601
www.crcpd.org

FDA/CDRH
5600 Fishers Lane Rockville, MD 20857
www.FDA.gov

FDA/CDRH/Mammography
1350 Piccard Drive Rockville, MD 20850
www.FDA.gov/cdrh/mammography

Fluke Biomedical
6920 Seaway Blvd. Everett, WA 98203
www.flukebiomedical.com

Gammex-RMI
2500 W. Beltline Highway Middleton, WI 53562-0327
www.gammex.com

Healthcare Information and Management Systems Society (HIMSS)
230 East Ohio Street Suite 500 Chicago, IL 60611-3270
www.himss.org

Integrating Healthcare Enterprise (IHE)
www.ihe.net

National Council on Radiation Protection and Measurements
7910 Woodmont Avenue Suite 800 Bethesda,
MD 20814-3095
www.ncrp.com

National Electrical Manufacturers Association
1300 N. 17th Street Suite 1752 Rosslyn, VA 22209
www.nema.org

Radiological Society of North America, Inc.
820 Jorie Boulevard Oak Brook, IL
60523-2251
www.rsna.org

Society for Computer Applications in Radiology
10105 Cottesmore Court Great Falls, VA 22066
www.scarnet.org

The Joint Commission
1 Renaissance Boulevard Oak Brook Terrace, IL 60181
www.jointcommission.org

United States Department of Health and Human Services
200 Independence Ave S.W. Washington, DC 20201
www.hhs.gov

Bibliography

Adams H, Arora S: *Total quality in radiology*, Delray Beach, Fla, 1994, GR/St Lucie Press.

Adler A, Carlton R: *Introduction to radiography and patient care*, ed 4, St Louis, 2007, Elsevier.

Al-Assaf A, Schmele J: *The textbook of total quality in healthcare*, Delray Beach, Fla, 1993, GR/St Lucie Press.

American Association of Physicists in Medicine: *Basic quality assurance in diagnostic radiology*, Rep No 4, Chicago, 1978, The Association.

American College of Radiology Committee on Quality Assurance in Mammography: *Mammography quality control: radiologic technologists manual*, Reston, VA, 1999, American College of Radiology.

Anderson R: Darkroom disease: a matter of debate, *ASTR Scanner* 28(10):1, 1996.

Ball J, Price T: *Chesneys' radiologic imaging*, ed 5, Boston, 1989, Blackwell Scientific.

Balter S: Fundamental properties of digital imaging, *Radiographics* 13:129, 1993.

Bonnick S, Lewis L: *Bone densitometry for technologists*, Totowa, NJ, 2002, Humana Press.

Bushberg J, et al: *The essential physics of medical imaging*, Baltimore, 1994, Williams & Wilkins.

Bushong S: *Radiologic science for technologists: physics, biology, and protection*, ed 9, St Louis, 2008, Mosby.

Carlton R, Adler A: *Principles of radiologic imaging*, ed 4, Albany, 2006, Delmar.

Carroll Q: *Fuchs' principles of radiologic exposure*, ed 8, Springfield, Ill, 2007, Charles C Thomas.

Carter C, Veale B: *Digital radiography and PACS*, St Louis, 2007, Elsevier.

Curry T, et al: *Christensen's physics of diagnostic radiology*, ed 4, Philadelphia, 1990, Lea & Febiger.

Deming WE: *Out of the crisis*, Cambridge, Mass, 1986, MIT Press.

Forster E: *Equipment for diagnostic radiography*, Boston, 1985, MPT Press.

Gaucher E, Coggey R: *Total quality in health care*, San Francisco, 1993, Jossey-Bass.

Graham N: *Quality in health care*, Gaithersburg, MD, 1995, Aspen.

Gray J, et al: *Quality control in diagnostic imaging*, Baltimore, 1983, University Park Press.

Haus A, Jaskulski S: *The basics of film processing in medical imaging*, Madison, Wis, 1997, Medical Physics Publishing.

Hendee WR, Ritenour ER: *Medical imaging physics*, ed 4, New York, 2002, Wiley-Liss.

Hendrick RE, et al: *Mammography quality control*, Reston, VA, 1994, American College of Radiology.

Huda W, Slone R: *Review of radiologic physics*, ed 2, Philadelphia, 2003, Lippincott Williams & Wilkins.

Joint Commission on Accreditation of Healthcare Organizations: *Forms, charts & other tools for performance improvement*, Oak Brook Terrace, Ill, 1994, The Joint Commission.

Lam R: *Continuous quality improvement for hospital diagnostic radiology services I, II*, Albuquerque, 1994, American Society of Radiologic Technologists.

Lam R: *Processor quality control of radiographers*, Albuquerque, 1994, American Society of Radiologic Technologists.

Lederer W: *Regulatory chemicals of health and environmental concerns*, New York, 1985, Van Nostrand Reinhold.

Lorh KN: Outcomes measurement: concept and questions, *Inquiry* 25:37, 1988.

Mammography quality standards, 21 CFR part 900: *Fed Reg* 21:471, 1994.

McKinney W: *Radiographic processing & quality control*, Philadelphia, 1988, JP Lippincott.

McLemore J: *Quality assurance in diagnostic radiology*, St Louis, 1981, Mosby.

Meisenheimer C: *Improving quality*, ed 2, Gaithersburg, MD, 1997, Aspen.

National Council on Radiation Protection, Rep No 85, Bethesda, MD, 1986, The Council.

National Council on Radiation Protection, Rep No 99, Bethesda, MD, 1986, The Council.

National Council on Radiation Protection, Rep No 103, Bethesda, MD, 1989, The Council.

National Council on Radiation Protection, Rep No 105, Bethesda, MD, 1988, The Council.

National Council on Radiation Protection, Rep No 116, Bethesda, MD, 1993, The Council.

Obergfell A: *Law & ethics in diagnostic imaging and therapeutic radiology*, Philadelphia, 1995, WB Saunders.

Parelli R: *Principles of fluoroscopic image intensification and television systems*, Delray Beach, Fla, 1997, GR/St Lucie Press.

Samei E, et al: *Assessment of display performance for medical imaging systems*, 2004, Draft report of the American Association of Physicists in Medicine (AAPM), Task Group 18, Version 10, August 2004.

Siegel E, Kolodner R: *Filmless radiology (formerly computers in health care)*, New York, 1999, Springer.

Shepard C: *Radiographic image production and manipulation*, New York, 2003, McGraw-Hill.

Shleien B, Slaback L, Birky B: *Handbook of health physics and radiological health*, ed 3, Baltimore, 1998, Williams & Wilkins.

Thompson M, et al: *Principles of imaging science and protection*, Philadelphia, 1994, WB Saunders.

Tortorici M: *Medical radiographic imaging*, Philadelphia, 1992, WB Saunders.

Vyborny C, Schmidt R: Mammography as a radiographic examination: an overview, *Radiographics* 9:723, 1989.

Wentz G: *Mammography for radiologic technologists*, New York, 1992, McGraw-Hill.

Wolbarst A: *Physics of radiology*, Norwalk, Conn, 1993, Appleton & Lange.

Zandlerk A, et al: *Managing outcomes through collaborative care*, Chicago, 1995, American Hospital Publishing.

Glossary

Acceptance Testing Quality control testing performed on new equipment on delivery and installation.

Accuracy The extent to which a measurement is close to the true value.

Action The activity to achieve the desired outcome.

Active Matrix Array (AMA) A large-area (the size of conventional film/screen image receptors) integrated circuit that consists of millions of identical semiconductor elements deposited on a glass base that acts as the flat-panel image receptor.

Actual Focal Spot The actual area of the x-ray tube target from which x-rays are emitted.

Adverse Event A harmful or unintended incident that may occur during any diagnostic procedure.

Aggregate Data Indicator Quantifies a process or outcome related to many cases.

Agitation Stirring, swirling, or shaking of processing solutions.

As Low as Reasonably Achievable (ALARA) Philosophy of keeping radiation exposure to a minimum.

Amorphous Without form.

Analog-to-Digital Convertor (ADC) Device for converting an analog electronic signal into a digital electronic signal for processing by a computer.

Appropriateness of Care Whether the type of care is necessary.

Archival Film Film images made before 1974 and containing 20% more silver than film made afterward.

Archival Quality How well an image can be stored over time.

Artifact The appearance in a diagnostic image of anything that is not a part of the patient's anatomy.

Aspect Ratio The ratio of the width of the image displayed on a computer or video monitor to the height of the display.

Automatic Brightness Control (ABC) Also called *automatic brightness stabilization* (ABS), it is an electronic method of regulating fluoroscopic image brightness level for variations of patient thickness and attenuation.

Automatic Brightness Stabilization Electronic method of regulating fluoroscopic image brightness. Also known as *automatic brightness control.*

Automatic Exposure Control (AEC) Electronic system that terminates the x-ray exposure once an adequate amount of radiation has been emitted.

Automatic Gain Control Electronic method of regulating image brightness.

Avoirdupois Ounce Unit of weight in the English system more commonly known as the *standard ounce.*

Axial Resolution Minimum reflector spacing along the axis of an ultrasound beam that results in separate, distinguishable echoes on the display.

Background Radiation Radiation exposures from naturally occurring radioactivity and extraterrestrial cosmic radiation.

Bandwidth The range of frequencies that can be satisfactorily transmitted or processed by a system.

Base + Fog Inherent optical densities in film resulting from the tint added to the base of the film and silver grains not exposed to radiation.

Benchmarking Involves comparing one organization's performance with that of another.

Beryllium Window A portion of the mammographic x-ray tube where the useful beam exits.

Bioassay The laboratory determination of the concentration of a drug or other substance in a specimen.

Bit *Bi*nary dig*it*; the smallest unit of computer memory that holds one of two values, one or zero.

Brainstorming A group process used to develop a large collection of ideas without regard to their merit or validity.

Brightness Gain The degree of image brightness increase obtained with an image intensifier.

Bromide Drag Decrease in optical density caused by halides being deposited on trailing areas of the film during automatic processing.

Cause-and-Effect Diagram A causal analysis tool. Also known as a *fishbone chart* or *Ishikawa diagram.*

Center of Rotation (COR) The fulcrum, or pivot point, of tomographic equipment motion.

Central Tendency The central position of a sample frequency.

Channeling A potential problem in certain metallic replacement silver recovery units whereby the fixer forms a straight channel that reduces efficiency.

Charge-Coupled Device (CCD) A two-dimensional electronic array for converting light patterns into electronic signals.

Chatter Artifact that appears as bands of increased optical density that occur perpendicular to film direction because of inconsistent motion of the transport system, usually the result of slippage of the drive gears of drive chain.

Chemical Activity How well the processing solutions per-form their desired function.

Chemical Impurity The presence of a chemical or other substance that normally should not be present.

Chi-Square A statistic test for an association between observed data and expected data represented by frequencies.

Chromatography Any one of several processes for separating and analyzing various gaseous or dissolved chemical materials.

Cinefluorography The recording of a fluoroscopic image onto motion picture film.

Collimator (1) A device that regulates the area of x-ray beam exposure. (2) A device for improving image resolution in nuclear medicine procedures.

Comparator A portion of an automatic exposure control system that compares the amount of radiation detected with a preset value.

Compression Applying pressure to a body area to reduce part thickness.

Computed Radiography (CR) A process of creating a digitized radiographic image using a photostimulable phosphor.

Concurrent Data Data collected during the time of care.

Consumer An individual who chooses to comment or complain in reference to an examination including the patient or representative of the patient (e.g., family member or referring physician).

Continuity of Care The degree to which the care is coordinated among practitioners or organizations, or both.

Continuous Variables Variables that have an infinite range of mathematic values.

Contrast Indicator Value obtained during sensitometric testing, which indicates film contrast.

Contrast Resolution The ability of an imaging system to distinguish structures with similar transmission as separate entities.

Contrast Scale The change in linear attenuation coefficient per computed tomographic number relative to water.

Contrast-to-Noise Ratio (CNR) The ratio between the image contrast to the amount of image noise (both quantum mottle and/or electronic); can be used to describe image quality.

Control Chart A modification of the trend chart in which statistically determined upper and lower control limits are placed.

Coulomb per Kilogram International System of Units radiation intensity equivalent to 3876 roentgens.

Count Rate Measurement of the activity of a radioactive substance.

Counts per Minute A measure of the decay rate of ionizing emissions by radioactive substances.

Critical Path Documents the basic treatment or action sequence in an effort to eliminate unnecessary variation.

Customer A person, department, or organization that needs or wants the desired outcome.

Darkroom Area protected from white light where films are processed.

Data Set The information or measurements that were acquired by evaluating the particular sample.

Daylight System A system for loading and unloading film from image receptors outside of a darkroom.

Densitometer Electronic device for measuring the optical density of a film.

Deficit Reduction Act Federal legislation enacted in 2005 to help reduce Medicare and Medicaid spending.

Depth of Visualization Depth into a patient or phantom at which signals from scattered echoes can create an image.

Detector Also known as the *sensor*, it is a radiation detector that monitors the radiation exposure at or near the patient and produces a corresponding electric current that is proportional to the quantity of x-rays detected.

Developer A processing solution responsible for conversion of the latent image to a manifest image in film.

Dichotomous Variables Variables that have only two values or choices.

DICOM *D*igital *I*maging and *C*ommunications in *M*edicine, a standard used for transferring digital images in diagnostic imaging.

Digital Fluoroscopy Computerized enhancement of fluoroscopic images.

Digital Imaging and Communications in Medicine (DICOM) A system of computer software standards that allows different digital imaging programs to understand one another.

Digital Radiography (DR) A method of obtaining a digitized radiographic image utilizing an active matrix array.

Digital Subtraction Angiography An electronic method of enhancing visibility of vascular structures involving digital fluoroscopy.

Direct-to-Digital Radiographic (DDR) Systems Method of creating digital radiographic images, also known as *flat-panel* or *flat-plate imaging*; involves the installation of a flat-panel image receptor in the Bucky of a radiographic table or upright Bucky, which sends an electronic signal directly to a digital image processor.

Disintegrations per Minute (DPM) A measure of the rate of ionizing emissions by radioactive substances.

Dose Area Product (DAP) Measurement that incorporates the total dosage of radiation along with the area of field that is being used.

Dose Calibrator A component in nuclear medicine equipment for determining the amount of radionuclide.

Dual-Energy X-Ray Absorptiometry (DEXA) X-rays with two separate energies used to obtain bone density data.

Dwell Time The amount of time that the fixer solution is in contact with the active portion of the silver recovery device.

Edge Enhancement The enhancement of structure margins (edges) using digital processing techniques.

Edge Spread Function A graphic indication of image resolution.

Effective Focal Spot The area of the x-ray tube target that emits x-rays when viewed from the perspective of the image receptor.

Effectiveness of Care The level of benefit when services are rendered under ordinary circumstances by average practitioners for typical patients.

Efficacy of Care The level of benefit expected when healthcare services are applied under ideal conditions.

Efficiency of Care The highest quality of care delivered in the shortest amount of time with the least amount of expense and a positive outcome.

Electron Beam Computed Tomography (EBCT) A fifth-generation CT scanner design used in cardiac imaging.

Electrolysis A process in which an electric charge causes a chemical change in a solution or molten substance.

Emission Spectrum Graphic demonstration of the component energies of emitted electromagnetic radiation.

Energy Resolution The amount of variation in pulse size or spreading of the spectrum produced by a detector.

Extended Processing A method of film processing that extends the normal developer time to increase image contrast.

F-center Empty lattice sites in photostimulable phosphors where crystal electrons are trapped following exposure to x-ray energy.

Field Uniformity Refers to the even distribution of magnetic field strength in the region of interest.

File Transfer Protocol (FTP) A method for transferring files across a computer network.

Fill Factor The percentage of pixel area that is sensitive to the image signal (contains the x-ray detector). The fill factor for most current systems is approximately 80% because some of the pixel area must be devoted to electronic conductors and the thin film transistor (TFT).

Fixer Processing solution responsible for removal of undeveloped silver halide and hardening of the film emulsion.

Flood Replenishment A timed method of replenishing processing solutions with an automatic processor.

Flowchart A pictorial representation of the individual steps required in a process.

Flow Meter A device for measuring the volume of liquid flowing through it.

Fluorescence The type of luminescence that is desired for use in intensifying screens because it occurs when certain crystals emit light within 10^{-8} seconds after being exposed to radiation.

Flux Gain The gain in image brightness occurring with an image intensifier during fluoroscopy resulting from the high voltage across the tube.

FMEA (Failure Mode and Effects Analysis) A procedure for analysis of potential failure within a system, classifying the severity or determining the failure's effect upon the system, and help determine remedial actions to overcome these failures.

Focal Spot Blooming An increase in stated focal spot size, usually as a result of an increase in milliampere.

Focus Group Group dynamic tool for problem identification and analysis.

FOCUS-PDCA A quality management method developed by the Hospital Corporation of America.

Foot-Candle Measurement of illuminance: lumens per square foot = foot-candles.

Frequency The number of repetitions of any phenomenon within a fixed period.

Full-Width Half Maximum (FWHM) A measure of resolution equal to the width of an image of a line source at points where the intensity is reduced to half the maximum.

Fusion Imaging A combination of two images such as PET and CT.

Gamma Camera A device used for image acquisition in many nuclear medicine procedures.

Gas-Filled Detector A category of radiation detector consisting of a gas-filled chamber.

Geiger-Müller (GM) Meter A survey meter used mainly for radiation protection purposes as a survey instrument and an area monitor.

Geiger-Müller Tube A type of gas-filled radiation detector.

Green Film Film that has not been processed.

Grid Latitude The margin of error in centering the central ray of the x-ray beam to the center of the grid.

Half-Value Layer The amount of filtering material that reduces the intensity of radiation to one half of its previous value.

High-Contrast Resolution The ability to resolve small, thin black-and-white areas.

High-Contrast Spatial Resolution The minimum distance between two objects that allows them to be seen as separate and distinct.

High-Frequency Generator A type of x-ray generator that dramatically increases the frequency of alternating current sent to the x-ray tube.

HIPAA (Health Insurance Portability and Accountability Act) Enacted in 1996 (also known as the Kennedy-Kassebaum Act or Public Law 104-191) to simplify healthcare standards and save money for healthcare businesses by encouraging electronic transactions.

Histogram A data display tool in the form of a bar graph that plots the most frequent occurrence of a quantity in the center.

Histogram Error Improper optical density resulting from selection of an incorrect preprocessing histogram in a cathode-ray system (such as using an adult histogram when radiographing a pediatric chest).

Homogenous Phantom A device used in quality control testing that is uniform in thickness and density.

Horizontal Distance Measurement A quality control test for ultrasound equipment requiring measurements taken perpendicular to the sound beam axis.

Humidity A measurement of the relative level of moisture in the air.

Hydrolyzed Reduced Technetium A type of technetium-99m used in radionuclide imaging.

Hydrometer A device for measuring specific gravity.

Hyporetention A residue of fixer components remaining on a film after processing.

Illuminance The brightness of light projected on a given surface, measured in lux or foot-candles.

Image Compression A reduction of the space required to store or time required to transfer a digital image.

Image Enhancement The use of a computer to improve or enhance an image.

Image Intensifier An electronic device that brightens a fluoroscopic image.

Image Inversion Allows the converting of a negative image (standard radiographic image) into a positive image (meaning a reverse of the negative image where white areas on the negative image are black on the positive image and vice versa).

Image Lag An image persisting on a cathode-ray tube even after termination of radiation.

Image Management and Communication System (IMACS) A computerized system for storing patient images and medical records.

Image Restoration A process in digital imaging whereby the final image is displayed.

Image Uniformity A uniform brightness level throughout the image when visualizing a homogenous phantom.

Incident Any occurrence that is not consistent with the routine care of a patient or the normal course of events at a particular facility.

Incident Light The emitted light from its source before striking the film.

Indicator A valid and reliable quantitative process or outcome measure related to one or more dimensions of performance.

Input Information or knowledge necessary to achieve the desired outcome.

Intensification Factor A measurement of intensifying screen speed.

Ion Chamber A type of gas-filled radiation detector.

K-edge The binding energy of K-shell electrons.

Kerma An acronym for kinetic energy released in matter, it measures the amount of kinetic energy that is released into particles of matter (such as electrons created during Compton and photoelectric interactions) from exposure to x-rays.

Kilowatt Rating A rating of power output for x-ray generators.

Latensification The increase in sensitivity of a film after it has been exposed to light or ionizing radiation (such as in a cassette during a radiographic examination) so that it can be as much as two to eight times more sensitive to subsequent exposure as an unexposed film (depending on the type of emulsion).

Latent Image An invisible image present after exposure but before processing.

Lateral Resolution A measure of how close two reflectors can be to one another perpendicular to the beam axis and still be distinguished as separate.

Law of Reciprocity Law stating that the amount of x-ray intensity should remain constant at a specific milliampere-second value despite the milliampere and time combination.

Level of Expectation A pre-established level of performance applied to a specific indicator.

Line Focus Principle A principle stating that the effective focal spot always appears smaller than the actual focal spot because of the anode angle.

Line Spread Function A graphic indication of image resolution.

Linear Tomography A type of conventional tomography whereby the x-ray source and image receptor undergo reciprocal motion in a straight line.

Linearity Sequential increases in milliampere-seconds should produce the same sequential increase in exposure rate.

Liquid Crystal Display (LCD) Flat-panel display form for monitors.

Locational Effect A variation in film quality caused by the sensitometric test film being inserted in different portions of the feed tray.

Look-Up Table (LUT) A table used to assign (transform) digital data into image brightness values.

Loss Potential Any activity that costs a facility either money or its reputation.

Low-Contrast Resolution Performance variable measuring the ability to image structures of similar density.

Luminance The amount of luminous intensity emitted by a source of light.

Luminescence The emission of light resulting from x-rays exiting the patient, which energize the phosphor crystals. It can occur by one of two different processes, fluorescence or phosphorescence.

Magnification Electronic digital zoom with software manipulation that can reduce the need to take additional magnification views, as with film/screen mammography.

Mammography Quality Standards Act (MQSA) Federal legislation mandating quality standards for all mammographic procedures.

Manifest Image The final visible image.

Matrix Size The number of pixels allocated to each linear dimension in a digital image.

Mean The average set of observations.

Mean Computed Tomography Number Average pixel value calculated by dividing the total computed tomography value by the total number of pixels in a sample.

Median A point on a scale of measurement above which are exactly one half of the values and below which are the other half of the values.

Metallic Replacement A method of silver recovery from used fixer solution.

Minification Gain An increase in brightness with image intensifier tubes as a result of the difference in size between the input and output phosphors.

Mobile X-Ray Generator A smaller-size x-ray generator mounted on wheels that can be transported to various locations.

Mode The one value that occurs with the most frequency.

Modulation Transfer Function A graphic or numeric indication of image resolution.

Molybdenum-99 The parent element of technetium-99m.

Multichannel Analyzer A specialized scintillation detector that can select specific energy levels for detection.

Multifield Image Intensifier A specialized image intensifier that allows for magnified fluoroscopic images.

Nit A unit to measure luminance, equivalent to candela per square meter.

Noise Random signals or disturbances that interfere with proper image formation or demonstration.

Nuclear Regulatory Commission (NRC) Federal agency that enforces radiation safety guidelines.

Nyquist Frequency The highest spatial frequency resolved by an imaging system, measured in line pairs per millimeter (lp/mm).

Objective Plane The region remaining relatively sharp in detail during tomographic procedures.

Occupational Safety and Health Administration (OSHA) Federal agency that oversees the workplace environment.

Optical disk A large-capacity digital data storage device used to store digital images.

Orthicon A type of television camera tube.

Orthochromatic A type of film that is sensitive mainly to light in the green portion of the visible light spectrum.

Oxidation/Reduction Reaction A chemical change in which electrons are removed (oxidation) from an atom, ion, or molecule, accompanied by a simultaneous transfer of electrons to another atom, ion, or molecule (reduction). Also known as *redux*.

Panchromatic A type of film that is sensitive to all wavelengths of the visible light spectrum.

Pareto chart A causal analysis tool that is a variation of a histogram.

Phantom A quality control test tool used to simulate human tissue or body parts or demonstrate certain image characteristics.

Phosphorescence Delayed emission of light—often called *afterglow* or *lag*—not desired for use in intensifying screens that occurs when certain crystals emit light sometime after 10^{-8} seconds after exposure to radiation.

Photodetector An electronic device used for detecting photons of light, x-rays, or gamma rays.

Photoemission The emission of electrons from a material after exposure to light or other ionizing radiation.

Photofluorospot A method of recording static images during fluoroscopy.

Photometry The study and measurement of light.

Photomultiplier Tube (PMT) A device used in many radiation detection applications that converts low levels of light into electronic pulses.

Photon The smallest quantity of electromagnetic energy.

Photopeak The peak amplitude on an oscilloscope display.

Photostimulable Phosphor A barium fluorohalide material used to capture radiographic images in computerized radiography (CR) systems.

Picture Archiving and Communication System (PACS) A computerized system that stores patient images to allow access from remote locations.

Pincushion Distortion A type of distortion in image-intensified images caused by the projection of a curved image onto a flat surface.

Pixel Abbreviation for picture elements. Small cells of information that make up the digital image on a computer monitor screen.

Pixel Size The size of the picture element found in the matrix of a computer-generated image; the smaller the pixel size, the greater the spatial resolution.

Plumbicon A type of television camera tube.

Pluridirectional Tomography A specialized type of tomographic unit that allows for multiple-direction motion of the x-ray source and image receptor.

Point Spread Function A graphic demonstration of image resolution.

Population Any group measured for some variable characteristic from which samples may be taken for statistical purposes.

Portable X-Ray Generator A type of x-ray generator that is small enough to be carried from place to place by one person.

Positron Emission Tomography (PET) An imaging technique whereby a positron-emitting radionuclide is administered to a patient, and the result is the release of photons by an annihilation reaction.

Postprocessing A manipulation of the image data in the memory of the computer, before the image is displayed on a monitor.

Precipitation A process whereby silver particles are made to settle out of a used fixer solution.

Process An ordered series of steps that help achieve a desired outcome.

Psychrometer An instrument used to measure relative humidity.

Pulse Height Analyzer (PHA) A device that accepts or rejects electronic pulses according to their amplitude or energy.

Quality Assurance An all-encompassing management program used to ensure excellence.

Quality Control The part of the quality assurance program that deals with techniques used in monitoring and maintenance of technical systems.

Quality Improvement Team A group of individuals who are responsible for implementing the solutions that were derived by a focus group.

Quantum Mottle Image noise caused by statistical fluctuations in the number of photons creating the image.

Radionuclide Impurity The presence of other substance (s) in the radiopharmaceutical for nuclear medicine procedures.

RAID *R*edundant *a*rray of *i*nexpensive *d*isks, a computer storage medium with rapid image access time and fault tolerance.

Receiver Operating Characteristic (ROC) Curve A curve that plots the true-positive fraction versus the false-positive fraction and is used to evaluate imaging performance.

Reciprocity The amount of x-ray intensity should remain constant at a specific milliampere-second value despite the milliampere and time combination.

Recirculating Electrolytic A type of electrolytic silver recovery device that recirculates fixer back into the processor after silver reclamation.

Rectification The process of converting an alternating current (AC) into a direct current (DC).

Refresh Rate This refers to how many times each second that a video or computer monitor rewrites or updates the image on the display (also known as the frame rate or vertical scan frequency) of the monitor.

Region of Interest (ROI) A specified region of the image that is selected for display or analysis.

Relative Conversion Factor Measures the amount of light produced by the output phosphor per unit of x-radiation incident on the input phosphor.

Relative Speed A relative number indicating the speed of an intensifying screen imaging system.

Reliability The accuracy, dependability, or validity of the data that has been collected.

Repeat Analysis A data collection of repeat images to determine the cause of the repeats so they may be prevented in the future.

Reproducibility The same technique setting should always create the same exposure rate at any time.

Resonance Frequency (1) The frequency for which the response of a transducer to an ultrasound beam is a maximum. (2) In magnetic resonance imaging, the frequency at which a nucleus absorbs radio energy when placed in a magnetic field.

Risk Management The ability to identify potential risks to patients, employees, and visitors to the healthcare institution and institute processes that minimize these risks.

Roentgen The special unit of radiation exposure or intensity.

S Distortion An artifact that can occur in image intensifier tubes consisting of a warping of the image along an S-shaped axis.

Safelight A light source that does not fog film.

Safe Medical Devices Act (SMDA) Legislation of 1991 that requires a medical facility to report to the Food and Drug Administration any medical devices that have caused a serious injury or death of a patient (e.g., malfunctioning bed, nonworking defibrillator, nonworking pacemaker, malfunctioning radiation therapy unit) or employee. It also authorizes civil penalties to be imposed on healthcare workers or facilities that do not report defects and failures in medical devices.

Sample The number of items that are actually measured from a population.

Scan Image Uniformity The uniformity in brightness of an image created with a homogenous phantom.

Scatter Plot A graph that demonstrates a possible correlation between two variables.

Scintillation Crystal A sodium iodide crystal used in scintillation detectors.

Scintillation Detector A radiation detector consisting of a sodium iodide crystal coupled to a photomultiplier tube.

Scrap Exposed Film Exposed and processed film that is not of diagnostic use and is disposed of for silver recovery.

Screen Speed The amount of light that is emitted from an intensifying screen for a given amount of x-ray exposure.

Sensitivity Indicates the likelihood of obtaining a positive diagnosis in a patient with the disease.

Sensitometer An electrical device that exposes the film to a premeasured light source for quality control purposes.

Sensitometry The study of the relationship between the amount of radiation exposing a film and the optical density that is produced.

Sensor The radiation detector assembly in an automatic exposure control system.

Sentinel Event Indicator An individual event or phenomenon that is significant enough to trigger further review each time it occurs.

Serious Adverse Event An adverse event that may significantly compromise clinical outcomes or an adverse event for which a facility fails to take appropriate corrective action in a timely manner.

Serious Complaint A report of a serious adverse event.

Signal-to-Noise Ratio (SNR) Used to describe the relative contributions to a detected signal of the true signal and random superimposed signals or noise.

Single-Phase A type of x-ray generator with a single source of alternating current.

Single-Photon Emission Computerized Tomography (SPECT) A nuclear medicine procedure that creates cross-sectional images.

Six Sigma A management strategy that seeks to identify and remove the causes of errors in business processes.

Slice Position The relative position of the image section and the patient.

Slice Thickness The thickness of the image section.

Solarization A decrease in optical density with an increase in exposure. Also known as *image reversal*.

Solid-State Detector A radiation detector with silicon or germanium crystals.

Spatial Linearity The ability of a gamma camera system to produce a linear image with straight lines corresponding to the same straight lines of the bar pattern OR the amount of geometric distortion in the image as affected by the homogeneity of the main magnetic field and the linearity of the magnetic field gradients.

Spatial Resolution The ability of an imaging process to distinguish small, adjacent, high-contrast structures in the object.

Specificity Indicates the likelihood of a patient obtaining a negative diagnosis when no disease is present.

Spectral Matching The matching of film sensitivity with the color of light emitted by the intensifying screen.

Spectrum A display of electromagnetic energy on the basis of wavelength and frequency.

Specular Reflection A type of reflection coming from the surface of an electronic display that produces a mirror image of the light source creating it

Speed Indicator The step closest to 1 above the base + fog on a sensitometric test film.

Standard Deviation The amount of variance in a sample.

Static Electricity Electrical charges created by friction, which can cause artifacts on unprocessed film.

String Test A quality control test for Doppler ultrasound equipment.

Sulfurization A buildup of sulfur on the electrodes in an electrolytic silver recovery unit as a result of incorrect amperage setting.

Supplier One who provides goods or services.

Synergism The action of two agents working together is greater than the sum of the action of the agents working independently.

Target Composition Refers to the elemental composition of the x-ray tube anode.

Technetium-99m The isotope of technetium whose primary gamma ray has an energy of 140 kiloelectron volts.

Technetium Pertechnetate A radionuclide used in nuclear medicine procedures that consists of technetium-99m.

Temperature A measure of the average kinetic energy in atoms and molecules of matter.

Terminal Electrolytic An electrolytic silver recovery device in which the used fixer is removed for disposal.

The Joint Commission (TJC) A private agency (formerly known as JCAHO) responsible for accreditation of healthcare systems.

Thin-Film Transistor (TFT) Switches for each pixel of an array connected to circuitry that allows all switches in a row of the array to be operated simultaneously.

Three-Phrase An alternating-current power source made up of three single-phase currents that are staggered by 120 degrees.

Threshold A pre-established level of performance applied to a specific indicator.

Time of Day Variability A possible variable in sensitometric testing in which test films are processed at different times during the day, varying in optical density.

Tissue Equalization Image processing that compensates for varying breast tissue densities so that the entire breast (from the chest wall to the skin line) can be visualized in a single image.

Thermoluminescent Dosimeter (TLD) A type of radiation detector with crystals such as lithium fluoride that release light when heated that is proportional to the amount of incident radiation.

Tomography A radiographic process whereby specific slices of the body are imaged.

Transmitted Light The amount of viewbox light that is transmitted through a film image.

Trend Chart A graph that pictorially demonstrates whether key indicators are moving up or down over a given period. Also called a *run chart*.

Troy Ounce A unit of weight used for precious metals such as silver; 14.58 troy ounces = 16 standard ounces.

Ultraviolet Radiation A type of electromagnetic radiation in between visible light and x-rays.

Uniformity Correction Flood A quality control procedure for nuclear medicine equipment.

Variance A numeric representation of the dispersion of data around the mean in a given sample.

Veiling Glare Glare caused by light being reflected from the window of the output phosphor in an image intensifier. Also known as *flare*.

Ventilation The process by which air is changed into and out of a specific area.

Vertical Distance Measurement A quality control test variable for ultrasound equipment measuring along the sound beam axis. Also known as *depth calibration accuracy*.

Vidicon A type of television camera tube.

Viewbox Illuminator An electronic device for viewing transparency images such as radiographs.

Vignetting A decrease in brightness toward the periphery of a fluoroscopic image when using an image intensifier tube.

Voltage Ripple The variation from the peak voltage through the x-ray tube in an x-ray generator.

Volume Replenishment A type of system in an automatic processor that replenishes a volume of solution for each film introduced.

Window Level A value in digital imaging that selects the level of the displayed band of values within the complete range.

Window Leveling A manipulation of the dynamic range, allowing for the selection of more or less shades of gray to enhance image contrast.

Window Width A value in digital imaging that selects the width of the band of values in the digital signal that can be represented as gray tones in the image.

Answers to Review Questions

Chapter 1

1. a
2. c
3. b
4. b
5. b
6. d
7. d
8. c
9. b
10. d

Chapter 2

1. a
2. a
3. b
4. a
5. c
6. a
7. b
8. c
9. c
10. c

Chapter 3

1. b
2. b
3. d
4. c
5. a
6. c
7. a
8. c
9. b
10. b

Chapter 4

1. d
2. b
3. a
4. a
5. b
6. b
7. d
8. c
9. d
10. b

Chapter 5

1. b
2. c
3. b
4. a
5. c
6. c
7. b
8. d
9. b
10. c

Chapter 6

1. c
2. a
3. b
4. b
5. a
6. d
7. b
8. c
9. d
10. c

Chapter 7

1. b
2. c
3. c
4. a
5. d
6. c
7. b
8. b
9. d
10. c

Chapter 8

1. a
2. b
3. c
4. d
5. c
6. b
7. d
8. b
9. c
10. c

Chapter 9

1. c
2. d
3. c
4. b
5. c
6. d
7. b
8. d
9. a
10. d

Chapter 10

1. d
2. c
3. d
4. b
5. c
6. d
7. a
8. c
9. b
10. b

Chapter 11

1. b
2. a
3. d
4. c
5. c
6. d
7. a
8. b
9. d
10. c

Chapter 12

1. c
2. c
3. b
4. b
5. a
6. b
7. a
8. b
9. b
10. c

Chapter 13

1. d
2. b
3. a
4. c
5. d
6. a
7. a
8. b
9. a
10. d

Chapter 14

1. c
2. c
3. d
4. b
5. b
6. c
7. c
8. b
9. a
10. a

Chapter 15

1. c
2. d
3. b
4. c
5. b
6. c
7. b
8. c
9. a
10. b

Index

Note: Page numbers followed by *f*
indicate figures; *t*, tables; and *b*, boxes.